FOUNDATIONS FOR GLOBAL HEALTH PRACTICE

FOUNDATIONS FOR GLOBAL HEALTH PRACTICE

LORI DIPRETE BROWN

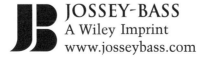

JOSSEY-BASS
A Wiley Imprint
www.josseybass.com

Registered Office
John Wiley & Sons, Inc., 111 River Street, Hoboken, NJ 07030, USA

Editorial Office
111 River Street, Hoboken, NJ 07030, USA

For details of our global editorial offices, customer services, and more information about Wiley products visit us at www.wiley.com.

Wiley also publishes its books in a variety of electronic formats and by print-on-demand. Some content that appears in standard print versions of this book may not be available in other formats.

Library of Congress Cataloging-in-Publication Data

Names: DiPrete Brown, Lori, 1961- editor.
Title: Foundations for global health practice/[edited] by Lori DiPrete Brown.
Description: Hoboken, NJ : Wiley, 2017. | Includes bibliographical references and index. |
Identifiers: LCCN 2017036459 (print) | LCCN 2017037373 (ebook) | ISBN 9781118603802 (pdf) | ISBN 9781118603635 (epub) | ISBN 9781118505564 (paper)
Subjects: | MESH: Global Health
Classification: LCC RA441 (ebook) | LCC RA441 (print) | NLM WA 530.1 | DDC 362.1–dc23
LC record available at https://lccn.loc.gov/2017036459

Cover images: ©everything possible/Shutterstock; ©studiocasper/iStockphoto
Cover design by Wiley

Set in size 9.6/13 and ITC New Baskerville Std by Aptara Inc., New Delhi, India

Printed in the United States of America

10 9 8 7 6 5 4 3 2 1

To the many people around the world who have welcomed me into their communities and their lives, shown me how small the world is, reminded me what is just, and revealed to me what is possible.
To my students who have made me a teacher and will rewrite this book someday.
To Kirk, Evan, Elise, and Kristen with so much love and gratitude.

CONTENTS

Part I   Global Health Concepts

Part II   Global Health Practice

Part III   Global Health Perspectives

LIST OF FIGURES, TABLES, AND BOXES

Figures

Tables

Boxes

Foundations for Global Health Practice began in 2006, in a small seminar room at the University of Wisconsin School of Medicine and Public Health in Madison, Wisconsin. I had come to academia relatively recently after working in the field of global health and development for the first 15 years of my career. A group of globally oriented educators from medicine, nursing, pharmacy, veterinary medicine, and public health, who were in the early stages of developing the global health enterprise at UW–Madison, encouraged me to teach a practical elective about global health fieldwork for their students.

The goal of the course was ambitious. Students came to the first class prepared to share their global health aspirations, and by the final class they were to present plans for how they would act on these goals through field study, research, or service. As we all quickly learned, for students to achieve these goals, they not only needed to receive good orientation on the foundations for global health practice from me as a teacher and experienced practitioner but also had to work together in teams with common interests and diverse skills and experiences, and they had to be proactive about their own learning. Over the years, the course engaged students from a broad range of fields—the previously mentioned health science professions, as well as agriculture, engineering, women's studies, nutrition, public policy, human ecology, and environmental studies.

In 2010, global health education efforts at UW–Madison extended to include a program of study for undergraduates. In my role with our campus Global Health Institute, I had the privilege of drawing lessons from our graduate education efforts to develop a curriculum for undergraduates in partnership with the College of Agriculture and Life Sciences. These curriculum development efforts had a profound effect on this book. The highly subscribed program has allowed me to work with hundreds of undergraduates over the past seven years. Their questions, insights, energy, and sheer numbers have been both exhausting and sustaining, and theirs were the faces in my mind as I worked on this book.

Andy Pasternak, senior editor at Jossey-Bass, approached me about this project at a time when the global health field was evolving quickly, and important goals for undergraduate education were being defined. The revision and renewal of the Millennium Development Goals as Sustainable Development Goals were in sight, governments around the world were embracing a Health in All Policies approach, the private sector was engaging in global health in new ways, and the conversation about linking environmental sustainability, ecosystem health, and planetary health had begun in earnest. These developments are reflected and represented in this book.

Beyond meeting academic standards, I have tried to make this a book that prepares students to enter this conversation as authentic scholars, professionals, and citizens. The core pedagogical principles are place-based knowledge; evidence-based practice; respectful dialogue; and diversity in terms of culture, identity, and academic discipline.

The expert voices included in this book represent leading universities, government, civil society, the private sector, and young leaders from around the world. This is intended to be the beginning of an increasingly inclusive conversation that can happen around the book in colleges and universities across the country. My hope is that instructors will use this as a framework and then include additional voices from their home institutions, local communities, and international partners.

How can course instructors use this book? This book enables faculty members from a variety of fields to lead an interdisciplinary global health course. Part 1 provides core content and framework, and part 3 provides essays and suggested reading to support guest lectures or special interests of students. The book can also support instructors who are interested in developing an immersive learning component of the course, or a summer experience with and for students. Part 2 can be used to guide this planning process, to do globally contextualized work in the local community or in communities around the world. Finally, the book provides support to instructors and academic advisors who are involved in helping students who are seeking internships, job placement, and graduate study.

How does this book fit into academic programs? This book is aligned with current competency frameworks for undergraduate public health education (Riegelman & Albertine, 2008) and civic competencies for undergraduates (Liberal Education and America's Promise, 2007; National Task Force on Civic Learning and Democratic Engagement, 2012). It can be used in undergraduate courses on global health and can fit well into undergraduate global health or public health majors, minors, and certificate programs. It can also be the basis for an elective course in majors such as agriculture, nutrition, engineering, nursing, social work, psychology, engineering, and education.

This book can also be used in the first year of public health master's programs to meet breadth requirements related to global health, and meets many accreditation criteria for these programs (Council on Education for Public Health, 2016). It can also support electives in health professions programs such as medicine, nursing, pharmacy, veterinary medicine, social work, public policy, and environmental studies. It is particularly useful to support students in developing graduate-level internships that are globally oriented.

A note to students: Whether your global health study is a first step toward a global health career or simply an interesting elective, I hope this book helps you develop a plan for lifelong global awareness and engagement. I hope that you have great conversations with your classmates that lead to friendships based on shared values and purpose; that you learn about other parts of your state, nation, and the world; and that in so doing you come to new insights about yourself and the places you call home. I hope that you will develop lifelong practices that reflect evidence-based inquiry, perspective taking, and a concern for the collective good, so that you can contribute to health and well-being in your own life, in your community, and in our world.

—Lori DiPrete Brown

References

Council on Education for Public Health. (2016, October). *Accreditation criteria: Schools of public health and public health programs.* Silver Spring, MD: Author.

Liberal Education and America's Promise. (2007). *College learning for the new global century.* Washington, DC: Association of American Colleges and Universities.

National Task Force on Civic Learning and Democratic Engagement. (2012). *A crucible moment: College learning and democracy's future.* Washington, DC: Association of American Colleges and Universities.

Riegelman, R., & Albertine, S. *Recommendations for undergraduate public health education.* (2008). Washington, DC: Association of American Colleges and Universities.

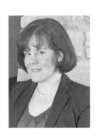

Lori DiPrete Brown, MS, MTS

Lori DiPrete Brown has been engaged in global health education at the University of Wisconsin–Madison for 14 years, where she serves as a distinguished faculty associate in the School of Medicine and Public Health as the associate director for education and engagement for the Global Health Institute at UW–Madison. DiPrete Brown began her career as a Peace Corps volunteer in Honduras, where she lived and worked in a residential program for teenage girls who had been orphaned or abandoned during childhood. Her subsequent global health practice, research, teaching, writing, and public speaking have focused on providing quality health care and social services that address the needs of women, children, and all people who are in highly vulnerable situations. DiPrete Brown has collaborated with international agencies including the US Peace Corps, USAID, the Pan American Health Organization, WHO, Care, and Save the Children. She has worked to strengthen systems of care in 15 countries around the world, including Costa Rica, Guatemala, Nicaragua, Chile, Mexico, Ecuador, Cameroon, and Ethiopia. DiPrete Brown holds degrees from Yale University, the Harvard School of Public Health, and the Harvard Divinity School. In 2012, she was awarded the UW School of Medicine and Public Health Dean's Teaching Award for her role in teaching and experiential learning in the health sciences. In 2016, she was awarded the Women's Philanthropy Council Champion Award for her efforts in advancing the status of women and gender issues at the University of Wisconsin–Madison. She blogs about global health and social change, and has written a novel about her work with young women titled *Caminata: A Journey.* Blog: http://globalhealthreflections .wordpress.com

CONTRIBUTORS

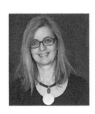

Araceli Alonso, PhD

Dr. Araceli Alonso is affiliated with the Department of Gender and Women's Studies and the School of Medicine and Public Health at University of Wisconsin–Madison, where she teaches global women's health and women's rights. She is also the founder and director of Health by All Means (HbAM), a global health initiative that started as Health by Motorbike (HbM), which provides a culturally and geographically sensitive model of integrated health promotion and disease prevention for women and girls living in remote and isolated communities around the world. Alonso is codirector of the UNESCO Chair on Gender, Well-Being and a Culture of Peace at the University of Wisconsin–Madison. She is also the director for gender, health, and clinical practice for UW's 4W Women and Wellbeing Initiative, where she directs STREETS (Social Transformation to End the Sexual Exploitation of Women and Children).

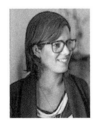

Fernanda Alonso, LLM, LLB

Fernanda Alonso is an associate at the O'Neill Institute. She holds a master of laws in global health law from Georgetown University and a bachelor of laws from the Instituto Tecnológico Autónomo de México (ITAM), Mexico City. Prior to joining the O'Neill Institute, Fernanda was the coordinator of the Drug Policy Program at the Centro de Investigación y Docencia Económicas (CIDE) in Aguascalientes, Mexico. There, she participated in legislative and policy projects for the Mexican government as well as in researching drug policy issues in Latin America. She also has experience as a legal policy advisor in other substance-control areas, including tobacco control and alcohol and food regulation.

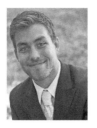

Michele Joseph Aquino, MS

Michele Aquino is a food scientist and sustainability specialist with expertise in agriculture and food manufacturing. After serving as an agriculture extension volunteer in the US Peace Corps, Michele completed graduate studies in sustainability management at the Earth Institute at Columbia University. At the time of this writing, Michele holds a private sector position working on global procurement strategy for organic and non-GMO foods. Michele also volunteers with a nonprofit organization that offers consulting for food and agriculture sector small businesses in developing economies.

James Kassaga Arinaitwe, MPH, MA

James Kassaga Arinaitwe is a global health and education advocate from Uganda. He is the cofounder and CEO of Teach For Uganda (TFU), a local nongovernmental organization that empowers young Ugandans to transform the nation's struggling education system. Prior to TFU, Kassaga worked for the Carter Center, Global Health Corps, Educate!, and BRAC. He's an Aspen Institute New Voices fellow, an Acumen global fellow, and a fellow at the African Leadership Network. Kassaga is an alumni of the Global Health Corps fellowship. His writings have been featured in *Al Jazeera,* NPR, Devex, the *Guardian,* and the *New York Times.* He is a graduate of Florida State University's College of Public Health & Policy and the SIT Graduate Institute's MA program in sustainable development and international policy. Website: http://www.jameskarinaitwe.com/writing/

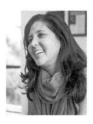

Ana Ayala, JD, LLM

Ana Ayala is the director of the global health law LLM Program at the O'Neill Institute for National and Global Health Law at Georgetown University. She focuses her work on global health security, which includes training legal, medical, and public health professionals to strengthen governments' ability to manage public health risks, and facilitating Global Health Security Agenda implementation through law.

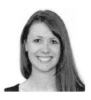

Alexis Barnes, MIPH

Alexis Barnes, the director of learning and training for GlobeMed, has been coordinating GlobeMed's education platform since January 2014. She has a diverse background working in various sectors of global development, including a position within the Chilean Ministry of Education, consulting for a capacity-building project in Uganda, and working in the International Grants Department for a public health organization. Most recently, Alexis completed a Global Health Corps fellowship in Uganda, working as a program manager for the Mpoma Community HIV/AIDS Initiative. That experience, coupled with a master's degree in international public health, drives her passion to be part of a movement and generation tackling underlying causes of social injustice.

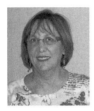

Linda C. Baumann, PhD, RN, FAAN

Linda Baumann is a professor emerita of the University of Wisconsin–Madison School of Nursing and School of Medicine and Public Health, and a fellow of the American Academy of Nursing and the Society of Behavioral Medicine. She received a BSN and MS in nursing from the University of Michigan and her PhD in psychology from the University of Wisconsin–Madison. Her expertise is in community health nursing, health behavior, and global health. Her research examines how beliefs about health and illness influence self-care behaviors, especially to promote diabetes self-care. She is a founding member of the UW–Madison Center for Global Studies and has led student field courses to Uganda, Cuba, Central America, and Thailand; she currently teaches in the masters of public health program. Professor Baumann has served as a consultant to the World Bank in Vietnam and in the West Bank for health workforce issues and health science programs. She is a Paul G. Rogers Society Global Health Research Ambassador and in 2012 was appointed to serve a four-year term on the US Preventive Services Task Force (https://www.uspreventiveservicestaskforce.org/).

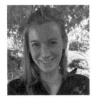

Sophie Broach

Sophie Broach is currently pursuing an MA in Global Affairs at Yale University's Jackson Institute. Previously, she worked in Laos for two years as an associate technical advisor for Population Services International, where she supported reproductive health and nutrition projects. She has also worked at the nonprofit Verité, where she carried out research on labor abuses, including violations of occupational safety and health standards. She holds a BA from Yale University.

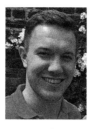

Evan DiPrete Brown

Evan DiPrete Brown graduated from Yale University with a degree in history. He is currently pursuing an MA in social sciences at the University of Chicago. His research focuses on sport, society, and culture.

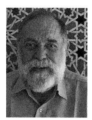

Richard Cash, MD

Dr. Richard Cash is a senior lecturer on global health in the Department of Global Health and Population at the Harvard T.H. Chan School of Public Health (HSPH). Cash and his colleagues conducted the first clinical trials of oral rehydration therapy in adult and pediatric cholera patients and patients with other infectious causes of diarrhea. For this work, he was presented the Prince Mahidol Award in 2006 and the Fries Prize in 2011. Other interests include scaling up health programs (as described in the book *From One to Many*), and health education and the development of public health institutions in LMICs. Cash is a visiting professor at a number of institutions in South and East Asia. He is also interested in research ethics in LMICs, and has conducted more than 60 workshops on research ethics in 15 countries.

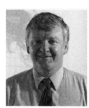

James F. Cleary, MD, FAChPM

Dr. Jim Cleary is a medical oncologist and palliative care physician trained at the University of Adelaide and the Royal Adelaide Hospital Australia. Since joining the University of Wisconsin–Madison faculty in 1995, he has been promoted to professor based on his development of clinical, education, and research programs in palliative care. His major focus is now on addressing the global lack of access to opioids in his work as director of the Pain and Policy Studies Group (PPSG) of the WHO Collaborating Center on Pain Policy and Palliative Care. PPSG interacts with over 40 countries and has been integrally involved in the International Pain Policy fellowship. Cleary serves on the *Lancet* Commission on Global Pain and Palliative Care and serves as chair for the American Society of Medical Oncology, where he collaborated on the development of resource-stratified guidelines on palliative care.

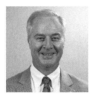

James Conway, MD

Dr. James Conway is a professor of pediatrics at the University of Wisconsin–Madison School of Medicine and Public Health, where he serves as director of the pediatric infectious diseases fellowship and as associate director for health sciences in the Global Health Institute. He has spent his career working and advocating for the prevention of vaccine-preventable disease, in the United States and abroad. He is a fellow of the American Academy of Pediatrics (AAP), and received an AAP Special Achievement Award in 2009 for his immunization projects. His interests include vaccine effectiveness, managing vaccine hesitancy, HPV vaccine initiatives, and the use of immunization registries. He is currently engaged in a new CDC/AAP collaboration, training pediatricians around the world as vaccine advocates.

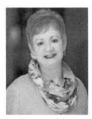

Mary Crave, PhD

Dr. Mary Crave has worked with extension and outreach programs at county, state, national, and international levels for 40 years. Her current focuses are on teaching outreach educators how to plan, teach, and evaluate programs, especially related to women and girls in agriculture, women's well-being, food security, participatory approaches, and youth development—in Africa and with the University of Wisconsin Extension. She credits her 10 years as a 4-H member in Wisconsin for not only introducing her to her profession but also making her the confident leader she is today. Crave holds degrees from the University of Wisconsin–Stout and the University of Wisconsin–Madison.

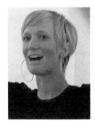

C. Perry Dougherty

Rev. C. Perry Dougherty is the executive director of Still Harbor, a group of spiritual leaders committed to offering comprehensive chaplaincy programs for social justice service and advocacy organizations. She is also an instructor at Harvard T.H. Chan School of Public Health and editor of *Anchor* magazine. She has more than 10 years of experience in organizational training and development. Perry brings an informed perspective on ministry, social justice, pedagogy, and learning to her work as a chaplain, facilitator, teacher, and writer. Perry is an ordained interfaith minister.

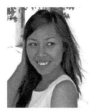

Devy Emperador, MPH

Devy Emperador is a global public health professional experienced in infectious disease research, laboratory capacity building, and project management in Sub-Saharan Africa. She served as a Global Health Corps fellow with the Infectious Diseases Institute in Uganda, a research fellow with the Division of Viral Diseases at the CDC in Atlanta, and a laboratory coordinator with the 2014–2015 CDC Ebola response in Sierra Leone. She joined University of California, San Francisco, in 2016 to manage a research trial that looks to improve HIV/AIDS testing and treatment adherence in southwestern Uganda. Devy is a graduate of Dickinson College and the UC Berkeley School of Public Health.

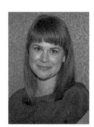

Jessica Evert, MD

Dr. Jessica Evert straddles international education and the medical profession. She served as the medical director of Child Family Health International from 2008 to 2013, when she was appointed to the executive director role. Evert is a member of faculty in the Department of Family and Community Medicine at the University of California, San Francisco, where she instructs in global health and community-based underserved care, and helped develop, as well as completed, the Global Health Clinical Scholars residency track. Evert is a graduate of the Ohio State University College of Medicine and is a longtime advocate for health-related international education quality and ethical standards.

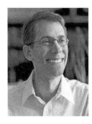

Eric A. Friedman, JD

Eric A. Friedman works at the O'Neill Institute for National and Global Health Law at Georgetown University, where he is project leader for the Platform for a Framework Convention on Global Health (FCGH), advocating for a global treaty grounded in the human right to health and aimed at closing health inequities. Along with the FCGH, he works on other right-to-health and global health projects. Before joining the O'Neill Institute, Eric was senior global health policy advisor at Physicians for Human Rights, where he focused on health systems, the global shortage of health workers, and HIV/AIDS. He holds a law degree from Yale Law School.

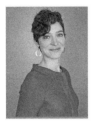

Sophia Friedson-Ridenour, PhD

Sophia Friedson-Ridenour holds a PhD from the University of Wisconsin–Madison in educational policy studies with a specialization in international and comparative education and a country expertise in Ghana, West Africa. Trained as an ethnographer, she collaborates with and works on multidisciplinary and mixed-methods projects across a range of sectors in international development, including education, health, agriculture, entrepreneurship, and governance. Thematically, her research across these sectors has focused on issues of one health, women and girls' inclusion and empowerment, community participation, global development policies, governance, and studying midlevel bureaucrats and middle-level actors. She has worked for the Center for Research on Gender and Women at UW–Madison and the African Gender Innovation Lab at the World Bank, and has collaborated on multiple research projects with scholars and practitioners from the Global Health Institute at UW–Madison.

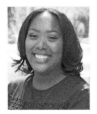

Angelina Gordon, MA

Angelina Gordon is director of communications, outreach, and diversity at the Global Health Fellows Program (GHFP) II, and oversees the communications and inclusion strategies that demonstrate USAID's thought-leadership in workforce development. She leads the project's outreach and diversity efforts by producing multimedia products for key audiences, including communities underrepresented in global health. Angelina previously served as knowledge management specialist with the Feed the Future Global Initiative, as well as senior specialist in knowledge management and documentation at Save the Children US. There she created the organization's first knowledge management strategy, which is still utilized. Angelina has worked in Africa and the Middle East and holds an MA in international development policy from Georgetown University.

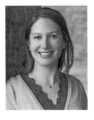

Katarina M. Grande, MPH

Katarina M. Grande is a public health practitioner focusing primarily on infectious disease surveillance, structural interventions, systemic poverty research, and HIV/AIDS program management. Globally, Katarina has worked with the CDC and PEPFAR in Tanzania, a USAID project as a

Global Health Corps fellow in Uganda, and an NIH research project in Malawi. Locally, she has worked for multiple city and state public health departments. She holds a BS in journalism and an MPH in environmental and global health. She currently works at the Wisconsin Division of Public Health's AIDS/HIV program as an epidemiologist.

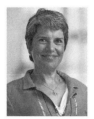

Cindy Haq, MD

Dr. Cindy Haq is a professor of family medicine and community health at the University of Wisconsin School of Medicine and Public Health. She is a champion for health equity and leads medical education programs to prepare health professionals to serve medically underserved communities. Haq has developed programs in Pakistan, Uganda, and Ethiopia and with governmental and nongovernmental organizations. She was the founding director of the UW Center for Global Health. She leads Training in Urban Medicine and Public Health (TRIUMPH) in Milwaukee, Wisconsin, to prepare medical students to become community-engaged physician leaders. She is a mother, grandmother, and teacher who delights in nurturing others to reach their highest potential.

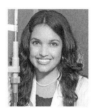

Luxme Hariharan, MD, MPH

Luxme Hariharan is a pediatric ophthalmologist who completed her ophthalmology training at the University of Pennsylvania and pediatric fellowships at the Bascom Palmer Eye Institute in Miami, Florida, and the Children's Hospital Los Angeles. She also has an MPH from Johns Hopkins, with an emphasis in global health and child health policy. Luxme's mission is to make sure that every child worldwide has the opportunity to develop his or her full visual potential and beyond. She is achieving this by bridging clinical and surgical care with policy, advocacy, and legislation for childhood blindness prevention both locally and globally.

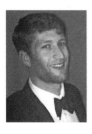

Andrew Hennessy-Strahs, JD

Andrew Hennessy-Strahs is a graduate of the UHC Chapel Hill School of Law, and is now an LLM student at Georgetown University Law Center. His interests include access to medicine and innovation of new medicines. He hopes to use an interdisciplinary approach to communicate with all stakeholders, across science, law, economics, and sociology.

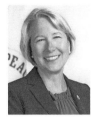

Carrie Hessler-Radelet, MS

Carrie Hessler-Radelet, the 19th director of the Peace Corps, was sworn in on June 25, 2014. Prior to this, she served as the agency's acting director and deputy director from 2010 to 2014. A member of a four-generation Peace Corps family, Hessler-Radelet began her career in international development as a Peace Corps volunteer in Western Samoa (1981–1983), teaching secondary school with her husband, Steve Radelet. She went on to spend more than two decades working in public health, focusing on HIV/AIDS and maternal and child health. During her time at the Peace Corps, Hessler-Radelet has led historic reforms to modernize and strengthen the agency to meet the challenges and opportunities of the 21st century. She spearheaded sweeping efforts to revitalize the volunteer recruitment, application, and selection process, resulting in record-breaking application numbers in 2015. Hessler-Radelet has also been instrumental in forging innovative strategic partnerships, such as Let Girls Learn, a powerful whole-of-government collaboration with First Lady Michelle Obama to expand access to education for adolescent girls around the world, and the Global Health Service Partnership, which sends physicians and nurses to teach in developing countries. Hessler-Radelet holds an MS in health policy and management from the Harvard School of Public Health and a BA in political science from Boston University. She and her husband have two children.

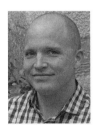

Eric Hettler, PE

Eric Hettler is a water resources engineering professional who has worked on complex water-related projects in North America and East Africa. He has experience working for both consulting engineering firms and international NGOs. His expertise includes the design and implementation of rural water supply and point-of-use water treatment programs and the planning and modeling of watershed-level projects. Hettler received his BS degree in civil engineering from Colorado State University, and he received his MS in civil engineering with an emphasis in water resources from the University of Minnesota. He was recently awarded his PE license from the National Society of Professional Engineers.

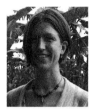

Laura E. Jacobson, MPH

Laura Jacobson received an MPH and certificate in global health from the University of Wisconsin–Madison. There she conducted qualitative research in rural Uganda on the role of mobile phone technology in strengthening the health system. In addition, she has contributed to academic, community-based, and government health services research on topics of patient–provider relationships, diversity in the workforce, access to cancer screening technology, and social entrepreneurship. She is most interested in how research can translate into lasting change for real people. Currently she consults on several public health–focused projects, including Oregon Health & Science University's Footsteps to Healing program for enhancing women's health in Ethiopia, and Hillside Health Care International for education and public health program development in rural Belize. She resides in Portland, Oregon, with her husband and son. Blog: https://lauraejacobson.com/

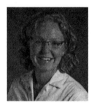

Gabrielle A. Jacquet, MD, MPH

Dr. Gabrielle A. Jacquet is the director of global health for the Boston Medical Center Emergency Medicine Residency Program and the assistant director of global health at the Boston University School of Medicine. Jacquet focuses on strengthening and standardizing global health in medical education. She is the founding course director for the Practitioner's Guide to Global Health, a series of three timeline-based, interactive, open-access courses to prepare trainees for safe and effective global health learning experiences. She is also the medical director for Child Family Health International, a 501(c)(3) that specializes in global health education.

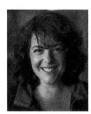

Nancy Kendall, PhD

Nancy Kendall is associate professor of educational policy studies at University of Wisconsin–Madison. Her research examines the consequences of national and international policies and funding streams directed at improving marginalized children's, communities', and states' well-being. She is affiliated with the African Studies Program, the Department of Gender and Women's Studies, the Development Studies Program, and the Global Health Institute at UW–Madison.

Kendall conducts comparative ethnographic research on US and global development education policies and their intersections with children's and families' daily lives. Research projects have examined Education for All, political democratization and educational governance, structural adjustment and education, US higher education, sexuality and HIV/AIDS education, and gender and schooling. Kendall has conducted extended research in Malawi, Mozambique, and the United States, and has conducted short-term research in Colombia, Kyrgyzstan, Tajikistan, and Zimbabwe. Kendall was a 2009 National Academy of Education/Spencer Foundation postdoctoral fellow, and has received research support from the Fulbright Foundation, Social Science Research Council, TAG Philanthropic Foundation, Wenner-Gren Foundation, WT Grant Foundation, and Lumina Foundation, among others. She is the author of *The Sex Education Debates* (University of Chicago Press, 2012) and has published in journals including *Compare, Comparative Education Review, Current Issues in Comparative Education, Educational Assessment Evaluation and Accountability, International Journal of Educational Development,* and *Sexuality Research and Social Policy.*

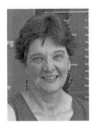

Connie Kraus, PharmD, BCACP

Connie Kraus directs the University of Wisconsin School of Pharmacy Office of Global Health and is a board-certified ambulatory care pharmacist, working throughout her career as a member of interdisciplinary health care teams. In 1993, she joined the faculty of UW, where she has developed numerous international collaborations resulting in educational opportunities for students, as well as research collaborations. She developed a clinical practice with the Department of Family Medicine and Community Health, where for more than 20 years she provided care at a clinic affiliated with a community health center. Kraus received her BS and PharmD degrees from the UW–Madison School of Pharmacy.

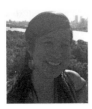

Carolina Kwok, BSc (PT), MPH

Carolina Kwok started her career as a physical therapist working with patients with neurological conditions. She worked with spinal injury teams in Nepal and worked with a community-based organization for people with disabilities in Cambodia. After attaining her MPH, she interned at the Pan-American Health Organization and started her global health career working in HIV research in Zambia, then in maternal health in Tanzania and tuberculosis in Africa and Asia. She started at the Clinton Health Access Initiative in 2014 to increase access to optimal MDR-TB drugs and diagnostics at sustainable prices.

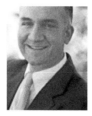

Alain B. Labrique, PhD, MHS, MS

Dr. Alain Labrique is the founding director of the Johns Hopkins University Global mHealth Initiative, a multidisciplinary center of excellence with over 140 projects engaged in mHealth innovation and research across the Johns Hopkins system. Labrique is lead investigator for several research projects measuring the impact of mobile information and communications technologies on improving maternal, neonatal, and infant health in resource-limited settings. Labrique was recognized as one of the top 11 mHealth innovators in 2011 by the Rockefeller Foundation and the UN Foundation and was a lead author on a Bellagio Declaration on mHealth Evidence. Labrique serves as an mHealth and technical advisor to several international and global health agencies and ministries of health, including the World Health Organization, GSMA, USAID, the mHealth Alliance, and HealthEnabled. Labrique serves as the current chair of the WHO mHealth Technical Evidence Review Group, a technical body convened to advise governments on mHealth investments. Labrique received a Presidential Excellence in Advising Award for teaching and mentoring students at the Bloomberg School, as he and his team strive to develop mortality reduction strategies for resource-limited settings.

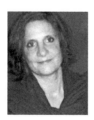

Teresa Langle de Paz, PhD

Dr. Langle de Paz is the codirector of the UNESCO Chair on Gender, Well-Being and a Culture of Peace at the University of Wisconsin–Madison and visiting professor and honorary fellow at the Department of Gender and Women's Studies. She is founder and codirector of a global educational feminist project, Women's Knowledge International (www.womensknowledge.org) (WKI), anchored at the Institute for Human Rights, Democracy and a Culture of Peace and Non-Violence (Demospaz), an institution founded and presided by former UNESCO general director Mr. Federico Mayor Zaragoza at Autonomous University of Madrid, Spain (www.demospaz.org). WKI's main premises are "making women's and feminist knowledge flow transnationally and intersectorially" and "bridging experiential knowledge and scientific research." Langle de Paz is also a member of the advisory board at the Foundation Women for Africa (www.mujeresporafrica.es). She has a doctorate in philosophy from Brown University and has been a professor of early modern Spanish literature and feminist theory at Lawrence University and the University of Houston in the United States and at Complutense University, International Menéndez Pelayo University, and Jaume I University in Spain.

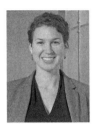

Katherine Leach-Kemon, MPH

As a policy translation manager at the Institute for Health Metrics and Evaluation (IHME) at the University of Washington, Katherine Leach-Kemon oversees the organization's work to bridge the gap between academic research and policy. To this end, she writes and contributes to the production of reports, infographics, and policy briefs; fosters collaboration with external organizations; and disseminates information to decision makers. Katherine originally came to IHME as a postgraduate fellow and has participated in the Institute's production of its *Financing Global Health* report since it was first published in 2009. Her work has been published in *The Lancet, Health Affairs,* and the *Journal of the American Medical Association.* Katherine received her MPH from the University of Washington.

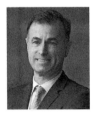

Keith Martin, MD, PC

Dr. Keith Martin is a physician, the founding executive director of the Consortium of Universities for Global Health (CUGH), a former six-term member of Parliament in Canada's House of Commons, and a member of the Queen's Privy Council for Canada. His main areas of interest are global health, foreign policy, security, international development, conservation, and the environment. Martin has been on numerous diplomatic missions, particularly in Africa, and has authored more than 160 published editorials.

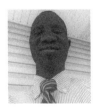

Augustino Ting Mayai, PhD

Augustino Ting Mayai is a South Sudanese demographic and development specialist with a PhD in sociology and development studies from the University of Wisconsin–Madison. Currently conducting health policy research in South Sudan and Ethiopia, he is also a research director at the Sudd Institute, the nation's premier think tank, and an assistant professor of public service at the University of Juba. His other professional experiences include working for the World Bank, UNICEF, UNFPA, the government of South Sudan (Office of the President), HTSPE, BlueForce, and the MSI.

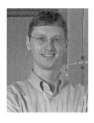

Sean McKee

Sean McKee specializes in policy translation for the Institute for Health Metrics and Evaluation (IHME) at the University of Washington in Seattle. His work in policy translation emphasizes explaining the often technical and arcane work of epidemiologists, health economists, and geospatial researchers to nonexperts in accessible and compelling ways. His work at IHME spans a range of topics including global burden of disease, evaluations, and resource tracking. His professional background includes time-managing, monitoring, and evaluating public health projects; managing a beer and wine store; and teaching college history.

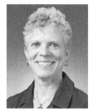

Janet Niewold, MS

Janet Niewold leads the University of Wisconsin–Madison global health field course Microenterprise and Health in Ecuador and is the founder and advisor for Wisconsin Without Borders Marketplace. She holds a lead role in UW's 4W initiative on women and microenterprise through the School of Human Ecology's Community Health and Wellbeing through Design and Microenterprise project. Janet has an MS in Latin American studies from UW–Madison. She operated her own business buying and selling artisan work from Latin America for over 20 years before bringing her expertise to UW–Madison.

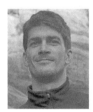

Kevin Orner

Kevin Orner is a PhD candidate in environmental engineering at the University of South Florida, where he studies nutrient and energy recovery from centralized wastewater treatment plants. After obtaining a BS in civil and environmental engineering with a certificate in technical communication from the University of Wisconsin–Madison in 2008, Kevin served for two years as a Peace Corps volunteer in Panama. In December 2011, he completed his MS in civil and environmental engineering at the University of South Florida. Kevin is an engineer in training (EIT) with engineering consulting experience.

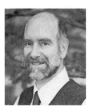

Jonathan Patz, MD, MPH

Dr. Jonathan Patz is a professor and the John P. Holton Chair in Health and the Environment at the University of Wisconsin–Madison, where he directs the Global Health Institute and has appointments in the Nelson Institute and the Department of Population Health Sciences. He is a long-standing expert on the health implications of global climate change. Patz served as a lead author on the Intergovernmental Panel on Climate

Change (IPCC) for 14 years, and cochaired the Health Expert Panel of the first US National Climate Assessment. He has taught and conducted research on climate change and its relations to health for nearly two decades.

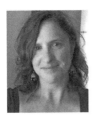

Louise Penner, PhD

Louise Penner is an associate professor of English at the University of Massachusetts Boston, where she teaches courses in 19th-century British literature and culture, and medical humanities. She is the author of *Victorian Medicine and Social Reform: Florence Nightingale among the Novelists* (Palgrave McMillan, 2010) and coeditor with Tabitha Sparks (McGill University) of *Victorian Medicine and Popular Culture* (Pickering and Chatto, 2015; reprinted by University of Pittsburgh Press, 2015).

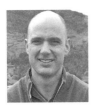

Giuseppe Raviola, MD, MPH

Dr. Giuseppe Raviola is an assistant professor of psychiatry and global health and social medicine at Harvard Medical School. He serves as director of mental health for Partners in Health, an international nongovernmental organization that builds health systems in 10 countries in close collaboration with local teams and ministries of health, and as director of the Program in Global Mental Health and Social Change at Harvard. Raviola's scholarly contributions center on the integration and application of quality improvement and public health approaches in innovating clinical practice, teaching, and research in the domains of psychiatry and global mental health.

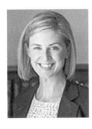

Sarah Roache, LLM, LLB

Sarah Roache is a senior associate at the O'Neill Institute for National and Global Health Law at Georgetown University. Sarah researches legal and policy interventions to reduce non-communicable disease risk factors, including tobacco and unhealthy foods. Sarah has also worked as a litigator, representing victims of tobacco-related diseases and thalidomide survivors.

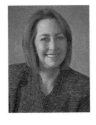

Sharon Rudy, PhD, BCC

Dr. Sharon Rudy, board-certified coach and board-certified counselor, is program director for the Global Health Fellows Program (GHFP) II at the Public Health Institute. Funded by USAID, the fellowship and internship program helps build the next generation of global health professionals. In her previous role as senior faculty at Johns Hopkins University Bloomberg School of Public Health, Rudy spent almost a decade working in Anglophone Africa designing, implementing, and evaluating national behavior change communication programs and client–provider interaction interventions. She has also worked in the Middle East, Africa, and Asia implementing performance improvement and training programs through IntraHealth, then based at the Medical School of the University of North Carolina, Chapel Hill. Rudy holds a PhD in counseling and organizational consulting and is a published author.

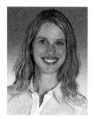

Trisha Seys Ranola, PharmD, CDE, BCGP

Trisha is a clinical assistant professor and the assistant director of the Office of Global Health at the University of Wisconsin–Madison School of Pharmacy, where she earned her degree in 2002, followed by a pharmacy practice residency at the William S. Middleton Memorial Veterans Hospital in 2003. She is currently a member of the Home Based Primary Care interdisciplinary team at the Madison VA clinic, which provides longitudinal care to veterans in their homes. She volunteered as a bilingual certified diabetes educator at a community health center, and continues her journey in global public health through her work in the Office of Global Health mentoring students and collaborating with international partners to form new educational programs and quality improvement research partnerships.

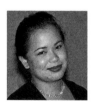

Sweta Shrestha, MPH

Sweta Shrestha is the assistant director for education for the University of Wisconsin–Madison Global Health Institute, where she serves as an advisor and instructional specialist for both the graduate and undergraduate certificates in global health and the associated field experiences. She was born in Nepal and immigrated with her family to the United States. Shrestha earned her bachelor's and her MPH from the UW–Madison School of Medicine and Public Health. She has worked on research and educational programs in multiple countries across South Asia and Africa, including Nepal, Sri Lanka, Uganda, Ghana, Ethiopia, and Zambia.

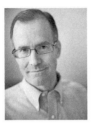

Brian W. Simpson, MPH, MA

Brian W. Simpson is editor-in-chief of the news website and weekday e-newsletter *Global Health NOW* (http://www.globalhealthnow.org/) and editor of *Hopkins Bloomberg Public Health* magazine, published by the Johns Hopkins Bloomberg School of Public Health. He also teaches science writing at Johns Hopkins University. Simpson earned an MA from the Writing Seminars at Johns Hopkins and an MPH from the Bloomberg School.

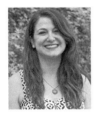

Alyssa Smaldino

Alyssa Smaldino is the executive director of GlobeMed. She studied public health at George Washington University (GWU), where she acted as copresident of GlobeMed and conducted internships with the GlobalGiving Foundation and National Institute of Mental Health. She began working for GlobeMed in July 2011 as the organization's first director of partnerships, during which time she conducted in-person capacity assessments with 50 grassroots organizations across 18 countries, provided leadership training to over 500 students, and started a program for grassroots leaders to develop new strategies for donor and volunteer relations. She became executive director in May 2015.

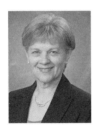

Karen D. Solheim, PhD, RN

Dr. Karen Solheim is a clinical professor and the director of undergraduate programs and the director of global health initiatives at the University of Wisconsin–Madison School of Nursing. She began global health work through service to encamped refugees and displaced persons in Thailand. Since then she has consulted on projects in Somalia, Cambodia, and India. She cofounded International Partners for Education, Inc., an organization that advocates social justice for orphaned and vulnerable children in Malawi. Solheim has developed and taught global health courses including experiences in Thailand, Malawi, Ireland, and Belize. She completed a postdoctoral traineeship in primary health care at the University of Illinois at Chicago College of Nursing Global Health Leadership Office, a WHO Collaborating Center for International Nursing Development in Primary Health Care.

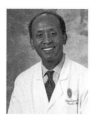

Girma Tefera, MD, FACS

Girma Tefera is a professor of surgery at the University of Wisconsin School of Medicine and Public Health. Since 2015, he has served as the medical director of the Operation Giving Back program at the American College of Surgeons. He is a native of Ethiopia and a medical school graduate from University of Pisa, Italy. He has worked in global health for over 15 years. His current focus is on providing leadership in global efforts to improve access to basic and emergency surgery for the billions of underserved people across the globe.

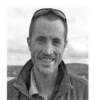

Jason Vargo, PhD, MPH, MCRP

Dr. Jason Vargo is an assistant scientist with the University of Wisconsin–Madison's Nelson Institute for Environmental Studies and the Global Health Institute. He works at the intersection of environmental urban planning and public health and explores the influence of urban design on healthy behaviors and safety, urban climate change, and the role of cities in global environmental change.

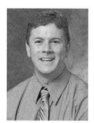

Kevin Wyne, PA-C, MPAS, MSc

Kevin Wyne is a faculty member at the University of Wisconsin Physician Assistant (PA) Program, where he is involved in many aspects of didactic and clinical education. He has worked clinically as an emergency medicine PA for the last 10+ years. Kevin is actively involved in global health work and coordinates service-learning experiences for health sciences students in Belize and Guatemala through the UW Global Health Institute. Areas of scholarly interest include the intersections between medicine and humanities, interprofessional medical education, extending health care to underserved areas, wilderness medicine, and incorporating technology into medical training.

ACKNOWLEDGMENTS

TEACHING IS a joy, a responsibility, and an honor. I feel so fortunate to have had the opportunity to teach as a member of the University of Wisconsin's rich interdisciplinary global health community. During my time with the Global Health Institute (GHI) at UW–Madison, I have had the privilege of collaborating with colleagues from public health, medicine, nursing, pharmacy, veterinary medicine, agriculture, engineering, environmental sciences, and more.

The GHI focus on sustainable global health has had a profound impact on my global health teaching and practice. I thank the following UW colleagues, many of whom are featured in these pages: Cindy Haq, Linda Baumann, Jim Conway, Connie Kraus, Chris Olsen, Jonathan Patz, Trisha Seys Ranola, Karen Solheim, and Betsy Teigland, who worked together to develop our graduate global health education programs that serve as a foundation for our campus-wide program. I also thank Sweta Shrestha, Pat Remington, Sherry Tanumihardjo, Susan Paskewitz, John Ferrick, Rick Keller, Josh Garoon, Devika Suri, Katie Freeman, and Robin Mittenthal for our wonderful shared work in UW's global health program for undergraduates.

I acknowledge the University of Wisconsin School of Medicine and Public Health, which has provided me with an academic home and supportive environment for my teaching and scholarship for over a decade. I am also grateful for the public health training I received at the Harvard School of Public Health and the Harvard Divinity School over 25 years ago. From working on child health and equity issues in Boston, to exploring linkages between health, faith, and human rights, to carrying out my first field studies in Nicaragua, Costa Rica, and Cameroon—I got the message that my work was important, that I could lead if I worked hard, and that well-being for all was possible. I am honored that I still have some connections to faculty and staff there, and can walk through those doors and feel 25 again!

I am particularly grateful to the global health leaders from around the world who have contributed chapters to this book. Amid the demands of global work, research activities, and their personal commitments, they have taken time to invest in the next generation of leaders.

I especially thank Katarina Grande and Laura Jacobson, who, in addition to offering their global health expertise and experience as authors, assisted me with editing the overall manuscript and in identifying authors from their networks who have made wonderful contributions to the book.

Finally, I thank the students who have studied with me over the years. Many have gone on to work as health care providers locally or globally, to study public health, or to serve in programs like the Peace Corps, AmeriCorps, or Teach for America. My life has been so enriched by knowing them, teaching them, and now having them as global health colleagues.

D URING THE past 25 years, global health study has evolved from a field defined by preventing the spread of infectious disease and medical service in poor countries to a dynamic interdisciplinary public health enterprise that fosters global collaboration to address disparities and maximize sustainable well-being across and within local, regional, national, global, and planetary geographies.

Foundations for Global Health Practice is an introductory text for undergraduate students from a broad range of disciplines who want to engage in global health practice in ways that are sustainable, ethical, and informed by current scholarship and practice. Global health activities have traditionally focused on infectious disease, population dynamics, and access to basic needs such as food and water, and it is important to sustain these commitments. Global initiatives have also worked to develop effective health care systems in low- and middle-income countries. It is essential to prepare students to build on success to date in these areas, through two-way partnerships that allow for comparative learning and mutual benefits in terms of quality, safety, access, and efficiency. Experiences from these lower-resource settings are important sources of global health innovation and improvement for all.

Concurrent with this progress in preventive and curative health care, the scope of global health has expanded to embrace the complex challenges and opportunities associated with globalization: new information technologies and increased environmental pressures due to increased human population and high-consumption lifestyles. Leaders in health care, government, civil society, and the private sector, as well as citizens themselves, have become increasingly aware of the need for all sectors to work together to enhance human health in ways that respect and protect the integrity and biodiversity of ecosystems, safeguard the health of our planet, and use resources in ways that are equitable and just. *Foundations for Global Public Health Practice* introduces core global public health concepts, presents principles and methods for effective engagement, and provides perspectives on critical issues from global health leaders.

Part 1 focuses on global health concepts. It begins with an invitation for students to take a leadership role in their own learning to develop a global perspective. It defines global health, identifies current challenges, and outlines systems, policies, and approaches that are in place to improve health and well-being. Further, it explores global health in the context of the Sustainable Development Goals (SDGs) and introduces students to such critical topics as global mental health, water and sanitation, agriculture and nutrition, climate change, and planetary health. Finally, it gives an overview of the role of information technology in global health and explores strategies related to scale-up of global health interventions.

Part 2 focuses on global health practice, providing guidance for global health engagement, including group field study, student internships, US-based global advocacy, and work on health disparities locally. It provides an overview of global health competencies, strategies for working with communities, and approaches to cultivating transformative leadership skills. It includes principles and models for global health field study courses that will be useful to instructors and students alike, provides guidance for student organizations, and offers some basic health and safety recommendations. Finally, it offers practical advice relating to identifying internships and jobs and developing a global health career.

Part 3 provides global health perspectives on a broad range of critical topics. This is a resource that can support self-study for students who want to pursue special interests or gain additional perspectives. These short chapters and the recommended readings included can also serve as a springboard that will allow course instructors to complement the text with guest lectures from faculty and community leaders who are engaged with global health disparities.

In summary, *Foundations for Global Health Practice* is designed as an introductory step toward transformative engagement in global health. Students will consider multisector strategies for sustainable health and well-being. They will be encouraged to understand health challenges, whether local or international, in a global and comparative context. Finally, and perhaps most important, they will be encouraged to be reflective about their engagement and gain a better understanding of the personal, local, and international implications of global citizenship in an interdependent world.

PART ONE

GLOBAL HEALTH
CONCEPTS

CHAPTER 1

DEVELOPING A GLOBAL PERSPECTIVE

Lori DiPrete Brown, MS, MTS

The teacher is no longer merely the-one-who-teaches, but one who is himself taught in dialogue with the students, who in turn while being taught also teach. They become jointly responsible for a process in which all grow.

—Paulo Freire

LEARNING OBJECTIVES

- Understand your responsibility to continually acquire and share global health perspectives and information as a contributing member of your learning community
- Identify and articulate the unique perspectives and experiences that you want to share within your community, and prepare to listen and learn from the perspectives and experiences of others
- Describe and access a variety of global health information sources that can inform global health work and study
- Consider literature and the arts as ways to inform and better understand health and well-being
- Create a personalized plan to use information sources, the arts, networks, and engagement to stay informed about global health

You are probably studying global health because you are interested in engaging with people from around the world, and you want, in some way, to be a partner for global change. You might be aware that, while 3.2 billion people had access to the Internet in 2015 (International Telecommunications Union, 2016), approximately 2.1 billion people, in spite of progress in recent decades, lack access to a safe water supply at home, and 4.4 billion lack safely managed sanitation (United Nations Children's Fund, 2016).

Foundations for Global Health Practice, First Edition. Lori DiPrete Brown.
© 2018 John Wiley & Sons, Inc. Published 2018 by John Wiley & Sons, Inc.

Further, 795 million people, nearly one in nine, are undernourished (Food and Agriculture Organization, 2015). You might be concerned about disease outbreaks such as the Ebola or Zika viruses, or you might find excitement in the possibility of polio eradication, which is within reach if political will and technical know-how can come together to address it. Perhaps you are interested in combating maternal and infant mortality, which will require strategies that combine health care with nutritional support and overall poverty reduction. You might be motivated by issues related to the environment and health, with an interest in sustaining human life and caring for the earth at the same time. You likely already know that these matters form the action agenda for your generation, and that addressing these problems is a complex enterprise. These challenges can be overwhelming, the barriers are formidable, and yet you want to engage, because advancing global health and well-being is important to you. You want to learn, and you think you have something to offer.

You may be a student who has traveled extensively, or you may be preparing for your first journey. Many of you will be studying places that are completely new to you, hoping to understand and embrace cultural differences while you find a way to make an impact. Some of you are exploring countries or regions that are somehow part of your own heritage, hoping that your special knowledge and connection will be an asset, as you bridge distance and generations to live a global life. Others may be preparing to engage with health challenges and disparities in your own country and community, bringing a new global lens to a familiar place. Still others are interested in working "everywhere," on issues that transcend national boundaries, such as infectious disease pandemics, the impact of climate change, and global resource scarcity. You aspire to work in the professions of health, education, engineering, agriculture, and governance. You are students of the biological sciences, the humanities and social sciences, the arts, and many other fields that can contribute to improved global health.

You and your classmates are motivated by many things, such as curiosity, a sense of justice, your faith, a spirit of adventure, a feeling of compassion and care for people, an interest in economic development, or a desire to foster peace or to promote the sustainability of our planet. You are part of a generation of students that has more access to information than any previous generation, and you are more interconnected than ever with other young people from a wide variety of backgrounds.

The geographic, disciplinary, and human terrain to be covered is vast, and the global health field is dynamic, with new challenges and perspectives and innovations emerging constantly. What does a student like you expect to learn in a global health class? What should you expect from your teachers? And what should they expect from you?

The study of global health can embrace the rich and diverse information available through a pedagogy of joint learning. Course leaders offer core content and structure to the inquiry, drawing on their own expertise as well as guest lectures from the campus and the community. Students contribute information and perspectives from their life experiences. In this way, the global health class is a rich learning experience for faculty members and students alike. Your study will be informed by many voices, many disciplines, and intergenerational perspectives.

This chapter provides guidance toward gaining global perspectives from within your classroom community, and outlines how you can use a broad range of information sources from health and social sciences research, the popular media, literature, music, and art to develop a global worldview. To explore these matters further, consider the following chapters in part 3: Brian Simpson's So You Want to Save the World? First, You've Got to Know It (chapter 21) and Louise Penner's reflection, The Importance of Narrative to Global Health Research and Practice (chapter 37). Self-directed reading during your global health course will help you identify your specific interests, talents, and passions. It will also allow you to be a deliberative and well-informed citizen advocate for improved health—both locally and globally, now and in the future.

Sharing Perspectives in a Diverse Learning Community

Most students agree that the most rewarding and educational aspect of global health learning is the experiential learning that is undertaken in communities around the world. It can be easy to overlook the fact that your classroom itself is a global learning opportunity. Lectures, readings, and discussion topics include many academic disciplines and regions of the world, and content should be inclusive of diverse perspectives in terms of race, gender, ethnicity, and sexual orientation, so that learning integrates the wisdom, knowledge, and experience of historically marginalized populations.

Perspective taking is an important skill related to social responsibility and professional and civic engagement both locally and globally. It can be defined as "taking seriously the perspectives of others: recognizing and acting on the obligation to inform one's own judgment; engaging diverse and competing perspectives as a resource for learning, citizenship, and work" (Dey and Associates, 2010, p. 1). The ability to learn from the perspectives of others, use evidence to support your own views, reconsider your opinions when presented with new information, and understand other points of view and maintain civil discourse with those who hold views different from your own are key components of perspective taking. Here we discuss some strategies for sharing diverse perspectives in your global health study.

Asking better questions. "Where are you from?" "What's your major?" "What is your religion?" "What political party do you belong to?" "Are you an athlete?" "Do you belong to a frat?" "What are you doing for spring break?" "Why are you studying global health?" These are questions that we often use to learn about others. Although there is nothing wrong with these questions in themselves, we can see that they are aimed at categorization and finding sameness, rather than being more open ended and allowing people to share differences. Much information is gained from these questions, but they may tempt us to apply stereotypes instead of experiencing people as individuals, and they may inadvertently lead to feelings of exclusion.

If our engagement is intended to purposefully increase inclusivity, share values and life experiences, and also learn from differences, then we might consider alternative strategies for asking questions. If we exchange or complement categorizing questions with questions that are open ended, and leave the type and degree of disclosure to the respondent, we can give people a chance to share what they know and want to share. Examples of these types of questions include, "What would you like our class to know about you?" "What knowledge and life experiences would you like to share in relation to today's topic?" "What do you hope to learn from others?" "Tell us more about your interests in global health."

Preparing to share your experiences. Preparing yourself for conversations about diversity in your own classroom is a great way to develop cross-cultural skills that will serve you well at home and abroad. Identify the unique life perspectives and experiences that you want to share, and take time to plan how you will frame your experience, what you want to disclose, what you do not want to disclose, what questions might arise, and how you will answer. It is important to balance risk-taking and vulnerability, which can lead to friendship and trust, with sensible and appropriate emotional boundaries. Fortunately, global health students generally have at least a semester together, and often share travel and immersion learning experiences as well, so there is time to share perspectives and to challenge each other gradually.

Listening and learning from others. Respectful and courteous listening, refraining from interrupting, and refraining from judging others are essential when you are sharing opinions and life experiences related to global health, especially when the topics are complex or controversial. It is important to try to consider the issue from the perspective of others and to formulate questions and comments accordingly. Listening strategies promote deeper sharing and understanding of different points of view. **Active listening** is the practice of listening to a speaker while providing feedback indicating that the listener both hears and understands what the speaker is saying (Grohol, 2016). Key strategies for active listening include listening with attention, refraining from interrupting, and allowing for pauses. It can also be helpful to prompt further conversations with phrases like "Tell me more" and other simple verbal encouragements. Restating or reflecting what you are being told is a good way to show that you understand and are listening. Also, following up with open questions can help share with more depth and detail.

One issue that can arise in classroom conversations about diversity is that students from historically marginalized groups are inadvertently put in the position of representing their entire group (which likely includes many distinct points of view) or having to do the work of educating teachers and other students about their experiences, without regard to balance, reciprocity, or appropriateness (Tilleczek & Ferguson, 2013). Instructors and facilitators can prevent this by setting ground rules with the group and monitoring and guiding the conversations. However, it is important for everyone in the group to make an effort to educate themselves alongside the group inquiry process and to consider intentionally what they would like to share and what they would like to learn.

Skills for discussion and debate. Global health conversations that explore a range of perspectives should lead to debate, differences of opinion, and sometimes difficult conversations. There is perhaps no better preparation for life and global citizenship. Points of view should be stated clearly and supported by evidence. Disagreement should be honest, civil, and respectful. Although you may find that you learn and change your mind as a result of discussion, the goal of these exchanges is not to reach consensus but rather to clearly understand the perspectives of others and to explore a range of opinions. If areas of disagreement reach an impasse, identify common ground and try to stay in a constructive conversation.

Sources of Global Health Information

In addition to bringing your rich life experiences to class, it is essential that you make a commitment to educating yourself and staying informed about global health topics, beyond assigned course readings. Global health study puts great emphasis on the public health academic literature, health statistics, epidemiology, and scientific evidence, as well as on anthropological and sociological research on the cultural and contexts that create health and disease. Also inclusive of perspectives from political science, economics, management, and implementation science, the public health literature is highly interdisciplinary. This section will discuss health statistics, the peer-reviewed academic literature, primary source documents, the gray literature, news media, nonfiction books, and general information sources to inform your global perspective.

Health Statistics

What is the leading cause of death in the world? What countries have the highest and lowest rates of infant mortality? How does the health status in countries with great per capita wealth compare to that in poorer countries? How are these health statistics changing over time? **Health statistics** include both empirical data and estimates related to health. Although it can seem arduous to memorize statistics for their own sake, an understanding of basic measures, and familiarity with the broad parameters of health statuses are essential to accurately characterize the human experience of our times. Global health practitioners should be able to access, cite, and interpret demographic and health statistics to answer questions like the preceding with data that are accurate and relevant. This skill will be important for research, advocacy, and practice.

The 2010 Global Burden of Disease Study, perhaps the most comprehensive study of its kind, reports ischemic heart disease as the leading cause of death globally, with an estimated seven million deaths in 2010 (Lozano et al., 2010). United Nations infant mortality estimates for 2015 indicated the lowest number of deaths per thousand infants in countries such as Iceland, Japan, Singapore, and Sweden (2), whereas Angola (96) has the highest rate of infant death in the world. The infant mortality rate in the United States is around 6 per 1,000; and more than 40 countries, most with lower per capita incomes, have better rates of infant survival than the United States (United Nations, 2015). Although these infant mortality rates reflect unacceptable levels of disparity, inequality, and inequity, there have been considerable successes in global health during the last 20 years. The global burden of disease data show that child mortality rates for children under five decreased by 60% from 1990 through 2010. Life expectancy overall increased by 12 to 15 years for men and women, reflecting lower rates of child mortality and other health improvements as well.

Data about mortality, morbidity, life expectancy, population, and other descriptive statistics are more available than ever before, allowing you to easily find answers to questions and to obtain a snapshot of the health status of populations in the countries where you will work or study. These statistics are valuable tools for research, practice, and advocacy because they can help characterize the frequency, severity, and importance of the health problems of individuals, communities, regions, and nations. We will explore these types of statistics in more depth in chapter 5.

It is important to know how to access and interpret health statistics and to be able to place them in a meaningful context with comparative data, both in terms of geographic comparisons and comparisons over time. In addition, chapter 5 provides a detailed overview of measures of disease burden and the Global Burden of Disease Study. Of course, health statistics are just the beginning of an in-depth inquiry, and complementary information about culture, economics, social conditions, and other factors will be needed to gain a thorough understanding of the disease burden, its causes, and strategies for prevention and treatment.

Peer-Reviewed Academic Literature

A **peer-reviewed journal** submits its research articles for outside review before publication. The specifics of the process may vary, with each journal following its own guidelines regarding manuscript submissions, the number of reviewers, review procedures, and the influence of reviewers' feedback (International Committee of Medical Journal Editors, 2010).

Generally, when a researcher submits an article to a peer-reviewed journal for consideration, an editor will review the submission, then identify and solicit peer reviewers.

(Often a double-blind process is used, whereby the authors and reviewers do not know each other.) Depending on the review, the journal may accept the article as is, request corrections and revisions, or reject the article. This expert review process increases the likelihood that what is published is accurate, well written, and appropriately referenced, and reflects new discovery.

In spite of the rigor of the peer-review process, there are several shortcomings in the production and dissemination of the peer-reviewed literature that limit its ability to realize its full potential to impact health and well-being. First, because health science research dollars are invested disproportionately, with only 10% of research dollars addressing the problems that face 90% of the population, there is a corresponding gap in the academic literature, which underrepresents health issues experienced by populations in low-income settings, including such conditions as malaria, tuberculosis, malnutrition, and infant and maternal mortality (Langer, Díaz-Olavarrieta, Berdichevsky, & José Villar, 2004). Second, because of the many challenges and barriers related to research capacity development at the individual and system levels, researchers from lower-income settings are underrepresented in the academic literature, leaving important gaps in the literature in terms of perspective, geographic representation, and representation of socially marginalized groups. Finally, leaders, researchers, and practitioners in low-resource settings may have trouble accessing the most recent research because of the difficulty of accessing print or electronic copies of the articles, language barriers (the literature is predominantly in English), or prohibitive subscription fees or copyright restrictions. Therefore, the discoveries reported in the peer-reviewed literature are not disseminated and adopted into practice as widely or as quickly as they should.

Efforts are under way to address all of these issues, as research-oriented grant-making agencies try to increase the focus on health disparities and low-resource settings, and investments in international training and partnerships work to strengthen global research capacity. Particularly notable is the open-access movement, which aims to make health information available worldwide free of charge. One leading and successful example is *PLoS Medicine*, a high-impact journal with open access and many globally focused articles. Another effort to increase access was initiated by the World Health Organization and a number of major health science journals in 2002. They established the Hinari Access to Research for Health program (see http://www.who.int/hinari/en/), which provides free access to more than 11,000 journals in over 100 low-income countries. This is not a full open-access model, as access may still be a challenge for some in higher-income countries; however, it removes barriers for many researchers who reside in low-income countries. Unfortunately, some countries with large health burdens and high levels of poverty, such as India, Pakistan, Indonesia, and China, do not receive free access benefits through Hinari, because they represent emerging markets for some of the major participating journals.

Another important source of health-related evidence in clinical, public health, and health equity research is Cochrane, a collaborative network that produces accessible health information. Established in 1993, Cochrane focuses on summarizing the most current health-related evidence through rigorous systematic review and synthesis of multiple articles on a given health topic. Initially, these analyses tended to prioritize English-language literature and higher-income countries, but the organization has grown decidedly international, with members from over 120 countries, and efforts are under way to provide more information in translation and to create more open access.

One example of a systematic review published by Cochrane, titled "Community-Based Supplementary Feeding for Promoting the Growth of Children under Five Years of Age in Low and Middle Income Countries" (Sguassero, Onis, Bonotti, & Carroli, 2012), illustrates these efforts to expand focus and to improve access and utility. In addition to making the full report available with open access, the Cochrane Library includes a detailed abstract in three languages (French, Chinese, and English) and the following helpful plain-language summary:

Under-nutrition is one of the underlying causes of childhood illness and death in low- and middle-income countries. Providing extra food to children or families beyond what they normally have at home is an intervention aimed at supporting the nutritional wellbeing of the target population. We included eight studies where the participants were randomly assigned to two groups: one group received the extra food and the other group was a control, either receiving no food or food with very low nutritional content. Although the impact of supplementary feeding on child growth appeared to be negligible, it is not possible to draw any conclusions until we have studies that involve larger numbers and do not allow assessors to know who is receiving the intervention. Although it is difficult to determine whether community-based supplementary feeding helps to promote the growth of children from birth to five years in low- and middle-income countries, it is obviously vital to continue to provide food, health care and sanitation to those who need them. (Sguassero et al., 2012, p. 2)

Which journals should you be reading to stay abreast of global health issues? The focus on the problems of low-income countries has been increasing in the leading high-impact journals, such as *The Lancet, Social Science and Medicine,* the *American Journal of Public Health,* the *New England Journal of Medicine,* and others. In addition, there are a number of journals that specifically focus on international or global health (see Box 1.1).

BOX 1.1

SELECTED GLOBAL HEALTH
PEER-REVIEWED JOURNALS

Bulletin of the World Health Organization

Global Health Action

Global Health: Science and Practice

Globalization and Health

Global Public Health

Health Promotion International

Health Services Research

International Journal for Equity in Health

International Journal for Quality in Health Care

International Journal of Health Services

Journal of the International AIDS Society

Lancet Global Health

New England Journal of Medicine

Public Library of Science Medicine (PLoS Medicine)

Tropical Medicine and International Health

As a student of global health, you should consider journals mentioned here and others as you determine which journals are most relevant for your interest areas. You can make it a habit to review the table of contents of selected publications and reading articles of most interest to you. In addition, you should identify journals that are aligned with your own regional or topical focus. In most cases, your university library already subscribes to journals of interest, and you can access the articles electronically and/or from off-site locations.

Primary Source Documents

Primary source documents can be defined as original documents (including translations) that were written during an experience or event and offer a personal testimony or observation, or constitute an official record of the event. These sources include charters, speeches, letters, diaries, interviews, autobiographies, and official records. Reports that discuss new research or findings as well as creative works can sometimes be considered primary sources; however, for the purpose of this inquiry, they are discussed separately later in this chapter. Primary sources are generally distinguished from **secondary sources** in that secondary sources interpret, summarize, or analyze primary sources. Secondary sources include textbooks, magazine articles, histories, criticism, commentaries, and encyclopedias, and are discussed later in this chapter.

Studying primary sources can familiarize you with the powerful ideas that have shaped global health practice. These sources can capture the aspirations of a generation, as does the following excerpt, still relevant today, from the 1978 Declaration of Alma-Ata, sponsored by WHO and UNICEF and signed by 134 countries:

> The Conference strongly reaffirms that health, which is a state of complete physical, mental and social wellbeing, and not merely the absence of disease or infirmity, is a fundamental human right and that the attainment of the highest possible level of health is a most important world-wide social goal whose realization requires the action of many other social and economic sectors in addition to the health sector (Declaration of Alma-Ata, 1978).

Quotes from speeches, letters, diaries, interviews, and autobiographies are also important global health primary sources. These sources provide testimony and an original voice, and capture the essence of key events or issues, both past and present, with great authenticity. Box 1.2 offers some examples of global leaders who have made statements of critical importance in relation to global health and well-being. Their statements inspire us, challenge us, and succinctly frame or reframe global health work.

BOX 1.2

BRINGING GLOBAL HEALTH TO LIFE WITH PRIMARY SOURCES

Thomas Jefferson. This message from the third president of the United States to Dr. Edward Jenner, who discovered the smallpox vaccine, was excerpted from a letter written at Monticello on May 14, 1806. Although small pox was not completely eradicated until 1979, Jefferson foresaw this eventual outcome over 150 years earlier.

> SIR,—I have received a copy of the evidence at large respecting the discovery of the vaccine inoculation which you have been pleased to send me, and for which I return you my thanks. Having been among the early converts, in this part of

the globe, to its efficiency, I took an early part in recommending it to my countrymen. I avail myself of this occasion of rendering you a portion of the tribute of gratitude due to you from the whole human family. . . . You have erased from the calendar of human afflictions one of its greatest. Yours is the comfortable reflection that mankind can never forget that you have lived. Future nations will know by history only that the loathsome small-pox has existed and by you has been extirpated. (May 14, 1806)

Nelson Mandela. A prominent leader of the South African anti-apartheid movement who was imprisoned for 27 years and then rose to serve as South Africa's first black president from 1994 to 1999, Nelson Mandela addressed the world in 2005 in his "make poverty history" speech with these words (BBC, 2005).

Like slavery and apartheid, poverty is not natural. It is man-made and it can be overcome and eradicated by the actions of human beings. And overcoming poverty is not a gesture of charity. It is an act of justice. It is the protection of a fundamental human right, the right to dignity and a decent life. While poverty persists, there is no true freedom.

Rigoberta Menchú. An indigenous Guatemalan woman, Menchú rose to global prominence for her efforts to give voice to the experience of her people as they struggled for land rights and social justice. Menchú won the Nobel Peace Prize in 1992 and continues to be active on topics related to indigenous rights, improved health, and social change in Guatemala and around the world. Her famous words underscore the power of testimony and story, and the relationship between individual and collective identity.

My name is Rigoberta Menchú. I am 23 years old. This is my testimony. I didn't learn it from a book and I didn't learn it alone. I'd like to stress that it's not only my life, it's also the testimony of my people. . . . My story is the story of all poor Guatemalans. My personal experience is the reality of a whole people. (Menchú, 1984)

Paul Farmer. Dr. Paul Farmer is best known for his work in Haiti, where he has been a partner in championing the health service needs of communities and improving health systems for three decades. Although he has published extensively on health equity and human rights in the peer-reviewed and popular press, his capacity to articulate his values about equity and justice succinctly and in personal terms are reflected in this quote.

Since I do not believe that there should be different recommendations for people living in the Bronx and people living in Manhattan, I am uncomfortable making different recommendations for my patients in Boston and in Haiti. (Clyne, 2000)

Gro Brundtland. Former prime minister of Norway and the first (the only, at this writing) woman to receive that honor, Gro Brundtland is a physician and public health expert who played a leading role in spearheading global efforts to link health, environmental sustainability, and the importance of addressing climate change. One of the forces behind the 1993 Earth Summit, she conveyed the depth of our interconnectedness with regard to health and well-being with these words.

In a globalized world, we all swim in a single microbial sea. (Brundtland, 2001)

Primary sources can inspire and give voice to a moment or a generation. They can also reveal, with marked candor, attitudes of ignorance, implicit bias and prejudice, or intent to do harm. For example, a senior USAID official was reported to disfavor any treatment of HIV/AIDS except for nevirapine for mother-to-infant transmission. His reason, given in spite of his own extensive experience in Africa, was quoted as follows:

> [Africans] don't know what Western time is. You have to take these [AIDS] drugs a certain number of hours each day, or they don't work. Many people in Africa have never seen a clock or a watch their entire lives. And if you say, one o'clock in the afternoon, they do not know what you are talking about. They know morning, they know noon, they know evening, they know the darkness at night. (Donnelly, 2001)

Fortunately, these biases, which can be understood as reflections of biases and blind spots of some in the medical and development establishments, did not prevail, and the George W. Bush administration went on to pass an expansive plan to treat AIDS in Africa (PEPFAR; see https://www.pepfar.gov).

In another example, primary sources in the form of direct quotes from tobacco industry leaders leave little room for doubt about the intent to ignore the harms associated with cigarette smoking. A Rothmans Exports public affairs manager, in an era when the harms of smoking cigarettes had been well documented, described the African setting as follows:

> It would be stupid to ignore a growing market. I can't answer the moral dilemma. We are in the business of pleasing our shareholders. We have a very strong feeling that if no one had heard of cigarettes in Timbuktu, then a Rothmans billboard would not mean anything. All we are doing is responding to a demand. (Quoted in Bates & Rowell, 1998, p. 72)

A Rothmans representative in Burkina Faso referenced the health profile of the country in justifying promotion of cigarettes there, implying that health risks related to cancer later in life are not important because of the shorter life expectancy. He said, "The average life expectancy here is about forty years, infant mortality is high: the health problems which some say are caused by cigarettes just won't figure as a problem here" (quoted in Bates & Rowell, 1998, p. 72).

Primary sources can provide you with authentic perspectives on global health issues and events, from historical context and accuracy, to testimony, to powerful words that reframe perspectives, to points for critique that can foster change, accountability, and justice. Studying and referencing primary sources are important for the credibility and rigor of your research, practice, and advocacy.

The Gray Literature

The term **gray (or grey) literature** was defined at the Twelfth International Conference on Grey Literature in Prague in 2010 as "the manifold document types produced on all levels of government, academics, business and industry in print and electronic formats that are protected by intellectual property rights, of sufficient quality to be collected and preserved by libraries and institutional repositories, but not controlled by commercial publishers; i.e. where publishing is not the primary activity of the producing body."

The volume, quality, availability, and breadth of the gray literature have changed dramatically in recent years. With the growth of the Internet, the digitization of most documents, and the dramatically increased literature search capability around the world, the challenges relating to accessing gray literature materials have been drastically reduced.

Examples of gray literature sources that could inform your global health engagement include working papers and technical reports prepared by governments or global health organizations, conference proceedings, annual reports, instructional materials, doctoral theses, blogs, websites, and newsletters. The gray literature is a great source for specific place-based information that may not be in the peer-reviewed literature. It is also a good source for instructional materials or for more in-depth discussion of topics that do not fit into an academic journal format. The gray literature is also more open, creating a space for a broad range of voices and perspectives. Although this is an asset, it is important to know how to evaluate the quality and reliability of gray literature sources and to be aware that these sources may have a positional slant, so it is important to explore a range of perspectives as you form your own views.

Place-Based Information: Going to Ethiopia? Chile? Thailand? Portugal? There are a number of gray literature sources that profile countries around the world so that you can prepare for your trip. Each of these sources has a slightly different focus. Whether you are planning to do field research, travel for cultural exchange, or partner with a local group for service-learning, reviewing a combination of these sources can enable you to quickly gain the contextual understanding that you need to get the most out of your experience.

BOX 1.3

RESOURCES FOR PREPARING A GLOBAL HEALTH COUNTRY PROFILE

For a quick overview, key facts, information about leaders, and a timeline of key historical events, consult the **BBC News Country Profiles** (http://news.bbc.co.uk/2/hi/country_profiles/default.stm).

The **CIA World Factbook** (https://www.cia.gov/library/publications/the-world-factbook/) provides a more detailed overview that includes geography, people, and society (basic health statistics are included here); an economic overview; description of key government sectors; and a summary of current transnational issues and challenges.

The **UNDP Millennium Development Goal (MDG) Country Reports** (http://www.undp.org/content/undp/en/home/librarypage/mdg/mdg-reports/) focus on the Millennium Development Goals and note progress over time. Regional information for comparison is also available.

World Health Organization (WHO) Country Reports (http://www.who.int/countries/en/) focus on health status, providing key statistics along with regional and global comparison data and useful graphs and charts. The site also includes information about the health workforce, service utilization, and risk factors, and special reports on alcohol and tobacco use.

The World Bank's Countries at a Glance (http://www.worldbank.org/en/country) features current news and overview articles, as well as links to world development indicators related to a broad range of health and development topics, ranging from school enrollment, water and sanitation statistics, and income, to climate change profiles that summarize changes in rainfall patterns. This source also provides regional summaries by geographic region and income level, and other groupings.

The Global Burden of Disease Study (http://www.healthmetricsandevaluation.org/gbd/country-profiles), covered extensively in chapter 5, is available in a highly interactive form that allows you to compare disease profiles by region, subregion, and sex and age groups. Country-specific summary profiles of the disease burden are also available.

The **Food and Agriculture Organization** (FAO; http://www.fao.org/countryprofiles/selectcountry/en/) provides thematic country summaries that review issues related to agriculture and nutrition for a given country, such as overall land and agricultural areas, rates of malnutrition, and Human Development and Global Hunger Indices.

Together these gray literature sources can provide you with an excellent country overview as well as a comparative understanding of that country within its geographic region and among other countries with similar characteristics.

Instructional Materials: Interested in Constructing a Biogas Latrine?

The gray literature is also a great source of instructional materials, how-to manuals, and practical field guides that can enhance your global health work. Many global assistance programs include as a program goal the sharing of tools and lessons learned. This allows them to have a broader impact and enhance their institutional reputations. Perhaps you are planning to do service-learning and would like to share information with partners about basic community development activities, such as planting a garden, making soap, planning health education activities, or building pit latrines. Although it is always essential to consider how to adapt project materials to the local context, you can find helpful resources that will provide a great deal of guidance on how to get started.

For example, to prepare for a latrine construction project, you could consult resources available through Engineering for Change (E4C, https://www.engineering forchange.org/), an organization committed to developing affordable and sustainable solutions to humanitarian challenges. Participating members include the American Mechanical Engineering Society and Engineers without Borders. The E4C Solutions Library includes a technical brief titled "Using Biogas Technology to Solve Pit Latrine Waste Disposal Problems." Written by Daniel Buxton of Practical Action, a UK-based organization devoted to using technology to address poverty, the brief includes design options, a discussion of application to different contexts, diagrams and flow charts, as well as attention to cultural and educational aspects and management for sustainability. This information is openly accessible and can facilitate the expansion and update of this technology in a range of settings.

Identifying and Evaluating Gray Literature Sources

Although the gray literature is a rich source of detailed information, it is important to learn how to access the material and also to evaluate its quality. Some of the gray literature is balanced, with the goal of informing, whereas other material may be more oriented toward persuading or advocating a point of view. Both kinds of material can be valuable; however, it is important to evaluate the accuracy and sources of the information you are reading and to be sure that you explore multiple perspectives as you define your own views.

Reviewing the affiliations and credentials of the authors and institutional sponsors can be helpful in determining the credibility of gray literature sources. It is also important to assess the quality of the writing and references. Your university likely has a librarian with expertise in health sciences, public health, or global health. It is wise to take advantage of this resource to learn to navigate the gray literature, both to learn new search skills and to ensure that your research for a specific project is thorough.

Newspapers, Magazines, Books, and Films

What are your current daily sources of news and information? Are they adequate to support and inform your interest in global health? As you prepare for global health engagement, it is important to be intentional and aware of how you monitor news and access general information. To be effective in global health work, you will need the contextual understanding and framework that familiarity with current events provides. With this preparation, you will be better able to share and discuss ideas with partners, develop contextually appropriate projects, and avoid social blunders, which, though often forgiven because you are a foreigner, are best avoided.

Newspapers, Magazines, and General Information Sources Although our first impulse may be to look for specialized sources of news related to global health, that strategy overlooks the very important fact that health and well-being, defined broadly, are central matters of concern for society. Whether you read them online or through news aggregators, or read them in print each morning, the headlines of your local and national newspapers are full of information related to global public health. Here you will find news stories about disease outbreaks, politics, war, peace, rights, and economic ups and downs. Beyond the front-page news of the day, in stories about food, water, and even the weather report, you will find information that informs global issues related to healthy diet, sustainable resource use, and climate change. Reading your local headlines through the lens of global public health concepts is a first important step toward developing a global worldview. If you are from a smaller town, you might also add to your reading a newspaper that has regional or national prominence, such as the *New York Times,* the *Washington Post,* the *LA Times,* the *Chicago Tribune,* or the *Miami Herald.*

If you have a specific country or geographic region of interest, you can identify a newspaper that is a good source of news coverage for the location where you will work or study. The BBC News country profiles mentioned earlier also list local newspapers. If you do not speak the language of the country, you can often find an online daily newspaper in English. You will also find useful material in leading news magazines, as well as magazines with more in-depth coverage of such topics as health, economics, science, nature, food, travel, and culture. Further, most established global health organizations are actively engaged in providing information to their members and the public. Including these sources in your regular reading is another effective way to stay informed about trends and new discoveries in global health. Last but not least, travel guides and maps, often thought of as tools to use during travel, can also help you answer basic and practical questions about people, places, and events, and will make your travel more efficient, effective, and safe.

With the many information sources available, it can be time consuming to find and read relevant articles from many sources. News aggregators, or news readers, allow you to choose the sources that you want to review and will feed them to your email or phone. By combining news sources from local, national, and international sources, you will be well positioned to stay abreast of key global health issues and to make connections between local issues and global trends. You may want to form an in-person or online discussion group or interest group to monitor global health news together and discuss the issues that arise.

Nonfiction Books and Documentary Films These sources allow for more depth and coverage than feature-length articles that you might see in other sources. Although some are purely factual, these sources often represent a point of view or experience, and are valued for their depth and comprehensiveness and for their effectiveness in communicating different perspectives on topics related to health and well-being.

BOX 1.4
SELECTED NONFICTION BOOKS ABOUT GLOBAL HEALTH

Nigel Crisp, *Turning the World Upside Down: The for Global Health in the 21st Century* (CRC Press, 2010)

Paul Farmer, *Pathologies of Power: Health, Human Rights and the New War on the Poor* (University of California Press, 2004)

William H. Foege, *House on Fire: The Fight to Eradicate Smallpox* (University of California Press, 2011)

Laura J. Frost and Michael R. Reich, *Access: How Do Good Health Technologies Get to Poor People in Poor Countries?* (Harvard University Press, 2009)

Fauziya Kassindja, *Do They Hear You When You Cry* (Delta, 1999)

Emily Mendenhall and Adam Koon (Eds.), *Environmental Health Narratives: A Reader for Youth* (University of New Mexico Press, 2012)

Stephanie Nolen, *28: Stories of AIDS in Africa* (Walker Books, 2007)

Ian Smillie, *Freedom from Want: The Remarkable Success Story of BRAC, the Global Grassroots Organization That's Winning the Fight against Poverty* (Kumarian Press, 2009)

Rickie Solinger, Madeline Fox, and Kayhan Irani (Eds.), *Telling Stories to Change the World: Global Voices on the Power of Narrative to Build Community and Make Social Justice Claims* (Routledge, 2008)

Devi Sridhar, *The Battle against Hunger* (Oxford University Press, 2008)

Roger Thurow and Scott Kilman, *Enough: Why the World's Poorest Starve in an Age of Plenty* (PublicAffairs, 2009)

Documentary films are a powerful way of getting informed and informing others. They possess an unparalleled capability to take the viewer into another world by using images, giving voice, and portraying real-life settings. Although there are many excellent, informative, and well-researched global health documentaries, you must be judicious about interpreting global health films and videos. Like text documents, they can be biased and inaccurate. They can inadvertently or intentionally leave out key information, and in some cases they can be exploitive of the people and places they are featuring. Thus, in evaluating these materials, it is important to consider whether credible fact-finding methods were used and whether the rights and dignity of the film's subjects were respected.

BOX 1.5
SELECTED FILMS RELATED TO GLOBAL HEALTH

Feature-Length Films

Contagion

Dirty Pretty Things

The Insider

The Kingdom

The Motorcycle Diaries

Traffic

Waltz with Bashir

Documentary Films

Big Sugar

The Body Beautiful

Chasing Ice

Dark Days

The Day My God Died

Donka: X-Ray of an African Hospital

Even the Rain

First Do No Harm: A Qualitative Research Documentary

Flow

Girl Rising

Grace under Fire

Living in Emergency: Stories of Doctors Without Borders

The People Paradox: World in the Balance

Rx for Survival

Sicko

Unnatural Causes

The White Helmets

Literature and the Arts

In addition to gathering factual and contextual information from a variety of sources to inform your global health work, you can also learn a great deal about the meaning of health and life and the aspirations of the people you are working with by learning about their stories, song, and art. This kind of study is enriching and enjoyable, and will enable you to gain understandings that will help you with your work. Further, learning about the local culture is an important way to express respect for that culture. This is especially true when working with populations that have experienced poverty, war, injustice, or social marginalization. Just as it is important to understand health data, economics, and political history, so it is important to be familiar with the great novels, poems, and works of art that are part of the story and identity of the people you hope to work with.

Fiction

Although current trends slightly favor nonfiction sources, seen as "true," over fiction as ways to learn about people and places, it is sometime the case that the creative arts—

fiction, poetry, music, and the visual arts—can express truths and nuances in ways that nonfiction cannot. It is a wonderfully rich and enjoyable way to explore the human experience from a variety of perspectives.

One example of a fictional work that is informative about global health is Abraham Verghese's acclaimed novel, *Cutting for Stone.* Set in a hospital in Ethiopia, it is the story of twin boys, with two fathers, two mothers, two countries, and one woman they both love. The boys are attached at birth, share a bed during their boyhood, and then, through life events that are shaped by many forces—global migration, revolution, love, human weakness, and chance—they are separated by miles, oceans, time, and their own differences. The story unfolds through the eyes of one of the twins, Marion, as he tries to understand and reconstruct the truth of his past. In addition to telling a rich human story of a family over several generations, the book is full of observations about health, illness, and what it means to provide medical care in a resource-limited setting.

The excerpt included here illustrates how a brief passage of fiction can have many layers, conveying subtle truth and foreshadowing events in ways that scientific description cannot. It portrays Sister Mary Joseph Praise, the boys' birthmother, an Indian nun and nurse, as she ministers to Dr. Thomas Stone, who is stricken with dysentery on a boat that is traveling from Madras to Ethiopia. During this scene, he is a stranger to her, but later she will work tirelessly with him and for him, as he performs fistula surgery in Ethiopia, and she will bear his sons. As the scene opens, the sister is confronted with the severity of the doctor's condition; she is afraid that she does not know enough about medicine.

But she knew how to nurse. And she knew how to pray. So, praying, she eased off his shirt which was stiff with bile and spit, and she slid down his shorts. As she gave him a bed bath, she was self-conscious, for she'd never ministered to a white man before.... The sinewy muscles of his arms bunched together fiercely at his shoulder. Only now did she notice that his left chest was smaller than his right; the hollow above his collarbone on the left could have held a half cup of water, what that on the right was only a teaspoon. And just beyond and below his left nipple, extending into the armpit, she saw a deep depression.... She touched there and gasped as her fingers fell in, not meeting the bony resistance.... Within that depression his heart tapped firmly against her fingers with only a thick layer of hide intervening. (p.19)

In addition to portraying what it must have been like to care for seriously ill patients on a boat, this scene reveals a trace of the colonial context in which it takes place, and uses bodily description to foreshadow the future intimacy between the nun and the doctor. In describing Dr. Stone's physical asymmetry, the writer begins to expose his complex and contradictory persona—that of a doctor who is completely engaged and devoted to saving human lives, yet unable or unwilling to form emotional relationships. Thus novels like *Cutting for Stone* can tell an important story that conveys human truths and at the same time be an important source for learning about health and disease, history and social context.

BOX 1.6

SELECTED WORKS OF FICTION RELATED TO GLOBAL HEALTH

Unity Dow, *Far and Beyon'*

Unity Dow, *Saturday Is for Funerals*

Helen Dunmore, *The Betrayal*

Amitav Ghosh, *The Calcutta Chromosome*

John Le Carré, *The Constant Gardener*

Ian McEwen, *Solar*

Zakes Mda, *The Heart of Redness*

Gregory David Roberts, *Shantaram*

Bob Shacochis *The Woman Who Lost Her Soul*

Abraham Verghese, *Cutting for Stone*

Nick Wood, *Azanian Bridges*

A. B. Yehoshua, *Open Heart*

Visual Arts, Poetry, and Music

Works of art that address human suffering and well-being can both help you explore and understand specific cultural contexts and lead you toward more transcendent ideas and truths about human reality and possibility.

One example of art that engages with these issues is *La Serie de las Manos,* 12 large paintings of hands that hang together at the Guayasamin Foundation. (See images

at http://guayasamin.org/index.php/obra/la-edad-de-la-ira/95-serie-de-las-manos.)
The artist, internationally acclaimed Oswaldo Guayasamin of Ecuador, felt that people
express a great deal with their hands, and in *La Serie de las Manos* he gave expression
to suffering he had seen around the world, and especially to the experiences of the
disenfranchised indigenous population in his own country. Each pair of hands embodies a different aspect of suffering, and is titled accordingly. The titles express a sort of
anatomy of suffering: insatiable hunger, then begging, then the kind of suffering that
leaves you silent, then fear, sorrow, anger, terror, and screams. Perhaps most profoundly
moving is the turn the series takes at that point. After presenting suffering in these raw,
painful forms, Guayasamin introduces tenderness as the key turning point, then follows
with prayer, mediation, hope, and finally solidarity and protest. This suggests dimensions of protest that are often overlooked: the just rage that is at the foundation of protest as deep, mindful, loving resistance to injustice. One can contemplate the images in
relation to what a mother experiences in the death of a child, or to the experience of an
entire people subjected to famine, drought, floods, or war.

Stories, images, poetry, and art provide powerful ways to understand the world.
What are the most important novels, poems, movies, and works of art in the country
that you will be visiting? How do those stories inform local conceptions of health and
well-being? What can you learn about health and well-being from music, food traditions,
community celebrations, and other cultural practices? Exploring these questions will
enrich your global experience and help you to be a more effective partner for change.

Chapter Summary

For global health education to be effective, you must be an active and contributing partner in the teaching and learning that occurs in your global health course. The academic
global health literature is a necessary but not sufficient source for acquiring broad contextual knowledge about global cultures and society. You should master use of health
data, the academic literature, primary sources, and the gray literature to learn more
about the regions and health topics that you hope to study. You should also monitor the
news media and engage with literature and the arts to develop breadth and depth of
understanding in relation to the culture, geography, history, and politics of the settings
where you hope to work. You should be prepared to share perspectives and life experiences and learn from the perspectives and life experiences of others. This chapter
outlines various sources of information that can help you form a global worldview, and
gives examples of how they can be valuable for global health study. Before proceeding
with further study, take the time to develop a personalized plan to seek out global health
information with the hope that, over time, this will become a lifetime habit. Taking an
active role in your global health education in this way is the first step on a path toward
global civic engagement.

Review Questions

1. What would you like the members of your learning community to know about your global health interests, perspectives, and life experiences? How will you prepare to listen and learn from others?
2. Why are you studying global health? How will it inform your future as a person, professional, and citizen?
3. List three to five information sources you will use to prepare yourself to make contributions to the group. Please include at least three different kinds of information sources.
4. Select one global health resource to share with your class or discussion group. What did you learn from it? What type of source is it? Why is it important?

Key Terms

Active listening

Gray literature

Health statistics

Peer-reviewed journal

Perspective taking

Primary source

Secondary source

References

Bates, C., & Rowell, A. (1998). *Tobacco explained: The truth about the tobacco industry . . . in its own words. Action on Smoking and Health.* Retrieved from http://www.who.int/tobacco/media/en/TobaccoExplained.pdf

British Broadcasting Corporation. (2005, February 3). In full: Mandela's poverty speech. Retrieved from http://news.bbc.co.uk/1/hi/uk_politics/4232603.stm

Brundtland, G. H. (2001, July 2). Address at the 24th Session of the Codex Alimentarius Commission, Geneva, Switzerland. Retrieved from http://www.fao.org/WAICENT/OIS/PRESS_NE/PRESSENG/2001/pren0143.htm

Clyne, C. (2000, April). The potential for global health solidarity: HIV through the eyes of a physician on the front lines—The *Satya* interview with Paul Farmer. *Satya.* Retrieved from http://www.satyamag.com/april00/farmer.html

Declaration of Alma-Ata, International Conference on Primary Health Care. (1978, September 6–12). Alma-Ata, USSR. Reprinted in *Development, 47*(2), 159–161.

Dey, E. L., & Associates. (2010). *Engaging diverse viewpoints: What is the campus climate for perspective taking?* Washington, DC: Association of American Colleges and Universities.

Donnelly, J. (2001, June 7). Prevention urged in AIDS fight. *Boston Globe,* p. A8.

Food and Agriculture Organization. (2015). State of food insecurity in the world in brief. Retrieved from http://www.fao.org/3/a-i4671e.pdf

Grohol, J. (2016). Become a better listener: Active listening. *Psych Central.* Retrieved from http://psychcentral.com/lib/become-a-better-listener-active-listening/

International Committee of Medical Journal Editors. (2010). Uniform requirements for manuscripts submitted to biomedical journals: Writing and editing for biomedical publication. *Journal of Pharmacology & Pharmacotherapeutics, 1*(1), 42–58.

International Telecommunications Union. (2016, June). ICT facts and figures. Retrieved from http://www.itu.int/en/ITU-D/Statistics/Documents/facts/ICTFactsFigures2016.pdf

Jefferson, T. (1806, May 14). *Thomas Jefferson to Edward Jenner.* [Letter]. *The Thomas Jefferson Papers Series 1.* Library of Congress, Washington, DC.

Langer, A., Díaz-Olavarrieta, C., Berdichevsky, K., & José Villar, J. (2004, October). Why is research from developing countries underrepresented in international health literature, and what can be done about it? *Bulletin of the World Health Organization, 82,* 10.

Lozano, R., Naghavi, M., Foreman, K., Lim, S., Shibuya, K., Aboyans, V., . . . Murray, C.J.L. (2010). Global and regional mortality from 235 causes of death for 20 age groups in 1990 and 2010: A systematic analysis for the Global Burden of Disease Study 2010. *The Lancet, 380,* 2095–2128.

Menchú, R. (1984). *I, Rigoberta Menchú: An Indian woman in Guatemala.* London, United Kingdom: Verso.

Sguassero, Y., Onis, M., Bonotti, A. M., & Carroli, G. (2012). Community-based supplementary feeding for promoting the growth of children under five years of age in low and middle income countries. *Cochrane Database of Systemic Reviews, 6.* CD005039. doi:10.1002/14651858. CD005039.pub3

Tilleczek, K., & Ferguson, H. B. (Eds.). (2013). *Youth, education, and marginality.* Waterloo, Ontario: Wilfrid Laurier University Press.

Twelfth International Conference on Grey Literature: Transparency in Grey Literature, GreyTech Approaches to High Tech Issues. (2010, December 6–7). Prague, Czech Republic. (Accessed from conference CD-ROM)

United Nations. (2015). Levels and trends in child mortality. Retrieved from http://www.un.org/en/development/desa/population/publications/mortality/child-mortality-report-2015.shtml

United Nations Children's Fund. (2016, April). Water, sanitation and hygiene. Retrieved from https://www.unicef.org/wash/

Verghese, A. (2009). *Cutting for stone: A novel.* New York, NY: Knopf.

CHAPTER 2

WHAT IS GLOBAL HEALTH?

Lori DiPrete Brown, MS, MTS

Health is the state of complete physical, mental and social wellbeing and not merely the absence of disease or infirmity.
—World Health Organization, 1946

LEARNING OBJECTIVES

- Define global health and understand it as an evolving concept
- Identify current health challenges and sources of disparities in health
- Understand basic measures, concepts, and methods of categorizing illness associated with assessment of global disease burden
- Describe the scope of global health practice
- Consider health and well-being through the lens of the social-ecological model and the social determinants of health

In 1946, the constitution of the World Health Organization (WHO) defined health as the state of complete physical, mental, and social well-being. Current articulations of global health are grounded in this historical and visionary definition, and also are informed by more recent paradigms that emphasize multisector approaches and the interconnected health of humans, animals, and the environment.

This chapter discusses global health, provides an initial introduction to how health status is measured, and profiles current health priorities. It also presents an overview of global health practice and discusses risk factors and social determinants of health.

Foundations for Global Health Practice, First Edition. Lori DiPrete Brown.
© 2018 John Wiley & Sons, Inc. Published 2018 by John Wiley & Sons, Inc.

Global Health: An Evolving Concept

The meaning and scope of the term *global health* are still evolving in both theory and practice. Related terms, such as *international health, tropical medicine, public health,* and, more recently, *global public health,* are sometimes used interchangeably with global health. A definition of global health suited to the 21st century must embrace the full range of disease conditions and risk factors that impact individual and community health, and must be relevant both locally and worldwide in its reach. To grasp the breadth and scope of global health, it is helpful to first correct some frequent misconceptions by discussing what global health is not, and then to pose some fundamental questions about the nature and purpose of global health.

Global Health Is Not Limited to Activities of the Health Sector and Provision of Health Care Services

Although increasing access to quality medical care is one aspect of global health, health status is the product of many interwoven factors, and such global health improvements as improved water and sanitation; health education; increased access to safe, nutritious food; and built environments that support healthy and sustainable lifestyles. Physicians, nurses, and pharmacists make important contributions to the health and well-being of communities, but the same can be said of engineers, teachers, farmers, and entrepreneurs.

For example, education programs can address health directly with lifesaving information, and they can also enhance health indirectly, through the overall improvements in quality of life that education affords. There is a high correlation between maternal education and maternal mortality. In a study that included 24 low-income countries, mothers with only 1 to 6 years of formal education were twice as likely as women with 12 years of schooling to die in childbirth (Karlsen et al., 2011). This and other correlations between educational status and quality of life suggest that education is essential and foundational for improvements in global health and development (see Kendall, chapter 36).

Similarly, access to water, basic sanitation, and adequate food and nutrition are essential components of global health. Again, these sectors rival health care services for importance and potential impact. Estimates indicate that at least 9.1% of the global disease burden and 6.3% of all deaths can be prevented with water, sanitation, and hygiene interventions (Prüss-Üstün, Bos, Gore, & Bartram, 2008) (see Hettler, chapter 8). Meanwhile, at least 3.1 million children die with malnutrition as the underlying cause. This accounts for nearly half of all deaths in children under the age of five. Another 165 million children experience stunted growth, with the associated suffering and developmental consequences (Black et al., 2013) (see Aquino, chapter 9).

The laudable effort to establish global consensus about health and well-being as a worldwide social goal can be undermined if appropriate improvements in health care access and quality are distorted by **medicalization**, or an overemphasis on medical rather than public health, social, or infrastructure solutions. Medicalization can be understood as a process that "would over-emphasize the role of health care to health; define and frame issues in relation to disease, treatment strategies, and individual behavior; promote the role of medical professionals and models of care; find support in industry or other advocates of technologies and pharmaceuticals; and discount social contexts, causes, and solutions" (Clark, 2014a). As the global health agenda shifts from a focus on infectious disease to one that also includes broader determinants of well-being, it is important to consider the potential harms and benefits of medicalization in relation to such topics as global mental health (Clark, 2014b), universal health coverage (Clark 2014d), and non-communicable diseases (Clark, 2014c). Analysis of the potential impact of medical framing in terms of social, community, and political action, as well as of the costs and benefits that can accrue to stakeholders in the medical establishment, government, civil society, and the private sector, are essential to the development of effective policies for global health and development.

Although it is important to attend to the potential distortions and dangers that can occur by medicalizing health and well-being, access to health care is widely acknowledged as a human right, and health care will and should continue to play a central role in global health efforts. However, the needs and strategies for medical collaboration have changed significantly over time. Rather than providing medical care directly to needy populations, international health providers engage in collaborative approaches to policy development and implementation and support efforts to build local capacity (see Conway, chapter 26; Tefera, chapter 30; and Hariharan, chapter 32). Despite continued shortages of health care in some parts of the world, global health efforts are increasingly favoring ownership by local providers and promoting education over short-term missions (Mitchell et al., 2013; Podda, 2010). Global health care involves collaboration among physicians, nurses, pharmacists, and a broad range of allied health professionals and paraprofessional workers, who all play vital roles in promoting health across the life course for individuals, families, and communities (see Baumann and Solheim, chapter 33; and Seys Ranola and Kraus, chapter 34). These collaborations continue to occur between high-income and low-income countries; increasingly, however, global health work is realized through partnerships and collaborations of leaders from low-income countries, often called south-south partnerships because the collaborators are geographically located in the **Global South**.

Global Health Is Not Just the Absence of Disease

As the WHO definition implies, global health efforts must go beyond disease prevention to encompass the full realization of human potential. Although global health efforts include successful immunization campaigns around the world and large-scale efforts to treat HIV/AIDS and tuberculosis, they also can include efforts to enhance psychological and social well-being, strategies to improve governance, and efforts to realize human rights and foster peace. Topics such as global mental health (see Raviola, chapter 7) and pain management to ensure a good quality of life during illness and at the end of life (see Cleary, chapter 31) are just two examples of areas that have been neglected in the past and will receive increased attention in the coming decades.

Global Health Challenges and Opportunities Are Not Limited to Lower-Income Countries

There are many health disparities in our interdependent world. The differences in health status between high-income countries and low-income countries can be shocking. For example, WHO cites infant mortality rates (IMRs)—that is, the number of infants who die between birth and the age of one per 1,000 live births—to be over five times higher in the Africa region, at a rate of 55 deaths per 1,000 births, than in the European region, which has a rate of 10 per 1,000 (WHO, 2017c).

However, it is important to be mindful of disparities within countries as well. For example, in 2013, overall IMR in the United States was 5.96, with a twofold difference between black infants (11.11) and white infants (5.06) (Mathews, MacDorman, & Thoma, 2015). Similarly, in China, when national IMR was 15 in 2007, urban areas experienced a rate of 7.7, whereas the IMR in rural China was 18.6 (Yanping et al., 2010).

A **health disparity** can be defined as "a particular type of health difference that is closely linked with social or economic disadvantage. Health disparities adversely affect groups of people who have systematically experienced greater social or economic obstacles to health based on their racial or ethnic group, religion, socioeconomic status, gender, mental health, cognitive, sensory, or physical disability, sexual orientation, geographic location or other characteristics historically linked to discrimination or exclusion" (US Department of Health and Human Services, 2008). Differences in health status noted within and across geographic areas, such as the ones described in the United States and China, should be analyzed with these factors in mind.

Finally, differences in health status among high-income settings are also worthy of note. Although we might expect that health rankings would closely mirror wealth rankings, this is not always the case. For example, despite high marks for health care quality, recent rankings place the United States at 19th in per capita income, but 41st in life expectancy. Further, there are 45 countries with lower IMRs than the United States (Central Intelligence Agency, 2016). Thus global health approaches might offer useful lessons from the health and social policies of other countries to improve health status in the United States.

Global Health Is Not a One-Way Street

The notion of global health work as charitable activity in which high-income countries provide assistance to low-income countries, or heroic individuals traverse the global to save people in need, is being displaced by models of mutual respectful engagement where citizens, leaders, and technical experts can work together in international partnerships and regional networks to achieve learning and innovations that benefit all partners in different ways. This open, multidirectional learning is the future of global health.

It is important to recognize that international collaboration in health has always led to two-way learning and benefits for all parties. However, traditional rationales, funding flows, and power dynamics in international health and global health work were based on the assumption that "developing countries" would benefit from expertise in "developed countries." The recognition that multidirectional learning does and should occur is long overdue. Mutual learning is sometimes called *frugal innovation, reverse-learning,* or *reverse innovation.* These terms are problematic, because they continue to presume a primary flow from north to south, rich to poor, and so on, but they are noted here because much good work in the literature is referenced under these terms. Some examples of the exciting innovations that arise when learning happens through a comparative systems approach include the adaptation of community health worker models from Brazil to North Wales, the development of highly effective and lower-cost surgical techniques across settings, and the development of new structures and processes for open innovation (Crisp, 2014). It is not an exaggeration to posit that all global health collaborations can and should have two-way learning and mutual benefits, some planned and some the unintended by-products of a creative and dynamic partnership.

What Does the "Global" in Global Health Mean?

Many students mistakenly believe that they must leave their home country to practice global health. I often begin my global health classes with a reminder that we are all in the world right where we are, and that a global perspective is possible, and in fact essential, if we are to exercise the responsibilities of national and global citizenship from our own communities. You do not have to travel, or live abroad, to think about health challenges from a global perspective or have an impact on global health. For example, US citizens might engage in a program of international engagement like the Peace Corps for a time, then return home to work in culturally diverse settings where their cultural knowledge or language skills help them to be more effective. Similarly, you don't have to leave home to be put in a position where you need to respond to a global health crisis. A flu outbreak in any part of the world can become a global epidemic in a matter of hours, as international travel enables the rapid spread of disease through the movement of international travelers, the transport of food and goods, and the migrations of birds, insects, and animals. You might work on global matters in a public health laboratory, at the Centers for Disease Control and Prevention (see Emperador, chapter 29), or through an advocacy organization, and have a global impact without leaving your hometown.

Even if you are not consciously or intentionally "practicing global health" in one of these ways, your lifestyle choices have an impact at the global level. For example, the high levels of per capita energy use in the United States and other high-income countries contribute to water shortages (see Hettler, chapter 8) and to climate change and the related global disruptions, including extreme weather, changing disease patterns, and impacts on biodiversity and food supply (see Patz and DiPrete Brown, chapter 10). Similarly, the choices that you make as a consumer have an impact on overall human resource use and determine what kinds of employment policies and business strategies will be sustained in our global economy.

There are many ways to think about the "global" part of global health. To some it means "international," to connote health matters of worldwide import that transcend national boundaries. It can also mean "holistic," contrasting itself with disease-specific notions of health. Further, theorists have suggested enlarging the "global" concept further to go beyond connection across solely geographic distance. They suggest using global to mean all-encompassing in other kinds of social, disciplinary, or economic spectra (Bozorgmehr, 2010).

For the purposes of this text, we will consider "global" to indicate that research and practice can occur anywhere, as long as health challenges are considered in light of local and global root causes and impacts and the relationships among them. Rather than understanding a global health focus as one that links "health here" and "health there," we can understand global health study and practice as a comparative and collaborative practice that necessarily begins in a specific local context; through a process of learning and exchange, the connections between well-being in that particular place, in other places, and everywhere become increasingly evident. Thus the global health journey involves growing understandings about the connections and relationships among all forms of life, human health, and care of the earth in all of these places, with implications for both worldwide and local action.

Is Global Health a Discipline? Where Can It Be Studied?

During the past 20 years, there has been a proliferation of global health departments, centers, institutes, and programs of study for health professional students and undergraduates. Further, global health research centers in academic medical centers and schools of public health have been established with support from the Fogarty Center and other sources.

In general, global health educational efforts are defined as interdisciplinary programs, with public health as a core discipline. Global health competencies have been articulated in a number of disciplines, and are discussed in detail in chapter 14.

The vast majority of global health programs have been developed in North America, responding to student demand for global opportunities and to the interests of academic institutions, driven by both altruism and financial incentive, in being part of research and implementation efforts supported by development assistance funds. Critics have expressed concern about this North American dominance and the associated human and financial resource allocations. Recommended reforms call for dismantling the "developing country/developed country dichotomy by generating global health leaders who can address developing and developed country priorities simultaneously wherever they are based" (Macfarlane, Jacobs, & Kaaya, 2008, p. 395).

Definitions of Global Health

In 2009, Koplan and colleagues defined **global health** as

> [an] area for study, research, and practice that places a priority on improving health and achieving equity in health for all people worldwide. Global health emphasizes transnational health issues, determinants, and solutions; involves many disciplines within and beyond the health sciences and promotes interdisciplinary collaboration; and is a synthesis of population-based prevention with individual-level clinical care. (Koplan et al., 2009, p. 1995)

This definition, which has well-being and equity as its cornerstones, is grounded in social justice philosophy, and implies the involvement of government, bilateral and multilateral cooperation, NGOs, civil society, and the private sector. Another important aspect of this definition is that although it has a strong focus on prevention and public health, it leaves no doubt about the fact that increasing the access to and quality of individual-level care is and should continue to be an important focus of global health activities.

Beaglehole and Bonita (2010) offer a more succinct and equally comprehensive definition of global health. They define global health as "collaborative transnational research and action for promoting health for all." This definition sets itself apart from unidirectional concepts, emphasizing the two-way collaboration and universal benefits of global health work.

A core group of deans of leading schools of public health have weighed in with the position that global health is public health (Fried et al., 2010). They argue that the public health field is conceptually and methodologically complete in its ability to address global health issues, and that integration of local and global perspectives can be realized under the public health umbrella.

In 1920, Winslow defined **public health** as

the science and the art of preventing disease, prolonging life, and promoting physical health and efficiency through organized community efforts for the sanitation of the environment, the control of community infections, the education of the individual in principles of personal hygiene, the organization of medical and nursing services for the early diagnosis and preventive treatment of disease, and the development of the social machinery which will ensure to every individual in the community a standard of living adequate for the maintenance of health. (Winslow, 1920, p. 30)

More recently and succinctly, the CDC Foundation (2017) has described public health as "concerned with protecting the health of entire populations. These populations can be as small as a local neighborhood, or as big as an entire country or region of the world."

Although global health work clearly fits within these parameters conceptually, the term *public health* has historically been associated with surveillance and action of the public sector at local, state, and national levels, and has sometimes been understood to exclude clinical medicine. Fried and colleagues (2010) underscore the Institute of Medicine's (2003) recognition of the need for multisectoral systems-based approaches. They emphasize that "the tenets of global public health highlight public health as a public good, benefiting all members of society. . . . [A] domestic focus on population health need not compete for attention with an international focus—in a global health system strengthening one strengthens the other" (Fried et al., 2010, p. 536).

Public health, with its breadth of methods and approach, is a core discipline for global health; yet, like all disciplines, it has boundaries. As our world becomes more globalized, technically complex, and interconnected, interdisciplinary approaches that go beyond public health must be engaged, including, for example, the study of culture, language, and the arts; research from behavioral and social sciences; and knowledge from medical or technical specialties related to information technology, environmental science, engineering, veterinary medicine, and others.

One Health

As we aim to articulate a global health concept that will be robust enough to endure in coming decades, an important contribution comes from the field of veterinary medicine. The American Veterinary Medical Association (AVMA, 2017) has put forth the concept of "one health," which is well aligned with global public health, but also offers unique elements. **One health** is defined as " the collaborative effort of multiple disciplines working locally and nationally and globally—to obtain optimal health for people, animals and our environment." From contributing to the preservation of biodiversity, to the tracking and management of infectious disease pandemics, to securing a more safe and efficient food supply, the one health approach plays a significant role in global health, and that role can be expected to increase.

Although issues related to the interface between humans, animals, and environments have always been central to the health of populations worldwide, current trends make them more important than ever. Growth trends indicate that the human population will reach 10 billion by 2100, and an overwhelming majority of these people will live in cities (see Vargo, chapter 38). There will be increasing demands on food and water supply, and projections estimate that an increase of 80% in animal production will be needed to meet the needs of the population in 2050. Further, the increased mobility of humans and animals and emerging **zoonotic disease** will continue to pose health threats to humans and animals alike (Rabinowitz & Conti, 2013). Given these challenges, it makes sense for public and global health perspectives to move beyond a single-species mind-set. Such a model could result in better ways to produce food animals, innovations in health care delivery to humans and their companion animals, and the use of animals and humans as sentinels of ecosystem health, for their mutual protection and the benefit of all.

Despite the simplicity and face validity of the one health concept, it has been difficult to put this interconnected thinking into practice systematically because of the challenges of working across disciplines. To date, the one health conversation has been represented principally in journals of veterinary medicine and microbiology (69%), with only 5% in public health and 4% in environmental sciences (Barrett & Bouley, 2015). Separate training, separate professional organizations, distinct surveillance systems, and distinct professional cultures create ongoing challenges for one health collaboration (Conrad, Meek, & Dumit, 2013). In addition to recommendations for integration within public health and the health sciences, there are also calls for integration with these fields and others, such as cultural anthropology (Wolf, 2015).

Will one health become an integral part of global health? While that effort continues as a work in progress, challenges related to planetary limits have become part of the global health conversation.

Planetary Health: Vital Signs to Guide Global Health and Development

As you read this text, you are perched between the Holocene epoch, a period of time that began about 11,700 years ago during which human civilization has grown and developed, and the Anthropocene, a period when human activities are recognized to have a substantial global effect on the earth's systems. Responding to the realities and possible risks of the pressures that human populations place on the earth, scientists have conceived of a framework of planetary thresholds and boundaries that define a "safe operating space for humanity" (Rockström et al., 2009).

The nine planetary boundaries that have been identified are global freshwater use, ocean acidification, land-system change, rate of biodiversity loss, chemical pollution, climate change, stratospheric ozone depletion, interference with the global phosphorus cycle, and interference with the global nitrogen cycle. Although a great deal of research is needed to determine appropriate thresholds in each of these areas and the interactive impacts that can occur among them, such thresholds can provide the global health community with some additional conditions and considerations as they work to determine how to deploy resources to improve health and to care for the earth.

Planetary health has been defined in relation to these planetary boundaries. The Lancet Commission on Planetary Health calls it "the achievement of the highest attainable standard of health, wellbeing, and equity worldwide through judicious attention to the human systems—political, economic and social—that shape the future of humanity and the earth's natural systems that define the safe environmental limits within which humanity can flourish" (Horton & Lo, 2015).

Planetary health concepts are not intended to displace those of public health or global health. Instead they offer different tools and guideposts to add additional dimensions to global efforts. At the planetary level, health challenges will be complex emergencies that are environmental in nature. They may be acute or unfold gradually over time. Even when some prediction is possible, there will not be certainty in terms of time and place. This requires new kinds of governance and response systems. In light of this science, the Lancet Commission recommends redefinition of prosperity to focus on "the enhancement of quality of life and delivery of improved health for all, together with respect for the integrity of natural systems," and calls for "urgent and transformative actions to protect present and future generations" (Whitmee et al., 2015, p. 1974).

These boundaries, and related safety thresholds, have practical significance for global health work. They can be thought of as vital signs for planetary health and sustainability. Personal health is monitored with such vital signs as temperature, heart rate, and blood pressure, with defined safe ranges and danger signs for each. The health of human populations is described by key measures such as life expectancy and IMR, and by other measures of well-being. Ecosystem health includes the health and integrity of animals, plants, and natural and built environments, each with its breaking point and signs of thriving. Similarly, planetary health can be monitored in terms of the nine boundaries, which can be understood as vital signs for the planet, with related safe planetary boundaries and danger thresholds.

Models have depicted the planetary boundaries (Rockström et al., 2009), articulated relationships between human health and support systems and specific threats like climate change (Myers & Patz, 2009), and related overall environmental health to planetary boundaries (Raworth, 2012). Figure 2.1 presents a conceptual map that illustrates how personal vital signs, human population vital signs, ecosystem vital signs, and planetary vital signs are embedded in each other and are interrelated. These relationships, though complex, can be studied and understood so that human and planetary health and well-being efforts are sustainable, reinforce each other, and avoid unintended consequences.

Carrying out global health work in alignment with and awareness of critical planetary health thresholds, and studying the relationships among vital signs at different levels, can make global health work more sustainable and effective, because by staying within the boundaries, we decrease the likelihood of major environmental disruptions.

FIGURE 2.1   Vital Signs for Human and Planetary Well-Being:
Achieving a Sustainable Balance

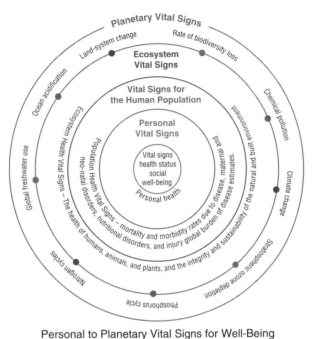

Personal to Planetary Vital Signs for Well-Being

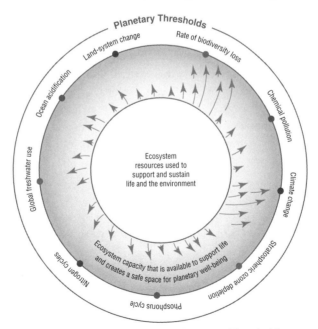

Sustaining Well-Being within Planetary Thresholds

By linking and integrating planetary thresholds and boundaries with health issues, people can see cobenefits between human and planetary health that may make them more likely to take action. For example, the need to feed the increasing human population will place additional stress on a number of planetary boundaries. Healthier plant-based diets, with the accompanying reduction in red meat consumption, could reduce chronic disease and at the same time alleviate pressures related to water use and other boundaries (Demaio & Rockström, 2015). Although it is sometimes presumed that health improvements require more resources, there are many cases where improvements to human well-being reduce resource use; in these cases improving vital signs for humans can have a positive impact on the vital signs for ecosystems and the planet. Public awareness and understanding of planetary thresholds and the relationships between the well-being of people, eco-systems, and the planet can lead to new ways of thinking and living on and with our earth. Just as individuals find ways to be healthier when they monitor vital signs like blood pressure and heart rate, so the human community can pay attention to planetary thresholds and work collectively toward planetary well-being and sustainability.

What Are the Challenges to Human Health?

At this writing, the world population clock records a global population of 7.47 billion people, and about 250 babies are born every minute. What are their odds for survival? Will their basic needs be met? What health conditions will they face?

Considering the complex and dynamic forces described earlier, it is hard to answer these questions with certainty. Tremendous strides in relation to child mortality and access to clean water and sanitation have been made since 1990. These gains could be offset by new setbacks, both foreseen and unforeseen, or further progress could be made, perhaps beyond what we can imagine, with increased political will and technological advances.

Box 2.1 offers a snapshot of current global health challenges, drawn primarily from recent WHO and United Nations (UN) sources. This overview provides a sense of the scale and comparative weight of the current challenges that face humanity—those living out their lives in very different conditions around the world, and those being born right this minute.

BOX 2.1
A SNAPSHOT OF GLOBAL HEALTH CHALLENGES

5.9 million children under 5 died in 2015 (WHO, 2017d).

An estimated **214 million women** in developing countries would like to delay or stop childbearing, but are not using any method of contraception (WHO, 2017b).

884 million people do not have access to basic drinking-water service, and **2.3 billion** do not have access to improved sanitation (WHO, 2017a, 2017i).

There were **2.1 million** new infections of HIV/AIDS in 2015, and **1.1 million** people died from this disease. By the end of that year, **37 million** people were living with HIV AIDS, and of these less than half, **17 million**, had access to treatment (Joint United Nations Programme on HIV/AIDS, 2016).

There were **10.4 million** new cases of TB and **1.8 million** deaths in 2015; **480,000** people developed multidrug-resistant TB, and 35% of deaths of people with HIV/AIDS were due to TB (WHO, 2017l).

Over **1 billion** people worldwide are affected by 18 neglected tropical diseases. Most impacted are populations living in poverty, without adequate sanitation and in close contact with infectious vectors and domestic animals and livestock (WHO, 2017h).

Among mental health challenges, **300 million** people suffer from depression, **60** million from bipolar disease, **47.5 million** from dementia, and **21 million** from schizophrenia (WHO, 2017g).

Over **600 million** adults are obese (BMI > 30), raising risk for chronic disease (WHO, 2016a).

Over **7 million** people die of tobacco use each year. Over **1 billion** people smoke worldwide, and up to half will die due to their tobacco use (WHO, 2017k).

Alcohol use causes an estimated **3.3 million deaths** each year, and at least **15.3 million** people suffer from drug use disorders (WHO, 2017f).

35% of women worldwide have experienced either intimate-partner violence or nonpartner sexual violence in their lifetime (WHO, 2016b).

Efforts to address these and other human health challenges must be carried out in a safe operating space for life—that is, one within the boundaries of planetary health. Thus care of the earth must be a framing value for global health. Global health efforts, wherever they take place, should foster health and well-being through evidence-based and sustainable practices—recognizing the interconnectedness of people, animals, and the environment—to promote health and well-being for all species and the earth itself.

Measuring Global Health Status

To prevent and treat disease and promote global health, it is important to understand basic measures that are used to monitor global health status.

Table 2.1 Top 10 Causes of Mortality in the World, 2015

Disease	Number of Deaths (millions)
Ischemic heart disease	8.76
Stroke	6.24
Lower respiratory infections	3.19
Chronic obstructive pulmonary disease	3.17
Trachea, bronchus, lung cancers	1.69
Diabetes mellitus	1.59
Alzheimer disease and other dementias	1.54
Diarrhoeal diseases	1.39
Tuberculosis	1.37
Road injury	1.34

Note: These causes of death accounted for approximately half of all deaths.

Source: "Top Ten Causes of Death," by the World Health Organization, 2017. Retrieved from http://www.who.int/mediacentre/factsheets/fs310/en/

Mortality and Morbidity

Mortality (death) and morbidity (illness) are the most common ways to measure the impact of disease. They can be expressed in terms of the total number of deaths or illnesses in a population (see Table 2.1) or as rates at which these events occur.

Mortality rates measure the rate at which people die due to a defined cause in a defined population over a defined period of time. Mortality rates for a given time period (usually a year) are expressed as a ratio, either deaths per 1,000 or deaths per 100,000.

When are the different denominators used? In general, mortality related to live births or overall death rates are expressed in deaths per 1,000. For example, an IMR of 5 indicates that, in a specified population, 5 infants per 1,000 die each year. The crude overall death rate for 2014 was 7.89, indicating that 7.89 people died for every 1,000 people in the global population that year. Death rates by condition, because they are relatively rare events, are generally expressed as the number of deaths per 100,000. For example, deaths due to cancer, diabetes, or other illness conditions are expressed this way. One exception would be during disease outbreaks with high mortality rates. In such cases, deaths per 1,000 might be used. For example, at the height of the Ebola outbreak, mortality rates were expressed in deaths per 1,000. It is important to note that maternal mortality rate (MMR), a very important sentinel indicator for global health that is often reported alongside IMR, is expressed as deaths per 100,000, whereas the complementary IMR is expressed as deaths per 1,000.

Morbidity refers to the presence of illness in an individual or population. It is usually described in terms of severity, duration, prevalence, and incidence. Severity refers to the risk of death and the degree of disability, pain, and suffering associated with the illness. Duration refers to the time between onset of disease and cure or death. **Prevalence** refers to the proportion of cases that are present in a population at a given moment in time or within a given time interval, and is often expressed as cases per 10,000 or 100,000. **Incidence** measures the number of new cases of the disease during a defined interval, usually 10,000 or 100,000 person-years. Incidence and prevalence are related in both simple and complex ways. The mathematical formula for incidence is simple: incidence multiplied by duration equals prevalence ($P = I \times D$). Yet the very simplicity of this formula is cause for caution in interpreting morbidity data.

Suppose you hear that the prevalence of HIV/AIDS, diabetes, or cancer is skyrocketing. This sounds like bad news. It might lead to calls for increased investment in prevention, or admonitions that the health care system is not doing its job. To be sure you understand what is happening, it is important to return to the simple formula. Prevalence increased because incidence, duration, or both aspects of morbidity increased. There are many possible interpretations to consider. People may be living longer because of improved care, as has been the case for HIV/AIDS, cancer, heart disease, and many other conditions. These positive developments increase prevalence as they increase life expectancy. In fact, even if the number of new cases decreased, prevalence might continue to rise depending on the comparative magnitude of the two changes. Alternatively, longer duration of illness does not always mean more life; it could also indicate that cures are taking longer than they should for nonfatal conditions, because of changes in health care access or antibiotic resistance. Increases and decreases in incidence should be interpreted with caution as well, but for different reasons. These increases can be explained by real increases in morbidity or by an increase in detection and recording. Again, positive action (increased detection and better record keeping) can lead to an apparently negative outcome. Alternatively, recording error can play a part in declines in incidence as well. As these examples illustrate, measures like incidence and prevalence should not be interpreted in isolation.

Case fatality ratio (CFR), which measures one aspect of the severity of an illness, is another important measure to consider in association with disease outbreaks. The CFR indicates the proportion of people who will die from an illness. Again, this is much more complicated that the simple definition of the measure implies. The CFR can vary greatly depending on how a case is defined (criteria for inclusion in the denominator), and also on the susceptibility to death in the population due to underlying health conditions such as malnutrition or other vulnerabilities. Responses to global pandemics, both by the scientific community and the general public, depend heavily on measures and perceptions related to the risk of death. For example, in 2009, a major outbreak of the novel H1N1 influenza occurred in Mexico City. Early reports suggested a very high CFR, and extensive measures were taken, in Mexico and globally, to prevent spread of this flu. In this case, CFR estimates were not reliable—a recent review documented 77 different estimates ranging from 1 to more than 10,000 deaths per 100,000 (Wong et al., 2013). The variation among sources stemmed from case definition, with estimates that depended on lab-confirmed cases ultimately leading to the lower and more accurate figures. Accurate CFR determined policy eventually, but not before the emergency response had other costs for citizens of Mexico and the world. Cases like the H1NI outbreak of 2009 are important opportunities to learn about optimal ways to use epidemiological information to respond in real time to novel global health challenges and the related uncertainties.

In summary, mortality, morbidity, and their associated measures are powerful tools. As you assess global health status, consider mortality, incidence, and prevalence information alongside an understanding of the local context and concurrent policies and practice.

Communicable Disease, Non-Communicable Disease, and Injury

Disease monitoring efforts often group specific disease conditions into categories so that they can understand the scale of larger trends and conditions that arise from similar causes. The Global Burden of Disease (GBD) Study, which will be discussed extensively in chapter 5, classifies over 300 specific diseases into three categories: (1) communicable, maternal, neonatal, and nutritional disease; (2) non-communicable disease; and (3) injury. Then, at a second level, the GBD clusters the diseases into the 20 disease categories listed in Box 2.2 (GBD 2015 Disease and Injury Incidence and Prevalence Collaborators, 2016).

BOX 2.2

GLOBAL BURDEN OF DISEASE STUDY—LEVEL 2 DISEASE CATEGORIES

Category 1: Communicable, Maternal, Neonatal, Nutritional

HIV/AIDS and tuberculosis

Neglected tropical disease and malaria

Maternal disorders

Neonatal disorders

Diarrhea, lower respiratory infections, other

Category 2: Non-Communicable Disease (NCD)

Cardiovascular

Neoplasms

Mental illness and substance abuse

Musculoskeletal disorders

Diabetes, urogenital, blood, and endocrine disease

Chronic respiratory illness

Digestive diseases

Neurological disorders

Cirrhosis

Other NCDs

Category 3: Injury

Unintentional injury

Transportation-related injury

Self-harm and violence

War and disaster

Communicable, Maternal, Neonatal, and Nutritional Disease (Category 1) **Communicable diseases** are infectious diseases that are contagious and that can be transmitted from one source to another by infectious bacteria or viral organisms. Transmission can occur through airborne viruses or bacteria, but also through blood or other bodily fluid. According to the 2015 GBD Study, the five leading causes of death from category 1 illnesses include lower respiratory infections, diarrheal disease, tuberculosis, HIV/AIDS, and neonatal preterm birth. Diseases like small pox and polio do not appear on the list as major killers because of successful vaccination campaigns during the past 50 years (see Conway, chapter 26). Such efforts need to be sustained as the fight against measles continues, polio eradication is within reach, and researchers continue to seek vaccines for other conditions.

Monitoring of communicable diseases also helps detect and respond to newly emerging and reemerging infectious diseases and virulent pandemics such as avian flu, the Ebola virus, and the Zika virus. Further, neglected tropical diseases must be monitored both to evaluate efforts to eliminate them and to track changing patterns of infection that could be associated with urbanization and environmental changes. Antibiotic resistance poses an additional challenge, increasing the dangers associated with conditions such as tuberculosis. Maternal, neonatal, and nutritional diseases are categorized with communicable diseases because so many of the causes of ill health in these populations are infectious.

Non-Communicable Disease A **non-communicable disease (NCD)** is a medical condition or disease that by definition is non-infectious and non-transmissible among people, and is attributed to a combination of genetic and lifestyle factors. Although NCDs may sometimes be referred to as chronic diseases, implying longer duration and slow progression, this is not completely accurate, as non-communicable causes may also result in a rapid death, as in the event of a sudden heart attack. Further, some communicable diseases (e.g., HIV/AIDS), when controlled with medications, take on the character of long-term chronic conditions as well, requiring ongoing management of symptoms across a longer life span. NCDs are responsible for over 60% of all death, overtaking communicable diseases in recent years. According to the 2015 GBD Study, the five leading causes of death from NCDs (category 2) were ischemic heart disease, cerebrovascular disease, chronic obstructive pulmonary disease, lower respiratory infection, and Alzheimer's disease. Mental illnesses (see chapter 7) are also included in the NCD category.

Injuries Injury is defined as "any unintentional and intentional damage to the body resulting from acute exposure to thermal, mechanical, electrical, or chemical energy that exceeds a threshold of tolerance in the body or from the absence of such essentials as heat or oxygen" (Society for the Advancement of Violence and Injury Research & Safe States Alliance, 2005). Intentional injuries can also be classified as acts of violence, defined by WHO (2017e) as "the intentional use of physical force or power, threatened or actual, against oneself, another person, or against a group or community, which either results in or has a high likelihood of resulting in injury, death, psychological harm, maldevelopment, or deprivation." Although the term *accident* is sometimes used in conjunction with injury, injuries, even unintentional ones, are rarely random. They are generally related to conditions or risk factors that are predictable and often preventable. According to the 2015 GBD Study, the leading five causes of death for injuries (category 3) were road injuries, self-harm, falls, interpersonal violence, and drowning. Prominent as a cause of death in all age groups, injury is a particularly important problem among 15- to 49-year-olds worldwide, for whom 3 of the 10 leading causes of death can be categorized as injuries, including road traffic accidents, self-harm, and interpersonal violence.

Global Health Transitions and Disease Burden

One of the expectations of global health and development efforts, both implicit and explicit, and dating back over a century, is that of demographic and epidemiological transition. The first aspect, **demographic transition**, predicts that improved conditions will lead to increased survival, especially among children; lower fertility rates; and an older age distribution. This demographic shift was to be accompanied by an **epidemiological transition**, where countries on the path to economic development would experience a shift in disease profile, from one burdened with infectious disease and mortality in the early years of life (GBD category 1 diseases and conditions), to one that experiences mostly NCDs (category 2 diseases and conditions) associated with the aging population, like the developed countries they emulated.

Although the infectious disease burden has generally decreased with development, it was never eliminated to the extent expected, leaving low-income countries to experience a **double burden of disease**. That is, they continue to address higher burdens of infectious disease, while at the same time putting systems in place to prevent and treat new burdens from NCDs (Dye, 2014).

In recent years, global health experts have identified a third layer of disease burden. The **triple burden of disease** refers to the disease burden associated with globalization and urbanization. All nations, individually and collectively, must prepare to deal with global pandemics, environmental degradation related to urbanization and population density, social disruptions and other problems associated with economic inequities, and the effects of climate change (Frenk & Gomez-Dantes, 2011). This third burden will be borne everywhere, but like the others, it takes a greater toll in lower-income settings.

Risk Factors

Although information about the burden of ill health due to disease is useful for planning medical care and certain public health efforts, there are some sources of ill health for which it is more useful to look at the underlying causes, or risk factors, when trying to assess, prevent, or treat disease. **Risk factors** can be defined as causes of disease and injury that may be malleable. Risk factor analysis of global burden allows us to complement what we know about the burden of specific diseases with knowledge about the impact of conditions that make people more vulnerable to disease in the first place. For example, we know that 21% of all deaths can be attributed to dietary risks (principally diets low in fruits and vegetables and high in sodium); another 20% can be attributed to high blood pressure; 13% are caused by tobacco use; and 12% of mortality can be attributed to air pollution (GBD 2015 Risk Factors Collaborators, 2016).

This knowledge allows us to address health challenges in new ways. For example, it suggests interventions such as health education and changes to policies related to the food system; strategies to curtail the desirability, availability, and use of tobacco; and regulations to maintain or improve air quality. In each of these examples, addressing one risk factor can have an impact on multiple diseases. Addressing risk factors, rather than individual diseases, can increase prevention and reduce severity and progression for a number of diseases at the same time.

The GBD Study classifies risk factors as behavioral, metabolic, environmental, and combinations of these three types. There are 77 risk factors in all. Environmental factors include those related to water and sanitation, air pollution, and occupational hazards. Behavioral risk factors include practices related to maternal and child malnutrition, tobacco use, alcohol and drug use, diet, low physical activity, unsafe sexual practices, and sexual abuse and violence. Metabolic risk factors are biological in nature and include cholesterol levels and body mass index (BMI) (GBD 2015 Risk Factors Collaborators, 2016).

Recently, the UN embarked on a worldwide risk factor approach to NCDs. In 2012, the UN held a high-level meeting to promote a strategy that addresses four common risk factors—tobacco use, poor diet, inadequate exercise, and excessive alcohol consumption—to reduce the incidence and severity of NCDs. Although high-tech treatments for NCDs can reduce death and disability, it is both better for individual health and more cost-effective to rely primarily on prevention as a long-term strategy to address these conditions.

Social Determinants of Health and the Social-Ecological Model

If health is a state of complete physical mental and social well-being and not just the absence of disease, then the conditions that lead to this state of well-being and thriving must be specified, and we need to begin with health, rather than illness.

The Social Determinants of Health

The **social determinants of health** are "the conditions in which people are born, grow, work, live, and age, and the wider set of forces and systems shaping the conditions of daily life. These forces and systems include economic policies and systems, development agendas, social norms, social policies, and political systems" (WHO, 2017j).

The most important social determinants will vary with the disease condition to be addressed and the population of focus. Box 2.3 lists the determinants of health developed by the Public Health Agency of Canada (2013). All of these determinants are backed up by evidence of a demonstrated relationship to health status.

BOX 2.3

SOCIAL DETERMINANTS OF HEALTH

Income and social status

Social support

Education

Social environment

Physical environment

Personal health practices and coping skills

Healthy child development

Biology

Health services

Gender

Culture

Social-Ecological Model

A **social-ecological model** is a framework that accounts for the multiple interrelated factors that facilitate or impede health and well-being. It is based on the fundamental idea that health is not determined solely by biological factors at the individual level, but rather that health is produced by interactions at the individual (age, sex, gender, race, biological factors), interpersonal (family and relationships), community (organizations and environmental factors), and societal (culture, economics, governance, etc.) levels. All of these levels offer opportunities to understand, prevent, and effectively respond to illness and disability.

Social-ecological models provide a robust lens for studying global health by graphically representing the social determinants of health and enabling you to visualize the relationships and interactions among the determinants. These models are useful for analyzing problems and root causes, and for planning multifaceted interventions to foster health. They can help you think about how health unfolds in different contexts, and how environment, behavior, genetics, culture, and policies can all influence health and well-being.

FIGURE 2.2   The Institute of Medicine Social-Ecological Model

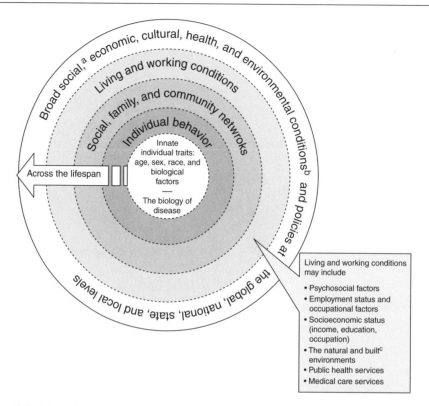

Living and working conditions may include

- Psychosocial factors
- Employment status and occupational factors
- Socioeconomic status (income, education, occupation)
- The natural and built[c] environments
- Public health services
- Medical care services

Notes: (a) Social conditions include, but are not limited to: economic inequality, urbanization, mobility, cultural values, attitudes and policies related to discrimination and intolerance on the basis of race, gender, and other differences; (b) other conditions at the national level might include major sociopolitical shifts, such as recession, war, and governmental collapse; (c) the built environment includes transportation, water and sanitation, housing, and other dimensions of urban planning.

Source: From *The Future of the Public's Health in the 21st Century,* by the Institute of Medicine, Washington, DC: The National Academies; 2003, p. 6. Reproduced with permission of the National Academy of Sciences.

The Institute of Medicine's social-ecological model (illustrated in Figure 2.2) is particularly well suited to a holistic and sustainable notion of global health because it maps health determinants at the individual and community levels, and extends outward to include political, cultural, economic, and global forces, and the global ecosystem. It allows us to see the connection between community well-being and care of the earth.

This holistic framework may seem theoretical, but a social-ecological perspective can have a real impact on the health care and social services that people need, especially those in vulnerable situations. Consider the case in Box 2.4: How would a social-ecological perspective lead to better care?

BOX 2.4

CASE STUDY: HEALTH AND WELL-BEING FOR TARASAI

Health Care for Tarasai

When Tarasai arrives at the health clinic, she seems fatigued, and complains of headaches and "not feeling well." The attending nurse recognizes Tarasai, who comes to the clinic frequently with her younger sister, who is very ill. The nurse guesses that the sister is in the later stages of HIV/AIDS. Taking this into account, the nurse screens Tarasai for HIV/AIDS and finds that she tests negative, which is good news. She recommends ibuprofen for headaches, which is available in the pharmacy for purchase. Tarasai seems too thin, and the nurse admonishes her about eating well and getting plenty of rest. She cautions her not to smoke or drink alcohol. She also uses the new educational materials that she has received from the Ministry of Health as part of a national healthy eating initiative to provide nutritional education. She reviews the "healthy plate" guidance with Tarasai, and gives her a pamphlet to take home for future reference. Tarasai is quiet throughout the visit and does not ask any questions. She says thank you softly as she leaves, and the nurse makes a mental note to follow up with Tarasai when she next visits the clinic with her sister.

More about Tarasai: A Home Visit

A local community group has been working with Tarasai since she lost both of her parents due to HIV/AIDS about four years ago. They make monthly visits to her home to provide food assistance and support. Tarasai has been caring for her brother and sister (now 9 and 6, respectively) since she was 10. Her grass-thatched home is spare, with a metal teapot and set of plates arranged neatly on a mud shelf, and thin bedrolls stacked in the corner. Outside there is no livestock or any trees for shade. The granary stands dilapidated and empty. During the household visit, two men from the homestead next door enter Tarasai's house without asking permission. They sit against the far wall and stare at Tarasai throughout the visit.

Tarasai does not attend school because she has to care for her siblings. Her brother does not attend because he does not have a uniform or school supplies; when he tried to attend in his only set of clothes, the other children made fun of him. Tarasai's sister does not attend school because she is regularly ill.

Tarasai spends between 5 and 10 days a month traveling to the health center with her sister. Because she is a child herself, Tarasai is not allowed to make health decisions for her younger sister, which has made access to needed care difficult.

The home visitors have been able to speak to Tarasai without the men present on only one occasion. During that visit, she burst into tears and could not be consoled. The visitors could not get her to calm down enough to speak to them. They stayed as long as they could, but had to move on to visit the other families on their list.

The home visitors believe that it is likely that the men take the food goods that the visitors bring to Tarasai and her siblings every month, and they fear that Tarasai is sexually abused as well.

Questions to Consider

What are the social determinants that are impacting Tarasai's health and that of her siblings?

What are the assets and challenges that she has at the individual, family, community, and societal levels?

What kinds of actions could the nurse or home visitors take to improve well-being for Tarasai?

Responses from a Social-Ecological Approach

Tarasai faces complex challenges. Consideration of the social determinants of health, and analysis using the social-ecological framework can help describe and understand her situation and needs, and determine some appropriate responses.

Using the social-ecological model to understand Tarasai's situation, we begin with individual and biological factors. She is a teenage girl who does not have any specific disease at this time, but she faces the risk of sexual violence because of her gender. It appears that her early childhood development was normal and healthy, but major life stressors began when her parents died.

Right now she does not appear to have effective social, family, or community networks. For various reasons, social institutions such as school and the health care system are failing her and her siblings; she has immediate neighbors who pose a threat; and the home visiting program, though well meaning, is not achieving its desired intentions for Tarasai.

Moving on to living conditions and the physical environment, it seems that Tarasai does not have a way to earn a living or make productive what appears to have been a formerly prosperous family farm. It is likely that the animal and seed stock her family might have had is now gone, and the environment was depleted when the trees were cut down to provide needed wood for cooking.

What could the nurse or home visitors have done for a girl like Tarasai? Clearly a multifaceted approach would be needed; there is no singular intervention that would make a difference for Tarasai. Neither the nurse nor the home visitors could have met all of Tarasai's needs, but they could have done more if their efforts had been informed by a social-ecological approach.

The nurse could have asked about family composition and found out that Tarasai, though a child, was the head of the household. Recognizing these stressors, the nurse might have suggested some kind of psychosocial support or mental health assessment. If she had understood the risk of violence and sexual violence, and reporting mechanisms were in place, a physical exam might have led her to discover and begin to address those problems. If she had asked about access to financial resources, she might have learned that Tarasai could not afford ibuprofen. If she had asked about how Tarasai was coping and what kind of help she needed, she might not have spent her limited time on health education on the basics of healthy eating, but instead would have focused on access to food or some other self-care strategies.

The home visitors also could have done more. First and foremost, they could have used their own social networks to address the immediate issue of personal safety for Tarasai and her siblings. From the information given, we can't conjecture about exactly what could or should have been done, but there are many possible responses. Was there a relative in a nearby town who could help? Was there a village leader or legal authority to appeal to? Could their own organization respond? They also could have assisted with access to school and social services. Education could have been an extremely helpful form of social support for all three children. The visitors could have served as navigators, dedicating one of their monthly visits to a meeting at school. Similarly, assisting with access to health care and possibly helping with clinic visits are other sources of support. They could also have taken steps to make sure that the food they were providing was used appropriately.

Source: The health care visit was developed as a hypothetical teaching case. The home visit is based on an actual ethnographic account found in Kendall and O'Gara, 2007.

As this case illustrates, when information about health status is combined with an understanding of the social-ecological context, it is possible to respond more effectively as a health care provider. Some health challenges may be best addressed by other sectors, such as school-based programs; interventions from the agricultural and food system; or coordinated care efforts among the myriad actors in government, the private sector, and civil society.

Chapter Summary

Global health efforts engage researchers and practitioners from a range of fields, as well as citizens themselves, in working toward health and well-being for all in the context of environmental sustainability—from personal to planetary health. Global disease burden is measured in terms of morbidity and mortality, for a range of conditions that are classified as communicable disease, maternal and neonatal disorders, nutritional disease, non-communicable disease, and injury. It is important to understand that there are health disparities within and between countries. There is now a great deal of reliable health data that both describe these differences and relate disease burden to risk factors that can be changed to reduce the burden of disease. A range of social determinants of health, such as income, education levels, and social and physical environment, can serve as opportunities to improve health from outside the health sector. A social-ecological model can serve as a useful framework for systematic assessment of health challenges and for the development of multifaceted solutions. It takes a whole society to foster health and well-being, and global health, as a concept and field of practice, has this goal as its central aim.

Review Questions

1. What does health mean to you? As you consider the holistic concept of health outlined here, which aspects would you like to learn more about so that you have a broad understanding of health? Which particular aspects would you like to study in more depth?
2. How can you use data about global health status in your work? Consider the global health challenges outlined in this chapter. Which do you think are the most important and why?
3. Think of some examples from your global health reading, the news, or other sources where efforts are under way to improve health by addressing one of the social determinants. What is the proposed strategy? How does it propose to improve health? Use the social-ecological model to analyze the strengths and weaknesses of the approach as proposed.

Key Terms

Case fatality ratio
Communicable disease
Demographic transition
Double burden of disease
Epidemiological transition
Global health
Global South
Health disparity
Incidence
Medicalization
Morbidity
Mortality rate
Non-communicable disease (NCD)

One health

Planetary health

Prevalence

Public health

Risk factor

Social determinants of health

Social-ecological model

Triple burden of disease

Zoonotic disease

References

American Veterinary Medical Association. (2017). One health—It's all connected. Retrieved from https://www.avma.org/KB/Resources/Reference/Pages/One-Health.aspx?utm_source= vanity&utm_medium=avma-legacy&utm_campaign=one-health&utm_term=direct-entry &utm_content=onehealth

Barrett, M. A., & Bouley, T. A. (2015). Need for enhanced environmental representation in the implementation of one health. *Ecohealth, 12*, 212–219. doi:10.1007/s10393-014-0964-5

Beaglehole, R., & Bonita, R. (2010). What is global health? *Global Health Action, 3*. doi:10.3402/ gha.v3i0.5142

Black, R. E., Victora, C. G., Walker, S. P., Bhutta, Z. A., Christian, P., de Onis, M., ... Maternal Child Nutrition Study Group. (2013). Maternal and child undernutrition and overweight in low-income and middle-income countries. *The Lancet, 382*, 427–451. doi:10.1016/ s0140-6736(13)60937-x

Bozorgmehr, K. (2010). Rethinking the "global" in global health: A dialectic approach. *Globalization and Health, 6*. doi:10.1186/1744-8603-6-19

CDC Foundation. (2017). What is public health? Retrieved from https://www.cdcfoundation .org/what-public-health

Central Intelligence Agency. (2016). Country comparisons. Retrieved from https://www.cia.gov/ library/PUBLICATIONS/the-world-factbook/rankorder/2102rank.html on Jan 5, 2017.

Clark, J. (2014a). Medicalization of global health 1: Has the global health agenda become too medicalized? *Global Health Action, 7*. doi:10.3402/gha.v7.23998

Clark, J. (2014b). Medicalization of global health 2: The medicalization of global mental health. *Global Health Action, 7*. doi:10.3402/gha.v7.24000

Clark, J. (2014c). Medicalization of global health 3: The medicalization of the non-communicable diseases agenda. *Global Health Action, 7*. doi:10.3402/gha.v7.24002

Clark, J. (2014d). Medicalization of global health 4: The universal health coverage campaign and the medicalization of global health. *Global Health Action, 7*. doi:10.3402/gha.v7.24004

Conrad, P. A., Meek, L. A., & Dumit, J. (2013). Operationalizing a one health approach to global health challenges. *Comparative Immunology Microbiology and Infectious Diseases, 36*, 211–216. doi:10.1016/j.cimid.2013.03.006

Crisp, N. (2014). Mutual learning and reverse innovation—Where next? *Globalization and Health, 10*. doi:10.1186/1744-8603-10-14

Demaio, A. R., & Rockström, J. (2015). Human and planetary health: Towards a common language. *The Lancet, 386*, E36–E37. doi:10.1016/s0140-6736(15)61044-3

Dye, C. (2014). After 2015: Infectious diseases in a new era of health and development. *Philosophical Transactions of the Royal Society B–Biological Sciences, 369*(1645). doi:10.1098/rstb.2013.0426

Frenk J., & Gomez-Dantes, O. (2011). The triple burden: Disease in developing nations. *Harvard International Review, 33*(3), 36–41.

Fried, L. P., Bentley, M. E., Buekens, P., Burke, D. S., Frenk, J. J., Klag, M. J., & Spencer, H. C. (2010). Global health is public health. *The Lancet, 375*, 535–537.

GBD 2015 Disease and Injury Incidence and Prevalence Collaborators. (2016). Global, regional, and national incidence, prevalence, and years lived with disability for 310 diseases and injuries, 1990–2015: A systematic analysis for the Global Burden of Disease Study 2015. *The Lancet, 388*, 1545–1602.

GBD 2015 Risk Factors Collaborators. (2016). Global, regional, and national comparative risk assessment of 79 behavioural, environmental and occupational, and metabolic risks or clusters of risks, 1990–2015: A systematic analysis for the Global Burden of Disease Study 2015. *The Lancet, 388*, 1659–1724.

Horton, R., & Lo, S. L. (2015). Planetary health: A new science for exceptional action. *The Lancet, 386*, 1921–1922. doi:10.1016/s0140-6736(15)61038-8

Institute of Medicine. (2003). *The future of the public's health in the 21st century.* Washington, DC: National Academies.

Joint United Nations Programme on HIV/AIDS. (2016). Fact sheet 2016: Global statistics—2015. Retrieved from http://www.unaids.org/sites/default/files/media_asset/UNAIDS_FactSheet_en.pdf

Karlsen, S., Say, L., Souza, J. P., Hogue, C. J., Calles, D. L., Gulmezoglu, A. M., & Raine, R. (2011). The relationship between maternal education and mortality among women giving birth in health care institutions: Analysis of the cross sectional WHO Global Survey on Maternal and Perinatal Health. *BMC Public Health, 11.* doi:10.1186/1471-2458-11-606

Kendall, N., & O'Gara, C. (2007). Vulnerable children, communities and schools: Lessons from 3 HIV affected areas. *Compare: A Journal of Comparative Education, 3*(1), 5–21.

Koplan, J. P., Bond, T. C., Merson, M. H., Reddy, K. S., Rodriguez, M. H., Sewankambo, N. K., … Consortium of Universities for Global Health Executive Board. (2009). Towards a common definition of global health. *The Lancet, 373*, 1993–1995. doi:10.1016/s0140-6736(09)60332-9

Macfarlane, S. B., Jacobs, M., & Kaaya, E. E. (2008). In the name of global health: Trends in academic institutions. *Journal of Public Health Policy, 29*, 383–401. doi:10.1057/jphp.2008.25

Mathews, T., MacDorman, M., & Thoma, M. (2015). Infant mortality statistics from the 2013 period linked birth/infant death data set. *National Vital Statistics Reports, 64*(9), 1–29. Hyattsville, MD: National Center for Health Statistics.

Mitchell, K. B., Giiti, G., Kotecha, V., Chandika, A., Pryor, K. O., Hartl, R., & Gilyoma, J. (2013). Surgical education at Weill Bugando Medical Centre: Supplementing surgical training and investing in local health care providers. *Canadian Journal of Surgery, 56*(3), 199–203. doi:10.1503/cjs.028911

Myers, S. S., & Patz, J. A. (2009). Emerging threats to human health from global environmental change. *Annual Review of Environment and Resources, 34*, 223–252. doi:10.1146/annurev.environ.033108.102650

Podda, A. (2010). Aims and role of Novartis Vaccines Institute for Global Health (NVGH). *Global Vaccine Research Forum, 2*(2), 124–127. doi:10.1016/j.provac.2010.07.003

Prüss-Üstün, A., Bos, R., Gore, F., & Bartram, J. (2008). *Safer water, better health: Costs, benefits, and sustainability of interventions to protect and promote health.* Geneva, Switzerland: World Health Organization.

Public Health Agency of Canada. (2013). What makes Canadians healthy or unhealthy? Retrieved from http://www.phac-aspc.gc.ca/ph-sp/determinants/determinants-eng.php#unhealthy

Rabinowitz, P., & Conti, L. (2013). Links among human health, animal health, and ecosystem health. *Annual Review of Public Health, 34,* 189–204.

Raworth, K. (2012). A safe and just space for humanity: Can we live within the doughnut. *Oxfam Policy and Practice: Climate Change and Resilience, 8*(1), 1–26.

Rockström, J., Steffen, W., Noone, K., Persson, A., Chapin, F. S., Lambin, E., … Foley, J. (2009). Planetary boundaries: Exploring the safe operating space for humanity. *Ecology and Society, 14*(2), art. 32. Retrieved from http://www.ecologyandsociety.org/vol14/iss2/art32/

Society for the Advancement of Violence and Injury Research & Safe States Alliance. (2005). Injury and violence prevention glossary. Retrieved from http://c.ymcdn.com/sites/www .safestates.org/resource/resmgr/imported/Glossary.pdf

US Department of Health and Human Services. (2008). The Secretary's Advisory Committee on National Health Promotion and Disease Prevention objectives for 2020. Phase I report: Recommendations for the framework and format of Healthy People 2020. Retrieved from http:// www.healthypeople.gov/sites/default/files/PhaseI_0.pdf

Whitmee, S., Haines, A., Beyrer, C., Boltz, F., Capon, A. G., Dias, B., … Yach, D. (2015). Safeguarding human health in the Anthropocene epoch: Report of the Rockefeller Foundation-Lancet Commission on planetary health. *The Lancet, 386,* 1973–2028. doi:10.1016/ s0140-6736(15)60901-1

Winslow, C. (1920). The untilled fields of public health. *Science, 51*(1306), 23–33.

Wolf, M. (2015). Is there really such a thing as "one health"? Thinking about a more than human world from the perspective of cultural anthropology. *Social Science & Medicine, 129,* 5–11. doi:10.1016/j.socscimed.2014.06.018

Wong, J. Y., Kelly, H., Ip, D.K.M., Wu, J. T., Leung, G. M., & Cowling, B. J. (2013). Case fatality risk of influenza A(H1N1pdm09): A systematic review. *Epidemiology, 24*(6). doi:10.1097/ EDE.0b013e3182a67448.

World Health Organization. (2016a, June). Obesity and overweight. Retrieved from http://www .who.int/mediacentre/factsheets/fs311/en/

World Health Organization. (2016b, November). Violence against women. Retrieved from http://www.who.int/mediacentre/factsheets/fs239/en/

World Health Organization. (2017a, July). Drinking water fact sheet. Retrieved fromhttp://www .who.int/mediacentre/factsheets/fs391/en/

World Health Organization. (2017b, July). Family planning/contraception fact sheet. Retrieved from http://who.int/mediacentre/factsheets/fs351/en/

World Health Organization. (2017c). Global Health Observatory data: Infant mortality. Retrieved from http://www.who.int/gho/child_health/mortality/neonatal_infant_text/en/

World Health Organization. (2017d). Global Health Observatory data: Under-five mortality. Retrieved from http://www.who.int/gho/child_health/mortality/mortality_under_five_ text/en/

World Health Organization. (2017e). Health topics: Violence. Retrieved from http://www.who .int/topics/violence/en/

World Health Organization. (2017f). Management of substance abuse: Facts and figures. Retrieved from http://www.who.int/substance_abuse/facts/en/

World Health Organization. Mental disorders. (2017g, April). Retrieved from http://www.who .int/mediacentre/factsheets/fs396/en/

World Health Organization. (2017h). Neglected tropical diseases. Retrieved from http://www .who.int/neglected_diseases/diseases/en/

World Health Organization. (2017i, July). Sanitation. Retrieved from http://www.who.int/ mediacentre/factsheets/fs392/en/

World Health Organization. (2017j). Social determinants of health. Retrieved from http://www.who.int/social_determinants/en/

World Health Organization. (2017k, May). Tobacco fact sheet. Retrieved from http://www.who.int/mediacentre/factsheets/fs339/en/

World Health Organization. (2017l, March). Tuberculosis. Retrieved from http://www.who.int/mediacentre/factsheets/fs104/en/

Yanping, W., Lei, M., Li, D., Chunhua, H., Xiaohong, L., Mingrong, L., … Juan, L. (2010). A study on rural-urban differences in neonatal mortality rate in China, 1996–2006. *Journal of Epidemiology and Community Health, 64,* 935–936.

CHAPTER 3

GLOBAL HEALTH CARE SYSTEMS AND UNIVERSAL HEALTH CARE

Lori DiPrete Brown, MS, MTS

Every system is perfectly designed to get the results it gets.

—Paul Batalden

LEARNING OBJECTIVES

- Define a health care system and its functions
- Review three frequently used frameworks for describing health care systems—the WHO Building Blocks, the Flagship Framework, and the Health Systems in Transition Template—and consider examples of how they have been used
- Define universal health care
- Review recent progress toward realizing universal health care in low-income countries
- Understand the value of comparative approaches to health care systems and improvement

If health care is to realize its full potential in contributing to global health and well-being, health systems must be designed to deliver affordable, accessible, and effective care. One necessary condition for the development of such systems is a common definition of what health systems are, along with some tools to describe, evaluate, and compare systems. Once a clear conceptual framework is in place, health care professionals from around the world can learn from each other and work together to optimize the contribution that health care systems make to overall health and well-being. Such collaborations are more important than ever, as governments around the world, even from the poorest countries, work to heed the call for universal health care. This chapter provides an overview of health systems and health system models, as well as a brief summary of efforts to date to establish universal health care in low-income countries.

Health Systems and How They Work

A **health system** can be defined as people, institutions, and resources arranged together in accordance with established policies to improve the health of the population they serve while responding to people's legitimate expectations and protecting them against the cost of ill health (World Health Organization [WHO], 2000).

There are numerous models and frameworks to describe health systems, and some experts have argued that there is not one single approach that encompasses all aspects (van Olmen, Marchal, Van Damme, Kegels, & Hill, 2012). Here we will describe three that are frequently used: the WHO Building Blocks, the Flagship Framework, and the Health Systems in Transition Template. In addition to describing the models, we will provide some examples of how they are best used.

The WHO Building Blocks

The health system building blocks, first described in the 2000 WHO *World Health Report,* constitute a clear and easy-to-use model for describing health care systems. The model includes six system inputs that together produce access, coverage, quality, and safety. A care system with these attributes, in turn, produces outcomes of responsive care, improved health, efficiency, and social and financial protection.

As Figure 3.1 shows, the WHO model breaks the system down into six building blocks: service delivery, the health workforce, health information systems, access to essential medicines, financing, and leadership and governance.

FIGURE 3.1   WHO Health System Building Blocks

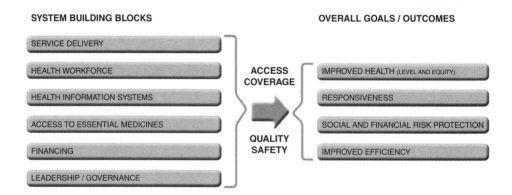

THE SIX BUILDING BLOCKS OF A HEALTH SYSTEM: AIMS AND DESIRABLE ATTRIBUTES

Source: Reproduced with permission of the World Health Organization.

One strength of this model is that it gives leaders, health care workers, and citizens an understandable model and clear language to talk about their experience in the health care system. Each of the building blocks is critical for the overall system to function, and they are distinct categories without a lot of overlap. This makes it easy to characterize and locate problems in complex systems and to identify possible starting points for quality improvement.

The interdependence of the blocks is very clear from this framework. Excellence in one area cannot make up for deficiencies in another. For example, increasing resources will not help if you do not have an adequately trained workforce. A highly trained workforce will not be effective if health professionals cannot find employment after graduation. With skilled workers in place, the system cannot work without medications, equipment, and supplies that are needed to provide essential health care. Consider the vital importance of health information systems, which are needed not only to provide safety and continuity for individual patients but also to monitor system performance and do health planning so that health care services offered are aligned with the disease burden for a given population.

The leadership and governance building block anticipates the need for system integration. It explores the idea of leadership for government services as well as stewardship within the overall sector. That includes regulatory bodies as well as making sure that the ministry of health services work well, protecting patients, anticipating and responding to disasters, and so on. The other building blocks cannot function effectively without leadership and governance.

The WHO Building Blocks model has been used extensively to design, describe, and evaluate health systems, further attesting to its utility. Here we present three different examples of how the WHO Building Blocks model can be used.

The Impact of Health Systems on Diabetes Care in Lower-Income Countries The WHO Building Blocks were used to study system impacts on diabetes care in selected low- and lower-middle-income countries. The clear structure of the building blocks allowed the researcher to find points of comparison and present a global picture that had meaningful insights despite the fact that different kinds of data were available for different countries. The same six countries (Mozambique, Zambia, Malawi, Nicaragua, Vietnam, and Kryrgystan) were studied for two of the building blocks (service delivery and access to medicines); analysis of some of the other building blocks (health information systems and leadership and governance) included analysis of a larger number of countries; still others (finance and workforce) drew insights from a smaller number of studies. In a landscape where systems and available data varied, the building blocks served as a framework and provided consistency to permit comparative analysis, and identification of model programs (Mozambique and Kryrgystan). The information assembled was then synthesized to identify common challenges (increased prevalence of diabetes and shortage of care capacity and medicine) and some promising interventions—namely, managing care at the primary care level and encouraging advocacy for essential medicine (Beran, 2015).

Preparing to Manage Non-Communicable Disease in Cambodia This district-level study focused on assessing preparedness for managing non-communicable diseases (NCDs) in Cambodia. Aware that the public health system and the building blocks model were oriented primarily toward communicable disease and maternal and child health, this study explored the capacity to respond to NCDs at the community level. This study interviewed health care providers, managers, and community members, using a questionnaire structured around the WHO Building Blocks. The results provided actionable information about system shortcomings. Most health care workers had not been trained in management of NCDs, medicines were not available, and service delivery models that were health-center based, rather than community based, were not responsive to the provision of ongoing care for chronic conditions. Interviews also indicated that some of the needed service delivery models were already in place for HIV care, so cross-learning within the Cambodian health care system was one recommended change strategy (Jacobs, Hill, Bigdeli, & Men, 2016).

The Feasibility of Health System Strengthening in Sudan This research focused on the perspectives of international health system experts working in South Sudan to assess the feasibility of strengthening the health system. In-depth qualitative interviews structured around the WHO Building Blocks were used to gather information. The study identified leadership improvements in management, information systems, and financial management, whereas health worker skills, service delivery capacity, and procurement of medicines were in need of improvement. Noting across-the-board negative impacts on the health system due to political instability, the study concluded that "A coordinated approach to balancing humanitarian need particularly in conflict-affected areas, with longer term development is required so as not to lose improvements gained" (Jones, Howard, & Legido-Quigley, 2015).

■ ■ ■

These examples illustrate the overall usefulness of the WHO Building Blocks model, despite difference geographic scopes and different methods. In each case, the building blocks enabled researchers to effectively describe systems, identify shortcomings, and specify potential action for improvement.

The Flagship Framework

The World Bank Flagship Framework, developed in the late 1990s by Hsiao, Berman, Reich, and Roberts (1997), discusses the health care system in terms of "controls" that can be manipulated to have system-wide impacts. As shown in Figure 3.2, the five

FIGURE 3.2 The Flagship Framework

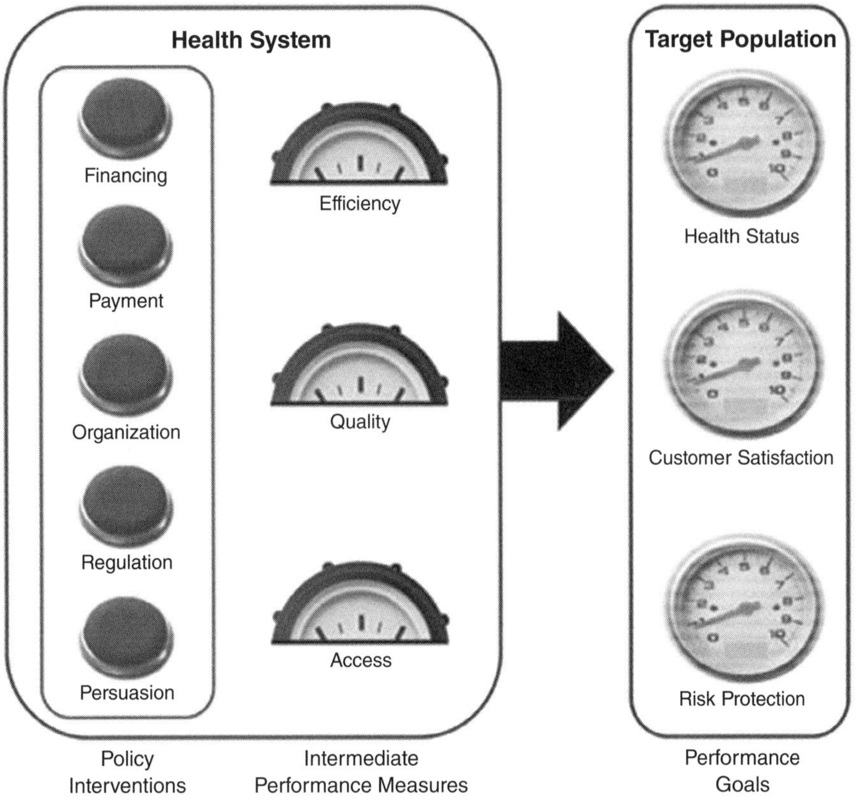

Source: From *Pharmaceutical Reform: A Guide to Improving Performance and Equity,* by Marc J. Roberts and Michael R. Reich, 2011. World Bank. © World Bank. https://openknowledge.worldbank.org/handle/10986/2353 License: CC BY 3.0 IGO

control knobs are financing, payment, organization and service delivery, regulation, and persuasion. Later articulations of the model also refer to politics, ethics, and values (Roberts, 2003). These controls influence access, quality, and efficiency, resulting in outcomes related to health status, satisfaction, and risk protection.

These control knobs can be explored with the following key questions (World Bank, 2011):

Financing: How is the health system funded? How are the funds allocated and spent?
Payment: How are health providers paid?
Organization: How are services organized and delivered?
Regulation: How are actors in the health system regulated?

Persuasion: How does the behavior of providers and patients influence the health system?
Politics: How does the history and political culture of the country influence the health system?
Ethics and values: What ethics and values are expressed in the health care system?

This model is harder to apply at the service delivery level and is intended for use by policymakers at the national and international levels. It is useful for system design and for planning systemic changes that create the conditions for improved quality, access, and efficiency. Recently, it has been used to provide guidance on pharmaceutical reform. The following description of the overall strategy, and an example of an application of the model, illustrate the usefulness of this model.

Guidelines for Pharmaceutical Reform The Guidelines for Pharmaceutical Reform are an international resource for policymakers. They use the Flagship Framework as an analytical tool, and present a broad range of policy options in each area (Roberts & Reich, 2011). The guidelines are intended to be advisory rather than directive, providing information for decision making to support national policymakers who have the best understanding of their own context. Leaders are trained and coached in the use of the guidelines. In addition to presenting the Flagship Framework as an analytical methodology, the guidelines include two in-depth case studies so that policymakers can learn from holistic analysis with a case method.

Barriers to Treatment of Chagas Disease in Mexico The Flagship Framework was used to provide policy analysis related to the care and treatment of chagas disease. Eighteen national policymakers were given in-depth semistructured interviews based on the Flagship Framework. The analysis revealed barriers to care and related them to the control knob that was most relevant. One important barrier to care was the exclusion of anti-trypanosomal medicines, effective for treatment, from the national formulary (regulation). Further, they found that chagas disease was not covered by health insurance (organization), and there were no clinical guidelines for treatment (organization). Effectiveness was also limited by low levels of providers' awareness about the disease (persuasion) (Manne et al., 2013).

The Health in Transition Template

The Health in Transition Template (HiTT) (Mossialos, Allin, & Figueras, 2007) was designed with high-income countries, principally in Europe, in mind. This approach relies on detailed descriptions of countries, all based on the same template or set of questions. Profiles are prepared by researchers with expertise in the methodology, in collaboration with country experts. The methodology is designed to make it easy to compare countries.

The Commonwealth Fund prepares annual profiles of international health care systems, employing the HiTT approach. In 2015, the report profiled 18 countries, including 9 in Europe (Denmark, England, France, Germany, Italy, Netherlands, Norway, Sweden, Switzerland) and 9 outside of Europe (Australia, Canada, China, India, Israel, Japan, New Zealand, Singapore, and the United States). Country profiles are organized around 11 questions (see Box 3.1), which reflect the content of the much more detailed template.

BOX 3.1

HiTT COUNTRY HEALTH SYSTEM PROFILES: KEY QUESTIONS

What is the role of government?

Who is covered and how is insurance financed?

What is covered?

How is the delivery system organized and financed?

What are the key entities for health system governance?

What are the major strategies to ensure quality of care?

What is being done to reduce disparities?

What is being done to promote delivery system integration and care coordination?

What is the status of electronic health records?

How are costs contained?

What major innovations and reforms have been introduced?

Source: Adapted from *International Profiles of Health Care Systems, 2015,* by E. Mossialos, M. Wenzl, R. Osborn, and D. Sarnak (Eds.), 2016. New York, NY: Commonwealth Fund.

These country profiles were designed to facilitate comparison, and the Commonwealth Fund report presents a number of comparative analyses, addressing finance and coverage, health care system indicators, and health system performance.

Comparing Finance and Coverage Finance comparisons describe the role of government, public system financing, and private insurance as well as characterize the design of benefits. The 2015 comparisons indicate, for example, that 9 of the 18 countries finance health care completely through taxation and government funds (Mossialos, Wenzl, Osborn, & Sarnak, 2016).

Comparing Health Systems The report includes 19 indicators that characterize spending, health care access and utilization, and the risk profile of the population. From this we can learn, for example, that the United States spends $9,000 per capita per year on health, whereas the cost in all other countries is below $6,400, and 11 countries are below $5,000 (Mossialos et al., 2016).

Comparing Performance Health care performance for 11 countries was measured in terms of waiting time for care, quality of care, avoidable deaths, immunization rates, and public perceptions about the health care system. This analysis revealed that the United States performed the best in relation to elder care, with 83% of patients saying that they had a treatment plan they could carry out in daily life, and 84% saying that they had access to a health care provider to answer questions between appointments. The United States also had the highest rate of avoidable deaths at 115 per 100,000, with the other 10 high-income countries ranging from 64 to 89. Perceptions about the health care systems were mixed across the board. In the United States, 25% of the population felt that the health care system worked well with minor changes, compared to 40%–63% for the remaining 10 countries. In all countries, a significant percentage of the population felt that fundamental changes to the health system were needed (33%–50%); however, fewer thought that the system needed to be completely rebuilt: 4%–12% in all countries except the United States, where 27% of people favored system overhaul (Mossialos et al., 2016).

The HiTT is most useful for high-income countries with complex systems. It is an excellent resource for cross learning among countries and for identification of policies and practices to improve quality, efficiency, access, and equity.

■ ■ ■

All three of the models presented here have strengths and unique benefits. The WHO model is most suited to the details of system design and to enabling change within the various building blocks. The Flagship Framework is more useful for policy development and macroeconomic analysis. The HiTT is useful if you are planning to work in one of the countries included in the study or if you are looking for ideas to apply in a country that has similar attributes in terms of health care system indicators, the health profile of the population, and income. All the models can help us find answers to the most important health system questions. Who is covered? What services are covered? How are services paid for? And, most important, how can we cover everyone?

Universal Health Care

Universal health care can be defined as a system of care in which all individuals and communities receive the health services they need without suffering financial hardship. The main characteristics of a universal health care system are that it creates conditions to cover all citizens, provides basic services (with progressive expansion), and is affordable to the population served. It includes the full spectrum of essential, quality health care, from health promotion to prevention, treatment, rehabilitation, and palliative care (WHO, 2016). It is important to note that universal health care does not mean completely free care, and it does not mean immediate access to all services. More often, a minimum package of essential services is provided at a cost that will not create a heavy financial burden.

In general, high-income countries have some form of universal health care. Here we describe the models that are in place and the different ways in which they provide and pay for services. In recent years, a number of low- and middle-income countries have made substantial process toward universal health coverage. Bolstered both by some positive experiences to date and by the inclusion of universal health care among the priorities for the recently adopted Sustainable Development Goals (see chapter 5), continued progress (despite current challenges) can be expected. Here we describe progress to date, with examples from Mexico, Rwanda, and Thailand.

Beveridge, Bismarck, and Universal Health Care

Although the frameworks presented in the previous section present many possible options for health system design, in practice, four different health system designs have dominated the landscape. These models are referred to as the Beveridge model, the Bismarck model, the national health insurance model, and the out-of-pocket model (Reid, 2009).

The **Beveridge model** is inspired by Britain's national health service. Examples of the model in practice include Britain, Italy, Spain, and Cuba. In these systems, health care is both provided and financed by the government through tax payments. Patients go to the clinic, receive care, and do not pay anything. If you are a student in the United States and find it hard to imagine this, think about how public schools or fire departments work. You can sign up and go to school without paying anything. And if there is a fire in your home, you can call the fire department, and they will help you for free. In the Beveridge model, medical treatment is a public service, and providers are government employees, so the government is controlling cost as the sole payer.

The **Bismarck model** is named for Otto von Bismarck of Germany, who invented the "welfare state"—a state in which government plays a key role in ensuring the well-being of its citizens. In this model, systems, providers, and payers are private, and citizens have insurance plans that are financed jointly by employers and employees through payroll deductions. Although there are similarities to a free-market system (because individuals make financial contributions and have choice of provider), everyone is covered, whether they are employed or not, and no one makes a profit. The government influences the system through policies and regulations. The Bismarck model is in place in Germany, Japan, France, Belgium, Switzerland, and a number of countries in Latin America.

In the **national health insurance model**, providers are private, but the payer is a government-run insurance program to which every citizen contributes. In these systems, the national insurance program collects the funds and pays all the bills; therefore, it has the ability to negotiate lower prices. These plans tend to reduce administrative complexity and costs, and governments have levers to control cost by limiting the medical services they'll pay for or by making patients wait to be treated. This model is exemplified by the systems in Canada, Taiwan, and South Korea, to name a few.

A number of countries do not have an organized system of paying for and providing health care services. By default these are classified as an **out-of-pocket model**. Although nearly all countries have some out-of-pocket expenses, these systems, generally found in low-income countries, rely on individuals to pay for most or all of their health care. In general, service provision in these settings is not organized either, so many people lack access both to care and to resources.

How does the United States fit into this typology? The answer is, it depends on who you are. In Reid's *The Healing of America* (2009), he presents a summary of the four models as they relate to care in the United States:

> These four models should be fairly easy for Americans to understand because we have elements of all of them in our fragmented national healthcare apparatus. When it comes to treating veterans, we are Britain or Cuba. For Americans over the age of 65 on Medicare, we are Canada. For working Americans who get insurance on the job, we are Germany. For the 15 percent of the population who have no health insurance, the United States is Cambodia or Burkina Faso or rural India, with access to a doctor available if you can pay the bill out of pocket at the time of treatment, or if you are sick enough to be admitted to the emergency ward at the public hospital. The United States is unlike every other country because it maintains so many separate systems for separate classes of people. All the other countries have settled on one model for everybody. This is much simpler than the U.S. system, and it's fairer and cheaper too. (Reid, 2009, pp. 20–21)

The US health care system has changed since the introduction of the Affordable Care Act in 2010, which aimed to increase access and affordability and to improve access to prevention services such as vaccination and screening (Koh & Sebelius, 2010)—in essence, to decrease the number of individuals falling into the out-of-pocket model of health care. Despite advances in coverage that have been achieved, the United States still stands out among high-income countries as the only one that has not arranged health care for all.

Universal Health Care and Low-Income Countries: Lessons for All

As already noted, universal health care is in place in most high-income countries, with the exception of the United States. Although there are challenges related to quality, efficiency, and coverage, and an ongoing need to adapt services to current needs, the foundations are in place; in general, health care improvements in these settings focus on stepwise gradual improvement, and system evolution rather than outright reform.

Meanwhile, many low- and middle-income countries have in recent years experimented with bold transformative efforts to make progress toward universal coverage. Among the countries that have made progress in this area are Argentina, Brazil, Chile, China, Columbia, Costa Rica, Ethiopia, Georgia, Ghana, Guatemala, India, Indonesia, Jamaica, Kenya, Kyrgyz Republic, Mexico, Nigeria, Peru, the Philippines, South Africa, Thailand, Tunisia, Turkey, and Vietnam. These countries have pursued strategies that focus on people living in poverty, by working to make care both more affordable and more accessible (Cotlear, Nagpal, Smith, Tandon, & Cortez, 2015).

Evaluations that looked at access to care as well as protection from financial hardship identified Brazil, Colombia, Costa Rica, Mexico, and South Africa as making the most successful strides, whereas progress was slower in Ethiopia, Guatemala, India, Indonesia, and Vietnam. In general, improvements came from increases in receipt of key health interventions, not from reductions in the incidence of out-of-pocket expenditure (Wagstaff, Cotlear, Eozenou, & Buisman, 2016). Here we describe three case examples of promising universal coverage efforts from Thailand, Mexico, and Rwanda.

Thailand: "30 Baht Treats All Diseases"

In 2001, Thailand introduced its 30 Baht Universal Coverage Program, which covers the entire population with the promise that patients would pay just 30 baht per visit for medical care. The campaign was simple and comprehensive, a high-risk all-at-once strategy (Hughes & Leethongdee, 2007). By 2012, coverage rates were 99.5% (World Bank, 2012), and accompanying health impacts included an increase in life expectancy to 74 years, and a drop in IMR to 11. Further, the disparity in IMR between richer and poorer populations in Thailand has been nearly eliminated (Sen, 2015). To hold these gains and address current health challenges, Thailand must continue to progress with attention to issues such as the geographic distribution of its health workforce and rising costs.

***Mexico: Achieving Universal Health Coverage through* Seguro Popular**   In 2003, Mexico introduced the *Seguro Popular,* a package of comprehensive health services. The program sought to improve financial protection and access for the 60 million Mexicans who did not have health coverage in 2002. By 2011, Mexico enjoyed health care coverage rates of 98%, with improved health care outcomes during that period. The data suggest that the improvements are correlated with the increased access to health care services; mortality in children under five dropped by 11% in the newly insured populations, and those who previously had insurance saw a smaller drop of 5%. Similarly, maternal mortality dropped by 32% in the *Seguro Popular* group, whereas previously insured women saw a lesser improvement of 3%. With the success in coverage and demonstrated health improvements, experts identify the need for further reforms related to system organization, and recommend Mexico as a country example with great implications for universal health care efforts in other low- and middle-income countries (Knaul et al., 2012).

Rwanda:* Mutuelles *for Community-Based Health Insurance   In 1999, Rwanda established *Mutuelles,* a community-based health insurance program based on annual member premiums. The program began with a pilot in 1999, at a time when 1% of the population had health coverage. In just five years, the program was scaled up to the national level, with standard packages and fees, and guidance about organization and delivery of services. After eight years, coverage had risen to 85%. After implementation of the program, Rwanda saw decreases in infant mortality and maternal mortality, and out-of-pocket spending on health care as a percentage of overall income dropped from 11.9% in 2000 to 7.7% in 2006. In 2012, 14 years after the program began, evaluators concluded that "Rwanda's experience suggests that community-based health insurance schemes can be effective tools for achieving universal health coverage even in the poorest settings. We suggest a future study on how eliminating *Mutuelles* copayments for the poorest will improve their healthcare utilization, lower their catastrophic health spending, and affect the finances of health care providers" (Lu et al., 2012).

■   ■   ■

Although all of these programs face challenges related to sustainability, cost, and quality, and continued success will require monitoring and ongoing improvement in financing, organization, and provision of services, these examples make it clear that improvement in health status through improved health care is a realistic goal for all countries. A comparative systems approach, through which countries at all income levels share experiences and learn from each other, can accelerate needed changes toward systems that are accessible, efficient, and effective.

Chapter Summary

Health systems are different, and those differences matter. The global movement toward universal health care requires an understanding of how to describe, evaluate, and transform health systems. Frameworks such as the WHO Building Blocks, the Flagship Framework, and the Health in Transition Template each do this in different ways.

Universal health care has been established in most high-income countries and is on the rise in low- and middle-income countries. As you work to improve global health in specific ways, it is important to return to a systems focus. In order to be an innovative collaborator in your global health work, ask yourself, "Who's covered?" "What's covered?" "How are these services financed?" Lessons from Thailand, Mexico, and Rwanda show that a comparative systems approach will generate a broad range options for health system improvement.

Review Questions

1. Consider a country where you would like to do global health work. Describe the health care system. How does it compare to the system in the United States or your home country?
2. What are the benefits of universal health coverage? What are the challenges? Do you think universal health coverage is a realistic global goal?

Key Terms

Beveridge model
Bismarck model
Health system
National health insurance model
Out-of-pocket model
Universal health care

References

Beran, D. (2015). The impact of health systems on diabetes care in low and lower middle income countries. *Current Diabetes Reports, 15*(4). doi:10.1007/s11892-015-0591-8

Cotlear, D., Nagpal, S., Smith, O. K., Tandon, A., & Cortez, R. A. (2015). *Going universal: How 24 developing countries are implementing universal health coverage reforms from the bottom up.* Washington, DC: World Bank Group. Retrieved from http://documents.worldbank.org/curated/en/936881467992465464/Going-universal-how-24-developing-countries-are-implementing-universal-health-coverage-reforms-from-the-bottom-up

Hsiao, W., Berman, P., Reich, M. R., & Roberts, M. J. (1997). *Background paper for Module II, Flagship Course, 1997*. Washington, DC: World Bank.

Hughes, D., & Leethongdee, S. (2007). Universal coverage in the land of smiles: Lessons from Thailand's 30 Baht health reforms. *Health Affairs, 26*, 999–1008. doi:10.1377/hlthaff.26.4.999

Jacobs, B., Hill, P., Bigdeli, M., & Men, C. (2016). Managing non-communicable diseases at health district level in Cambodia: A systems analysis and suggestions for improvement. *BMC Health Services Research, 16*. doi:10.1186/s12913-016-1286-9

Jones, A., Howard, N., & Legido-Quigley, H. (2015). Feasibility of health systems strengthening in South Sudan: A qualitative study of international practitioner perspectives. *BMJ Open, 5*(12). doi:10.1136/bmjopen-2015-009296

Knaul, F. M., Gonzalez-Pier, E., Gomez-Dantes, O., Garcia-Junco, D., Arreola-Ornelas, H., Barraza-Llorens, M., … Frenk, J. (2012). The quest for universal health coverage: Achieving social protection for all in Mexico. *The Lancet, 380*, 1259–1279. doi:10.1016/s0140-6736(12)61068-x

Koh, H. K., & Sebelius, K. G. (2010). Promoting prevention through the Affordable Care Act. *New England Journal of Medicine, 363*, 1296–1299. doi:10.1056/NEJMp1008560

Lu, C. L., Chin, B., Lewandowski, J. L., Basinga, P., Hirschhorn, L. R., Hill, K., … Binagwaho, A. (2012). Towards universal health coverage: An evaluation of Rwanda Mutuelles in its first eight years. *PLoS One, 7*(6). doi:10.1371/journal.pone.0039282

Manne, J. M., Snively, C. S., Ramsey, J. M., Salgado, M. O., Barnighausen, T., & Reich, M. R. (2013). Barriers to treatment access for chagas disease in Mexico. *PLoS Neglected Tropical Diseases, 7*(10). doi:10.1371/journal.pntd.0002488

Mossialos, E., Allin, S., & Figueras, J. (2007). *Health systems in transition: Template for analysis*. Copenhagen: WHO Regional Office for Europe on behalf of the European Observatory on Health Systems and Policies.

Mossialos, E., Wenzl, M., Osborn R., & Sarnak, D. (Eds.). (2016). *International profiles of health care systems, 2015*. New York, NY. Commonwealth Fund.

Reid, T. R. (2009). *The healing of America: A global quest for better, cheaper, and fairer health care*. New York, NY: Penguin Press.

Roberts, M. (2003). *Getting health reform right: A guide to improving performance and quality*. New York, NY: Oxford University Press.

Roberts, M., & Reich, M. (2011). *Pharmaceutical reform: A guide to improving performance and equity*. Washington, DC: World Bank.

Sen, A. (2015, January 6). Universal health care: The affordable dream. *Guardian*. Retrieved from https://www.theguardian.com/society/2015/jan/06/-sp-niversal-healthcare-the-affordable-dream-amartya-sen

van Olmen, J., Marchal, B., Van Damme, W., Kegels, G., & Hill, P. S. (2012). Health systems frameworks in their political context: Framing divergent agendas. *BMC Public Health, 12*. doi:10.1186/1471-2458-12-774

Wagstaff, A., Cotlear, D., Eozenou, P.H.V., & Buisman, L. R. (2016). Measuring progress towards universal health coverage: With an application to 24 developing countries. *Oxford Review of Economic Policy, 32*(1), 147–189. doi:10.1093/oxrep/grv019

World Bank. (2011). What is a health system? Retrieved from http://go.worldbank.org/2IJCRM6BG0

World Bank. (2012). Thailand: Sustaining health protection for all. Retrieved from http://www.worldbank.org/en/news/feature/2012/08/20/thailand-sustaining-health-protection-for-all

World Health Organization. (2000). *The world health report 2000: Health systems: Improving performance*. Geneva, Switzerland: Author. Retrieved from http://www.who.int/whr/2000/en/whr00_en.pdf

World Health Organization. (2016). Universal health care coverage fact sheet. Retrieved from http://www.who.int/mediacentre/factsheets/fs395/en/

CHAPTER 4

GLOBAL HEALTH POLICY AND THE SUSTAINABLE DEVELOPMENT GOALS

Lori DiPrete Brown, MS, MTS

Health . . . is a fundamental human right[,] and . . . the attainment of the highest possible level of health is a most important world-wide social goal whose realization requires the action of many other social and economic sectors in addition to the health sector.

—Declaration of Alma-Ata, September 1978

LEARNING OBJECTIVES

- Understand the goals and objectives of the Declaration of Alma-Ata and the Millennium Development Goals
- Become familiar with the Sustainable Development Goals, how all contribute to health, and, conversely, how health contributes to all of them
- Outline the goals and targets of Sustainable Development Goal 3, to ensure healthy lives and promote well-being for all people at all ages

The goal of "Health for All," the vision of Alma-Ata, has driven health and development initiatives for the past 40 years. This chapter traces the success, evolution, and revival of the notion that health is essential for, and to a degree synonymous with, human thriving. It reviews the Declaration of Alma-Ata, the Millennium Development Goals, and the Sustainable Development Goals (SDGs). The holistic approach of the SDGs and the current focus on universal health care represent a moment in which global health

Foundations for Global Health Practice, First Edition. Lori DiPrete Brown.
© 2018 John Wiley & Sons, Inc. Published 2018 by John Wiley & Sons, Inc.

policy has come full circle, returning to the principles the Declaration Alma-Ata originally promoted in 1978.

From Alma-Ata to the Millennium Development Goals

The following review of major initiatives and their underlying principles will explore the ways in which the focus of global health policy shifted and developed from 1978 to 2015. Although there has been a consistent focus on holistic health and reducing disparities, the way these policies are articulated has evolved in light of changing social, scientific, and environmental paradigms.

The Declaration of Alma-Ata, 1978

The **Declaration of Alma-Ata** promoted health as a worldwide social goal, and was endorsed by 134 countries in the midst of the Cold War. It laid out a set of premises and core principles, and focused on comprehensive primary health care for all as the strategy that would be most promising for achieving its goals. The Declaration affirmed health as a human right, spoke out against economic inequality, and underscored the responsibility of governments for providing health care. In its call for international cooperation, it both justified the human health focus as a necessary component of the new international economic order and denounced militarization, suggesting that working toward peace would allow for diversion of military expenditures toward health (Declaration of Alma-Ata, 1978).

The main emphasis of the document was to set forth the principles and promise of primary health care. The Declaration laid out not only the ends but also the means by which it would be realized. Thus the global community endorsed primary health care as a way to achieve the goal of "Health for all by the year 2000."

The Alma-Ata Approach: Comprehensive Primary Health Care

The concept of primary health care did not emerge at the conference, but rather was the product of a number of critical trends in the 1960s and 1970s. Single-disease approaches, also called vertical approaches, were unsuccessful in combating diseases such as malaria. At the same time, community-based approaches that were low-tech and had the potential to reach the world's disenfranchised poor seemed promising. Examples included the barefoot doctors in China and the village health care worker models that were being developed in medical missions and faith-based programs (Cueto, 2004).

According to the Declaration, **primary health care**

includes at least: education concerning prevailing health problems and the methods of preventing and controlling them; promotion of food supply and proper nutrition; an adequate supply of safe water and basic sanitation; maternal and child health care, including family planning; immunization against the major infectious diseases; prevention and control of locally endemic diseases; appropriate treatment of common diseases and injuries; and provision of essential drugs.

Further, primary health care "involves, in addition to the health sector, all related sectors and aspects of national and community development, in particular agriculture, animal husbandry, food, industry, education, housing, public works, communications and other sectors; and demands the coordinated efforts of all those sectors."

Selective Primary Health Care, 1979

The comprehensive approach to primary health care was criticized for being unrealistic, nonspecific, and too broad to be effective. Before it was possible to test the validity of this critique, the effort was reframed through a movement toward **selective primary health care** (Walsh & Warren, 1979). Selective primary health care described itself as an "interim strategy" and set achievable goals targeting causes of maternal and child mortality in developing countries. It gained momentum and led to programs that, rather than working comprehensively and holistically on multiple causes of ill health, focused on a cluster of lifesaving interventions for easily treatable conditions. UNICEF's GOBI-FFF program is one example of this. It focused community health workers' efforts on seven interventions: growth monitoring, oral rehydration therapy, breast-feeding, and immunization (GOBI), female education, family planning, and food supplementation (FFF).

Some proponents of the Declaration of Alma-Ata accepted selective primary health care as a useful interim measure, but others saw it as antithetical to the principles of Alma-Ata. Although it is easy to consider the Declaration of Alma-Ata as simply the first stage of a developing global policy initiative, it continues to form the basis of an approach to global health; in fact, the World Health Assembly reaffirmed the Declaration in honor of its 30th anniversary in 2009. Despite subsequent articulation of the Millennium Development Goals and now the Sustainable Development Goals, advocates of comprehensive primary health care have not reset their clocks, and instead express their aspirations for global health in terms of Alma-Ata: "Twenty years from now, at the half century of Alma-Ata, we could see a different world, with basic health care reaching many of the poorest families. However, to achieve this goal we need to revitalize the original revolutionary principles of Alma-Ata, sticking consistently to the core values of universal access for care, equity, community participation, inter-sectoral collaboration, and appropriate use of resources" (Lawn et al., 2008, p. 926).

The Millennium Development Goals, 2000

The United Nations (UN) Millennium Declaration articulated a holistic vision for human development, rather than just for health. It began with core values that included freedom, equality, solidarity, tolerance, respect for nature, and shared responsibility for worldwide economic and social development. It goes on to discuss goals in six different focus areas: peace, poverty, the environment, human rights, vulnerable populations, and Africa (UN General Assembly, 2000). Even though this declaration has been part of the public discourse for nearly 20 years, relatively few would be able to name these values or describe the aspirations set forth for each of these focus areas. Just as the broad and aspirational Declaration Alma-Ata was simplified to create an interim strategy, so too the Millennium Declaration led to the development of the Millennium Development Goals, which have become both yardstick and compass for governments, civil society, and health and development professionals for nearly two decades.

What Goals and Targets Developed out of the Millennium Declaration? The **Millennium Development Goals (MDGs)**, drawn from and based on the UN Millennium Declaration, are defined as the world's time-bound and quantified targets for addressing extreme poverty in its many dimensions—income poverty, hunger, disease, lack of adequate shelter, and exclusion—while promoting gender equality, education, and environmental sustainability. The MDGs, adopted by 189 nations, are eight goals that respond to the world's main development challenges, to be achieved by 2015.

BOX 4.1
THE MILLENNIUM DEVELOPMENT GOALS

Goal 1: Eradicate extreme hunger

Goal 2: Achieve universal primary education

Goal 3: Promote gender equality and empower women

Goal 4: Reduce child mortality

Goal 5: Improve maternal health

Goal 6: Combat HIV/AIDS, malaria, and other diseases

Goal 7: Ensure environmental sustainability

Goal 8: Develop a global partnership for development

Did the Health-Related MDGs Meet Their Targets? Although all these goals impact and are impacted by health, here we will take a closer look at those that are directly health related. For each, we will summarize what they aimed to do and what they actually accomplished.

Goal 4: Reduce Child Mortality MDG 4 aimed to reduce under-five child mortality by two thirds between 1990 and 2015. By 2015, child mortality decreased from 90 to 43 deaths per 1,000 live births. This is a substantial improvement, but failed to meet the MDG target of a drop of two thirds. Despite the fact that population has more than doubled, the number of deaths of children under five has declined from 12.7 million per year in 1990 to under 6 million in 2015 (United Nations Development Programme [UNDP], 2015).

Goal 5: Improve Maternal Health MDG 5 aimed to reduce the maternal mortality ratio by two thirds between 1990 and 2015, and wanted to achieve universal access to reproductive health services by 2015. The maternal mortality ratio has declined by 45 percent worldwide. There are still significant gaps in access to family planning worldwide, with over 200 million women who cannot access desired contraception (UNDP, 2015).

Goal 6: Combat HIV/AIDS, Malaria, and Other Diseases MDB 6 aimed to halt and begin to reverse the spread of HIV/AIDS by 2015 and to achieve universal access to treatment for HIV/AIDS. This goal also included halting and beginning to reverse the incidence of malaria and other major diseases. New HIV infections fell by approximately 40 percent between 2000 and 2013, from an estimated 3.5 million per year to 2.1 million. By June 2014, 13.6 million people living with HIV (less than half of those infected) were receiving antiretroviral therapy (ART) globally, an immense increase from just 800,000 in 2003. ARTs averted 7.6 million deaths from AIDS between 1995 and 2013. Regarding malaria, the global incidence rate has fallen by an estimated 37 percent, and more than 6.2 million malaria deaths have been averted. Between 2000 and 2013, the tuberculosis mortality rate fell by 45 percent, and 37 million lives were saved (UNDP, 2015). In the area of infectious disease, there has again been great success, but not all targets were met.

Were the MDGs Good for Health? What Worked, What Did Not?

The MDGs raised the profile of global health and mobilized assistance; and, as noted, they were associated with substantial health gains. There was considerable progress in low- and middle-income countries, though not all targets were met. However, like the selective primary health care interventions 20 years before, the MDGs realized their success in health through more targeted vertical approaches. This sometimes led to fragmentation of care, and there was sometimes incentive to pass over national health priorities in order to focus on the MDGs. Further, the MDGs overlooked a number of globally important health issues, including the burden of non-communicable diseases (NCDs, e.g., diabetes and cancer), mental health, and lack of access to universal health coverage.

Health in All Policies

Health in All Policies (HiAP) has been defined as "a network approach to policy-making throughout government—a whole-of-government approach with a focus on health—based on acceptance of different interests in the policy arena and the importance of building relationships among policy-makers to ensure policy outcomes" (Kickbush & Gleicher, 2012, p. 39). It emerged as "an innovation in governance in response to the critical role that health plays in the economies and social life of 21st century societies, to take governance beyond intersectoral action and healthy public policy" (p. 39). The HiAP approach recognizes that health is an important social goal and a fundamental human right, and that many determinants of health are located outside the health care sector. Factors such as economic opportunity, food systems, education, and the built and natural environment all impact health and can be leveraged to improve health in individuals and communities. HiAP strategies include integrated program evaluation and budgeting as well as policy and implementation efforts that utilize interagency committees, cross-sector action teams, and sustained opportunities for community participation (WHO & Government of South Australia, 2010). HiAP has been employed around the world, in both low-income and high-income settings. It will continue to be an important approach as countries work toward the Sustainable Development Goals.

The Sustainable Development Goals

When the term of the MDGs ended in 2015, there was a desire to realize the unfinished agenda of those goals and also broaden that agenda with new strategies to address the most extreme poverty and to integrate issues of environmental sustainability, from climate change to excess consumption. This agenda, set for 2030, aimed at eradicating poverty and transforming economies through sustainable development.

This ambitious agenda was the product of one of the most participatory consultations in history. The MDGs had demonstrated the power of a unified global agenda, and in order to have similar global focus for 2030, the UN appointed the High-Level Panel of Eminent Persons to make recommendations for the post-2015 agenda. This panel, made up of 27 international leaders, consulted with political leaders, multilateral organizations, and scholars from around the world. Panel members also listened to the perspectives of 5,000 civil society organizations from 20 countries, and 250 CEOs from 30 countries. Finally, they received input from hundreds of thousands of citizens directly, through interviews conducted face-to-face and on the Internet and mobile phones (UN, 2013).

This effort resulted in the **Sustainable Development Goals (SDGs)**, which include 17 goals with 169 targets covering a broad range of sustainable development issues. On September 25, 2015, the 193 countries of the UN General Assembly adopted the 2030 development agenda, titled *Transforming Our World: The Sustainable Development Agenda for 2030* (sustainabledevelopment.un.org/).

BOX 4.2

THE SUSTAINABLE DEVELOPMENT GOALS

1. End poverty in all its forms everywhere
2. End hunger, achieve food security and improved nutrition and promote sustainable agriculture
3. Ensure healthy lives and promote well-being for all at all ages
4. Ensure inclusive and equitable quality education and promote lifelong learning opportunities for all
5. Achieve gender equality and empower all women and girls
6. Ensure availability and sustainable management of water and sanitation for all
7. Ensure access to affordable, reliable, sustainable and modern energy for all
8. Promote sustained, inclusive and sustainable economic growth, full and productive employment and decent work for all
9. Build resilient infrastructure, promote inclusive and sustainable industrialization and foster innovation
10. Reduce inequality within and among countries
11. Make cities and human settlements inclusive, safe, resilient and sustainable
12. Ensure sustainable consumption and production patterns
13. Take urgent action to combat climate change and its impacts*
14. Conserve and sustainably use the oceans, seas and marine resources for sustainable development
15. Protect, restore and promote sustainable use of terrestrial ecosystems, sustainably manage forests, combat desertification, and halt and reverse land degradation and halt biodiversity loss

16. Promote peaceful and inclusive societies for sustainable development, provide access to justice for all and build effective, accountable and inclusive institutions at all levels
17. Strengthen the means of implementation and revitalize the Global Partnership for Sustainable Development

*Acknowledging that the United Nations Framework Convention on Climate Change is the primary international, intergovernmental forum for negotiating the global response to climate change.

Source: Transforming Our World: The 2030 Agenda for Sustainable Development, by the UN General Assembly, October 21, 2015. A/RES/70/1. Retrieved from http://www.refworld.org/docid/57b6e3e44.html

SDG 3: Healthy Lives

The health goal of the 2030 agenda can be summed up in a deceptively simple statement: "ensure healthy lives and promote well-being for all at all ages." Another way of saying "health for all," this goal builds on the past 40 years of focused efforts to meet basic health needs. The targets indicate a continuation of the MDG health agenda. SDG 3 makes reproductive health care more prominent, and addresses NCDs, substance abuse, road traffic accidents, and mental health. The call for universal health coverage has been emphasized as critical for making the whole health agenda possible.

BOX 4.3

SDG 3: ENSURE HEALTHY LIVES AND PROMOTE WELL-BEING FOR ALL AT ALL AGES

3.1. By 2030, reduce the global maternal mortality ratio to less than 70 per 100,000 live births
3.2. By 2030, end preventable deaths of newborns and children under 5 years of age, with all countries aiming to reduce neonatal mortality to at least as low as 12 per 1,000 live births and under-5 mortality to at least as low as 25 per 1,000 live births
3.3. By 2030, end the epidemics of AIDS, tuberculosis, malaria and neglected tropical diseases and combat hepatitis, water-borne diseases and other communicable diseases
3.4. By 2030, reduce by one third premature mortality from non-communicable diseases through prevention and treatment and promote mental health and well-being
3.5. Strengthen the prevention and treatment of substance abuse, including narcotic drug abuse and harmful use of alcohol
3.6. By 2020, halve the number of global deaths and injuries from road traffic accidents

3.7. By 2030, ensure universal access to sexual and reproductive health-care services, including for family planning, information and education, and the integration of reproductive health into national strategies and programmes

3.8. Achieve universal health coverage, including financial risk protection, access to quality essential health-care services and access to safe, effective, quality and affordable essential medicines and vaccines for all

3.9. By 2030, substantially reduce the number of deaths and illnesses from hazardous chemicals and air, water and soil pollution and contamination

3.a. Strengthen the implementation of the World Health Organization Framework Convention on Tobacco Control in all countries, as appropriate

3.b. Support the research and development of vaccines and medicines for the communicable and non-communicable diseases that primarily affect developing countries, provide access to affordable essential medicines and vaccines

3.c. Substantially increase health financing and the recruitment, development, training and retention of the health workforce in developing countries, especially in least developed countries and small-island developing States

3.d. Strengthen the capacity of all countries, in particular developing countries, for early warning, risk reduction and management of national and global health risks

Source: Transforming Our World: The 2030 Agenda for Sustainable Development, by the UN General Assembly, October 21, 2015, A/RES/70/1. Retrieved from http://www.refworld.org/docid/57b6e3e44.html

At this writing, the SDGs are relatively new. Are there too many goals and subgoals? Despite the intentions of integration, will they be implemented through focused vertical programs that address particular targets? Even with their comprehensive aims, there are important health issues that are not addressed. For example, the goals do not explicitly address the needs of people with disabilities, the health issues related to aging, or the need for pain management and palliative care at the end of life. Further, despite the focus on well-being and the broad interdisciplinary call of the SDGs, there is no mention of the arts, rest, or play as contributors to health and integral parts of well-being.

Health as an Integral Part of the SDG Agenda

Although the health goals in SDG 3 are comprehensive and ambitious, they alone do not express the role of health in sustainable development. Health is an integral part of the whole agenda and has special implications for each of the other 16 goals.

The graphic in Figure 4.1, prepared by the World Health Organization, shows how health overlaps with many, in fact all, of the SDGs, and how the whole agenda can be health enhancing. Combating hunger, ensuring access to water and sanitation,

FIGURE 4.1   Health and the SDG Agenda

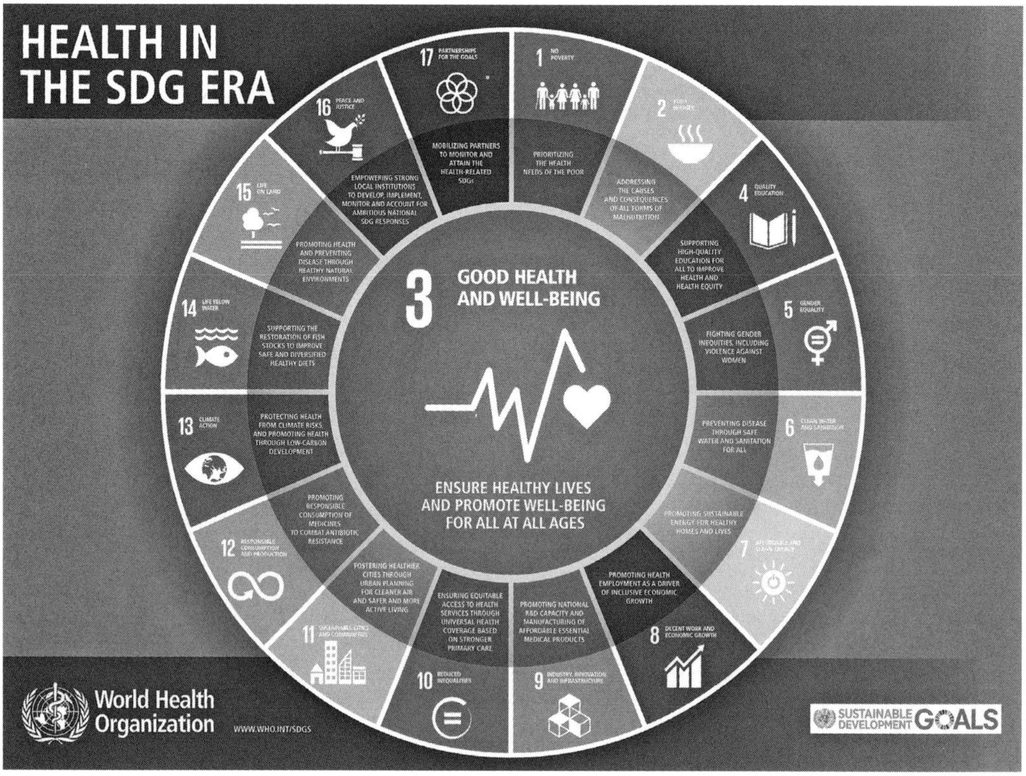

Source: From "Infographics on Sustainable Development Goals," World Health Organization, 2017. Retrieved from http://www.who.int/sdg/infographics/en/. Reproduced with permission of the World Health Organization.

education for all, and gender equality all have links to health that have been articulated since the Alma-Ata years. The SDGs, with their environmental and planetary focus in such areas as climate change, biodiversity, and clean air, open up the possibility of reinforcing known human health linkages in new ways, and identify new linkages that can exploited for the good of both human health and environmental health, now and in the future.

Chapter Summary

Worldwide efforts to collaborate on health and well-being include the Declaration of Alma-Ata, the United Nations Millennium Declaration, and the 2030 Agenda for Sustainable Development. Each of these has focused on health with broad principles and a gradually expanding list of targeted interventions. The Declaration of Alma-Ata championed primary health care at the community level and made great strides in child survival and maternal and child health. The Millennium Development Goals integrated the health goals within an overall approach to development. In addition to continuing progress on maternal and child health, the MDGs addressed new infectious diseases such as HIV/AIDS and the persistent problems of malaria and tuberculosis. The Sustainable Development Goals, developed through a highly participatory process, are comprehensive, touching on many new sectors and expanding the health goals to include NCDs, mental health, and other global challenges.

Key Terms

Declaration of Alma-Ata
Millennium Development Goals (MDGs)
Primary health care
Selective primary health care
Sustainable Development Goals (SDGs)

Exercise: Young Leaders Speak Out

Write a 300-word declaration titled "Global Health for the 21st Century: Young Leaders Speak Out." Use the declarations discussed in this chapter as models as you articulate your vision for the future of global health. Address the following:

What are the most important health problems we can address?
What kinds of actions could we take?

Review Questions

1. Consider the Declaration of Alma-Ata, the UN Millennium Declaration, and the Sustainable Development Goals. What do they have in common? How do they differ?
2. Discuss the health priorities in SDG 3. Are they responsive to current global health challenges as you understand them? What is most important? What is missing?
3. Beyond SDG 3, which goals are most important for health? Why?

References

Cueto, M. (2004). The origins of primary health care and selective primary health care. *American Journal of Public Health, 94*, 1864–1874. doi:10.2105/ajph.94.11.1864

Declaration of Alma-Ata, International Conference on Primary Health Care. (1978, September 6–12). Alma-Ata, USSR. Reprinted in *Development, 47*(2), 159–161.

Kickbush, I., & Gleicher, D. (2012). Governance for health in the 21st century. Geneva, Switzerland: World Health Organization.

Lawn, J. E., Rohde, J., Rifkin, S., Were, M., Paul, V. K., & Chopra, M. (2008). Alma-Ata 30 years on: Revolutionary, relevant, and time to revitalize. *The Lancet, 372*, 917–927.

Ottawa Charter for Health Promotion. (1986). *Canadian Journal of Public Health, 77*(6), 425–430.

United Nations. (2013). *A new global partnership: Eradicate poverty and transform economies through sustainable development. The report of the High-Level Panel of Eminent Persons on the post-2015 development agenda.* New York, NY: Author.

United Nations Development Programme. (2015). *Millennium Development Goals report.* Retrieved from http://www.undp.org/content/undp/en/home/librarypage/mdg/the-millennium-development-goals-report-2015.html

United Nations General Assembly. (2000, September 18). *United Nations Millennium Declaration, resolution adopted by the General Assembly,* A/RES/55/2. Retrieved from http://www.refworld.org/docid/3b00f4ea3.html

Walsh, J. A., & Warren, K. S. (1979). Selective primary health care: An interim strategy for disease control in developing countries. *New England Journal of Medicine, 301*, 967–974. doi:10.1056/NEJM197911013011804

World Health Organization & Government of South Australia. (2010). The Adelaide Statement on Health in All Policies: Moving towards a shared governance for health and well-being. *Health Promotion International, 25*, 258–260.

CHAPTER 5

GLOBAL HEALTH CHALLENGES FOR THE 21ST CENTURY
THE GLOBAL BURDEN OF DISEASE

Sean McKee, MA
Katherine Leach-Kemon, MPH

It is a capital mistake to theorize before one has data. Insensibly one begins to twist facts to suit theories, instead of theories to suit facts.

—Sir Arthur Conan Doyle

LEARNING OBJECTIVES

- Define global burden of disease
- Describe how the global burden of disease can inform decision making
- Introduce measures of global disease burden and articulate differences between years of life lost, years lived with disability, and disability-adjusted life years
- List data sources used to estimate the global burden of disease
- Understand what tools to use to explore the findings of the Global Burden of Disease Study
- Identify main findings from the study

When we think about health problems, any number of diseases may come to mind. We commonly hear about diseases that kill people, such as cancer and heart disease. But diseases that cause substantial suffering and prevent people from going to work or to school, such as back pain and depression, are not as widely discussed as major drivers of poor health. The Global Burden of Disease Study measures all of these types of health

Foundations for Global Health Practice, First Edition. Lori DiPrete Brown.
© 2018 John Wiley & Sons, Inc. Published 2018 by John Wiley & Sons, Inc.

problems, in terms of both premature death and disability. It also measures the burden-related **risk factors** that can cause diseases and injuries, such as poor diet, smoking, and unsafe water. Because governments have limited resources, understanding their countries' biggest health problems and risk factors is essential for ensuring that they are buying the most health for the money. This chapter defines the global burden of disease, discusses how it is measured, and provides an overview of main findings from the most recent Global Burden of Disease Study.

What Is the Global Burden of Disease?

Everyone, all over the world, deserves to live a long life in full health, yet disease and disability can decrease the duration or quality of life. This gap between optimal versus actual health is referred to as the *burden of disease*. The **global burden of disease** is the collective health gap caused by all disease and disability in the world. The Global Burden of Disease Study is an estimate of health gaps for a comprehensive set of disease and injury causes and for major risk factors, in world populations using all available mortality and health data and methods to ensure internal consistency and comparability of estimates.

To improve health, the world's decision makers and development partners and citizens need to make good decisions about how to allocate money, human resources, and attention to address health issues. And to do *that*, decision makers need accurate and accessible data on the harm that health problems cause across time, geography, age, and sex. They need mortality and morbidity data, and they need to be able to combine or compare disease burden across conditions, estimate burden in subpopulations, understand the impact of various risk factors, and understand these gaps in regional and global comparative contexts.

The Global Burden of Disease (GBD) Study enables scientists, policymakers, governments, and citizens to do all these things and more. The main metric of the GBD Study is **disability-adjusted life years (DALYs)**, the sum of years lost to early death and years lived with disability. One DALY equals one healthy year of life lost. This common metric can express cumulative as well as condition-specific disease burden. For example, Ministry of Health officials in Ethiopia who are developing priorities for community health workers can use GBD to express the total disease burden in their country, as well as to identify the burden associated with the top 10 causes of early death and disability in their country. The common unit of the DALY also enables them to compare or combine the burdens of morbidity and mortality for different conditions. Similarly, global advocates for specific diseases or conditions can use GBD findings to combine or rank disease burden across countries or for groups of countries, to educate donors and policymakers that, for example, in less developed countries, depression is one of the top three causes of disease burden among women ages 15 to 49 (Figure 5.1).

FIGURE 5.1   Leading Causes of Early Death and Disability among Women Ages 15 to 49 in Low Socio-demographic Index (SDI) Countries, 1990–2015

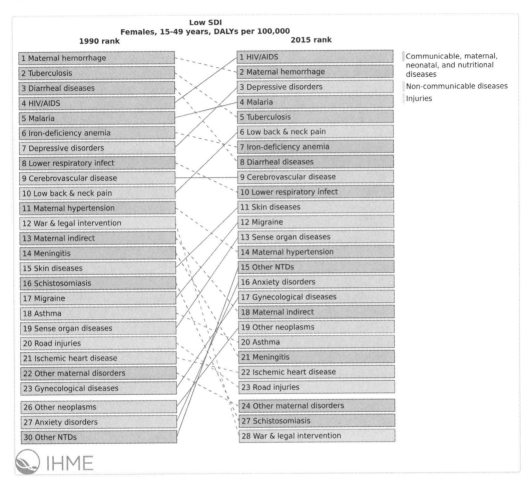

Low SDI
Females, 15-49 years, DALYs per 100,000

1990 rank	2015 rank
1 Maternal hemorrhage	1 HIV/AIDS
2 Tuberculosis	2 Maternal hemorrhage
3 Diarrheal diseases	3 Depressive disorders
4 HIV/AIDS	4 Malaria
5 Malaria	5 Tuberculosis
6 Iron-deficiency anemia	6 Low back & neck pain
7 Depressive disorders	7 Iron-deficiency anemia
8 Lower respiratory infect	8 Diarrheal diseases
9 Cerebrovascular disease	9 Cerebrovascular disease
10 Low back & neck pain	10 Lower respiratory infect
11 Maternal hypertension	11 Skin diseases
12 War & legal intervention	12 Migraine
13 Maternal indirect	13 Sense organ diseases
14 Meningitis	14 Maternal hypertension
15 Skin diseases	15 Other NTDs
16 Schistosomiasis	16 Anxiety disorders
17 Migraine	17 Gynecological diseases
18 Asthma	18 Maternal indirect
19 Sense organ diseases	19 Other neoplasms
20 Road injuries	20 Asthma
21 Ischemic heart disease	21 Meningitis
22 Other maternal disorders	22 Ischemic heart disease
23 Gynecological diseases	23 Road injuries
26 Other neoplasms	24 Other maternal disorders
27 Anxiety disorders	27 Schistosomiasis
30 Other NTDs	28 War & legal intervention

Communicable, maternal, neonatal, and nutritional diseases
Non-communicable diseases
Injuries

IHME

Note: Early death and disability are measured in disability-adjusted life years (DALYs). This figure uses GBD 2015 data. This figure comes from IHME's Global Burden of Disease Compare visualization tool, available at http://vizhub.healthdata.org/gbd-compare.

GBD researchers are increasingly delving deeper into local trends. For example, a policymaker in Mexico can use the study to understand which states are most heavily impacted by violence (Figure 5.2).

A worldwide collaborative effort to measure the impact of health problems on people, the GBD Study is coordinated by the Institute for Health Metrics and Evaluation (IHME) at the University of Washington in Seattle. It is the biggest study of global health issues in the world, using roughly 65,000 sources of data to produce more than

FIGURE 5.2   Early Death and Disability from Interpersonal Violence across Mexican States, 2015

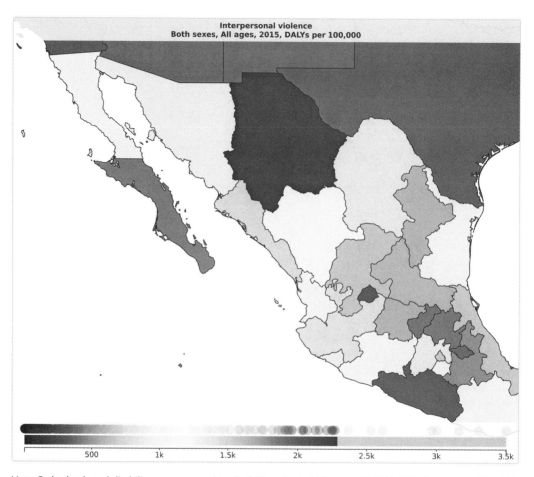

Note: Early death and disability are measured in disability-adjusted life years (DALYs). This figure uses GBD 2015 data. This figure comes from IHME's Global Burden of Disease Compare visualization tool, available at http://vizhub.healthdata.org/gbd-compare.

two billion results. As of 2017, those results include estimates for more than 400 diseases, injuries, and risk factors in 195 countries and territories from 1990 to the present. The GBD results are produced by a massive network of researchers, which includes over 2,500 collaborators working in more than 130 countries.

The GBD Study is updated and refined every year. Those refinements can include the addition of new data sources, adoption of new statistical techniques, inclusion of new diseases, and other improvements. Therefore, the estimates that make up the GBD Study improve with each yearly iteration.

The figures in this chapter come from GBD 2015, as those are the most recent estimates available as this book goes to press. Future updates to the GBD Study may include estimates that differ—usually slightly—from the figures cited in this chapter. The tools and URLs referenced in this chapter will always direct the user to the most recent GBD information, so users can be confident they are accessing the most up-to-date estimates available.

The History of the Global Burden of Disease Study

In the early 1990s, Drs. Christopher Murray and Alan Lopez, the GBD project's founders, realized that adding up all the deaths attributed to different causes by cause-specific advocacy organizations yielded a number three times greater than the number of global deaths per year. Further, there was no way to make apples-to-apples comparisons between diseases that cause death (mortality), such as cancer, and diseases that cause disability (morbidity), such as depression. In the GBD Study, disability is defined as short- or long-term loss of health.

To address these challenges, Murray and Lopez set about producing an independent estimate of worldwide deaths while also measuring the impact of nonlethal health problems. The resulting study, which provided a way to compare early death and disability caused by seemingly dissimilar health problems such as ischemic heart disease, road accidents, and depression, had a profound impact on health policy and agenda-setting throughout the world.

Following those initial efforts, the science behind the GBD project has been continually refined. The first major peer-reviewed GBD publications arrived in 1997, when *The Lancet* published a series of articles by the GBD project authors estimating mortality and disability around the world (Murray & Lopez, 1997). In 1998, the World Health Organization (WHO) established a Disease Burden Unit that published regular additions to the GBD estimates starting in 2000.

The GBD project took a leap forward in 2010. For the first time, collaborators revised estimates for the time from 1990 to the most recent year possible, replacing what had been a snapshot of global health with a comprehensive picture of health trends over time. The 2010 study also expanded its scope to 235 causes of death (up from 107), 67 risk factors (up from 10), 21 regions, and 20 age groups. Updates to the GBD Study in 2013 and 2015 also featured expanded sets of causes and risk factors. Starting with GBD 2015, the study will be updated on a yearly basis. GBD 2016 will include estimates for over 330 causes of disease and more than 80 health risk factors.

Since 2010, as the number of disease conditions and risk factors studied has grown, so too has the network of collaborators who produce the GBD Study. Coordinated by IHME (founded in 2007), GBD 2010 brought together work from 422 researchers around the world while making considerable advances in methods. GBD 2013 marked a leap forward, as did GBD 2015, which featured work by 1,870 collaborators (GBD 2013 Mortality and Causes of Death Collaborators, 2015). As of 2017, the collaborator network has grown to include more than 2,500 researchers in more than 130 countries.

How to Access and Use GBD Findings

There are several tools available via the IHME website that provide access to findings from the GBD Study and the data used in the study.

IHME provides pathways to data that it uses, but does not own, via the GHDx, which contains citations and source information for an enormous and ever-growing number of surveys, censuses, and other health-related data. Because the GHDx is searchable by country, data type, collecting organization, topic, and other characteristics, it is an excellent starting point for anyone seeking out data on the world's health. It can be accessed at http://ghdx.healthdata.org.

GBD estimates are available for download through the GBD Results Tool at http://ghdx.healthdata.org/gbd-results-tool. This web tool includes numerous ways to examine the GBD results by viewing and downloading estimates for different locations, diseases, risk factors, and so on. The tool allows for viewing the data in the form of text or graphs and for downloading data via .csv files.

In addition to GBD input data information and results, IHME hosts on its website GBD Compare (available at https://vizhub.healthdata.org/gbd-compare), a data visualization capable of generating compelling graphic representations of GBD estimates. These tools allow anyone to access and explore the full set of GBD estimates using maps, bar charts, tree maps, and other visuals.

Methods of Estimating Disease Burden

Completing each annual iteration of the GBD Study requires the compiling and analyzing of an enormous amount of data using complex estimation methods. Detailed descriptions of GBD 2015 methods, for example, are available in *The Lancet* (GBD 2015 DALYs and HALE Collaborators, 2016). Those papers, listed in the References section, are available free of charge on *The Lancet*'s website. The estimation methods used for each future iteration of the GBD Study will also be made freely available as those studies are published.

Data Sources

The data set used for the GBD estimates, which consists of all data to which collaborators could gain access, is immense. For the 2015 update to the GBD Study, for example, researchers compiled all available data on causes of death, injuries, and disease in 195 countries and nonsovereign states. The data used just for the creation of **years of life lost** (also known as YLL) estimates, for example, consisted of 43,134 unique sources. YLLs are an estimate of the average years a person would have lived if he or she had not died prematurely. Information from many different sources fed into the overall data set. In estimating causes of death, the GBD researchers depended on data derived from vital registration systems, death surveillance systems, censuses, surveys, hospital records, police records, mortuaries, and verbal autopsies (surveys that collect information from individuals familiar with the deceased about the signs and symptoms the person had prior to death, enabling researchers to deduce how that person died). Researchers then completed a multistep cleaning process. This involved removing erroneous codes, applying statistical techniques to compensate for biases in the data sources, standardizing coding for causes of health problems, and reassigning deaths from incorrect causes to correct ones. The end result was a huge, standardized data set.

Life Expectancy

The GBD methodology rests on an egalitarian principle: no matter where you are born, you deserve to live as long as a person born in a country with the highest life expectancy in the world. When estimating the time lost to health problems around the world, the starting point against which that estimate must be measured is life expectancy.

Using a life expectancy tied not to location but to the longest lifespan achieved by people serves two main purposes. First, it acknowledges that although geography holds an outsized influence on life expectancy and health outcomes, it ought not to, and that we must work to eliminate health disparities. Second, using a standard life expectancy sets a high bar for achievement in health improvement goals. It reminds us just how much life and potential are lost, for example, when a three-year-old child in Ghana dies from malaria, because it assumes that the life of that child held just as much potential as that of a child born in Japan.

Mortality

Estimating mortality by cause allows for the further estimation of years of life lost (YLLs), years lived with disability (YLDs), disability-adjusted life years (DALYs), and so on. Therefore, mortality estimation is one of the first major steps in the GBD calculations. After addressing data-quality issues, researchers used a variety of statistical models to determine the number of deaths from each cause. To ensure that the number of deaths from each cause did not exceed the total number of deaths estimated in a separate GBD demographic analysis, researchers applied a correction technique to ensure that estimates of the number of deaths from each cause do not add up to more than 100% of deaths in a given year.

Years of Life Lost

After producing estimates of the number of deaths from each cause, researchers then calculated **years of life lost** to premature death, or YLLs, for each cause of death. This calculation depends on the life expectancy standard discussed earlier, in which any death from a particular cause is attributed YLLs equal to the highest observed life expectancy minus the age of death—in other words, YLL = (highest observed life expectancy for age-of-death cohort)−(age at death). The YLL calculation, accordingly, places more weight on causes of death that occur in younger age groups. The YLLs attributed to a single death due to malaria are likely to be much higher than the YLLs for a single death due to ischemic heart disease, as malaria tends to kill young children and ischemic heart disease primarily affects older adults.

Years Lived with Disability

The estimation of **years lived with disability** (YLDs), which is the duration in years that an individual experiences disability due to a health condition, consists of three main steps: (1) establishing the prevalence and incidence of diseases, injuries, and sequelae (health states caused by a disease—for example, the blindness that can be caused by diabetes) related to disability; (2) assigning levels of severity to those disabilities; and (3) combining those two elements into one comprehensive measure of disability.

Researchers collected data from government reports of cases of infectious diseases, data from population-based disease registries for conditions such as cancers and chronic kidney diseases, antenatal clinic data, hospital discharge data, and many other sources. They then used this data, along with statistical models, to generate estimates of the prevalence of each disability-causing sequela.

To assign levels of severity to the disability sequelae, researchers used data from an open-access Internet survey and household surveys in Bangladesh, Peru, Tanzania, Indonesia, the United States, the Netherlands, Italy, Sweden, and Hungary, which were undertaken between 2009 and 2013. Survey respondents were asked to rate the severity of different health states. The results were similar across all surveys despite cultural and socioeconomic differences. Respondents consistently placed conditions such as mild hearing loss and long-term treated fractures at the low end of the severity scale, whereas they ranked acute schizophrenia and multiple sclerosis as very severe. The researchers used these survey results to generate disability weights, which are coefficients of severity attributed to each disability. Multiplying a disability weight by time results in a "discounted" amount of time that captures the amount of healthy life lost due to that disability.

After estimating the prevalence and incidence of disabilities and establishing the relative severity of those disabilities, GBD researchers could combine the two, calculating the overall amount of healthy life lost to each disability. Summing the time lost to specific disabilities can be used to calculate time lost to a specific disease that causes multiple disabilities, time lost by certain populations or age groups, or the overall burden of disability so that it might be compared to the overall burden of premature mortality.

Disability-Adjusted Life Years

With YLLs and YLDs calculated, the calculation of DALYs is relatively simple: YLLs and YLDs by cause are summed for each geographical location, age group, sex, and year. DALYs, therefore, contain within them the features inherent in both YLLs and YLDs. For example, DALYs, like YLLs, weight the life lost to diseases affecting children more than that lost to diseases affecting older adults. DALYs also allow you to make direct comparisons between diseases that are dissimilar in characteristics or severity. DALYs offer, for example, a way to compare the population-level burdens of colorectal cancer with those of low back and neck pain. DALYs also provide a way to capture the mortality and disability burden of diseases in one measure.

Risks

The health risk factor analysis in GBD estimates the number of DALYs that are caused by different risk factors. In order to do that, GBD researchers first compared the disease burden in a population exposed to a risk factor to the disease burden expected in a population with the lowest possible risk exposure. The difference between those numbers—the excess risk above the theoretical lowest risk scenario experienced by a population—was attributed to DALYs by cause for each age, sex, location, and year in the study. Performing that estimation task required a number of complicated steps—steps that GBD researchers (and interested parties critiquing the GBD project) continue to interrogate, refine, and improve.

It should be noted that the GBD risk factor analysis does not include analyses of every health risk faced by people. The GBD project focuses its risk analysis efforts on three risk categories for which methods and data currently allow credible analyses: behavioral, environmental/occupational, and metabolic risks.

Main Findings from the GBD Study

The GBD Study documents an important transition, which is sometimes called "the epidemiological transition" and refers to the shift, in terms of causes of death and disability, from communicable to **non-communicable diseases (NCDs)**. NCDs are medical conditions or diseases that are not caused by infectious agents. Overall, in that transition, children are more likely to see their fifth birthdays, and women are more likely to survive childbirth. People are living longer lives, but spending much of their lives coping with disabilities brought on by disease. Although geography continues to play a determinative role in the health risks faced by people around the world, it is clear that countries, health systems, and people of the world are shifting toward coping with the health problems long associated with the "developed" world.

People in the World Are Living Longer Lives, and Death Rates Are Declining

Global life expectancy at birth rose steadily between 1990 and 2015. The clear trend that emerges is one of steady improvement, although at different levels for each sex. Males around the world in 2015 continued to live shorter lives than females. Although life expectancy has improved around the world between 1990 and 2015, it remained the case that people in more developed countries can generally look forward to longer, healthier lives than people in less developed countries.

Mortality for Mothers and Young Children Is Going Down

It has long been clear to epidemiologists that improving the health of mothers and young children has huge positive effects on **population health**, or "the health outcomes of a group of individuals, including the distribution of such outcomes within the group" (Kindig & Stoddart, 2003). Young children have relatively delicate bodies and immune systems, but after age five, their resilience increases. Likewise, pregnancy and childbirth pose heightened health risks for women, but those risks are mostly reduced shortly after giving birth. Therefore, targeting efforts to help children and women survive these risks can have a substantial payoff down the road. That was, in part, the inspiration behind the United Nations Millennium Development Goals (MDGs).

The MDGs, focused on health, nutrition, and equity, set ambitious goals for child and maternal health to be achieved between 1990 and 2015. They proposed that the world reduce the under-five child mortality rate by two thirds and the maternal mortality ratio (the number of maternal deaths per 100,000 live births) by three quarters. Although the MDGs for maternal and child health were not met by all countries, the progress made toward those goals was immense. The mortality rate for children under five dropped by half between 1990 and 2015, with notable progress made in preventing deaths from diarrheal and lower respiratory infections. The global maternal mortality ratio dropped from 282 per 100,000 live births in 1990 to 196 per 100,000 live births in 2015—a 30% decrease. An even more ambitious set of goals, the Sustainable Development Goals (SDGs), has been established to build on and expand the gains made in pursuit of the MDGs.

The burden of high child and maternal death rates was, and remains, concentrated in the lower-Socio-demographic Index (see Box 5.1) countries of sub-Saharan Africa and South Asia. Figure 5.3 shows disease burden from neonatal disorders in 1990 and 2015. A great deal of progress was made between those years, with far fewer children being born with health problems, but it remains true that neonatal health is unequally distributed around the world.

BOX 5.1

THE SOCIO-DEMOGRAPHIC INDEX

The 2015 iteration of the GBD Study includes a new metric that further enhances comparability of health data: the **Socio-demographic Index (SDI)**. The SDI ranks development of geographic areas along a spectrum of development from 0 to 1. It is composed of rescaled average rankings of those areas' incomes per capita, average educational attainment, and fertility rates.

Countries that were previously referred to as "developing" have, in recent decades, begun to experience health problems more and more similar to those of countries previously referred to as "developed"—a process often referred to as "the epidemiological transition." In this transition, countries have longer life expectancies, declining deaths due to infectious disease, and increasing health problems due to NCDs (such ischemic heart disease or diabetes) and age-related disability. As countries become more similar in this way, it makes less sense to refer to them using the binary of "developed" and "developing."

Therefore, the GBD refers to countries by their SDI, a new indexing metric devised by the GBD team for the 2015 update. GBD researchers determined that a few factors that have been established by researchers as contributing to population health—a country's income per capita, average level of educational attainment, and fertility rate—could be combined to generate a simple but reliable metric. Classifying countries by SDI allows the creation of a fine-grained spectrum of development (instead of either-or) with which countries may be ranked. As expected, we generally find that countries at the top of the SDI rankings experience better population health, but that is not true in every case. There are some countries and regions in the world that have healthier populations (and some that are less healthy) than would be expected solely on the basis of SDI. It may be that by examining the countries whose health metrics outperform their SDI, health researchers can establish how to increase health regardless of SDI. That could decouple health from development, paving the way for all people at all levels of wealth to live life in full health.

FIGURE 5.3   Early Death and Disability Due to Neonatal Disorders, 1990 and 2015

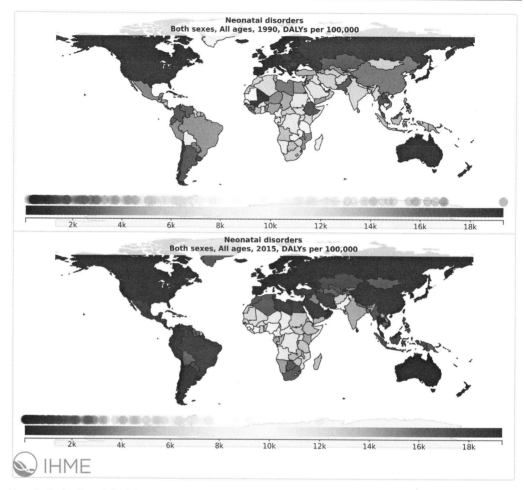

Note: Early death and disability are measured in disability-adjusted life years (DALYs). This figure uses GBD 2015 data. This figure comes from IHME's Global Burden of Disease Compare visualization tool, available at http://vizhub.healthdata.org/gbd-compare.

The Burdens of Communicable and Neglected Tropical Diseases Are Declining

The global health community has undertaken considerable efforts toward reducing the burden of communicable diseases. One of the MDGs was devoted to combating HIV/AIDS, tuberculosis, and malaria; the health-focused SDG proposes tackling those diseases plus neglected tropical diseases (NTDs) and hepatitis. Those efforts have borne results. The overall burden of communicable disease has gone down since 1990, driven mostly by improvements in low-, low-middle-, and middle-SDI countries.

Analyzing the different diseases in this category reveals a theme: burden from communicable diseases is concentrated in sub-Saharan Africa and South Asia in countries with low- and low-middle-SDI scores. Since 2000, the drop in communicable disease burden can be seen most prominently in the following disease groupings in sub-Saharan Africa: malaria, NTDs, HIV/AIDS, and tuberculosis.

Causes of Disease Burden Are Shifting from Communicable to Non-Communicable Diseases

Fewer people are dying today from communicable diseases such as lower respiratory tract infections, diarrheal diseases, and malaria than ever before. At the same time, NCDs that appear with age, such as Alzheimer's disease, hypertensive heart disease, and many cancers, are killing more people. Ischemic heart disease, stroke (cerebrovascular disease), and chronic obstructive pulmonary disorder remain near the top of the cause-of-death lists for 1990 and 2015 (see Figure 5.4).

FIGURE 5.4   Causes of Death per 100,000, Global, 1990 and 2015

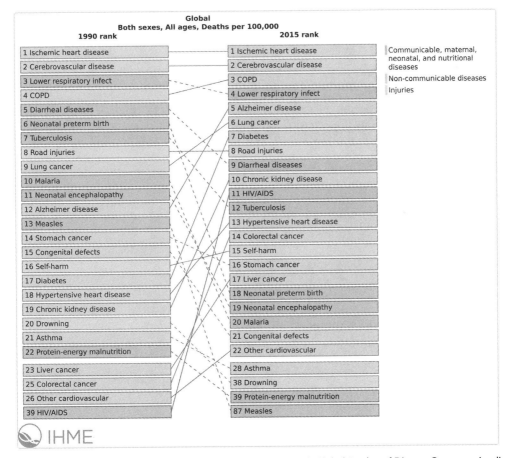

Note: This figure uses GBD 2015 data. This figure comes from IHME's Global Burden of Disease Compare visualization tool, available at http://vizhub.healthdata.org/gbd-compare.

These trends are hallmarks of an aging population. Surviving until age five greatly decreases a person's chances of dying from a communicable disease and therefore increases his or her chances of living into adulthood. And people who survive into adulthood tend to die from diseases like ischemic heart disease and stroke, thus these diseases' continuing high rankings on cause-of-death lists. It is also clear that the burden of several NCDs is increasing, such as diabetes and kidney disease, which have long been associated with more developed countries.

These changes in the leading causes of death do not take into account the amount of life lost. When examining the list of leading causes of YLLs in 1990 and 2015, it is clear that communicable, maternal, neonatal, and nutritional diseases still exact a heavy toll on human health (see Figure 5.5). (Communicable, maternal, neonatal, and nutritional diseases include diseases that primarily cause death and disability in

FIGURE 5.5   Causes of YLLs per 100,000, Global, 1990 and 2015

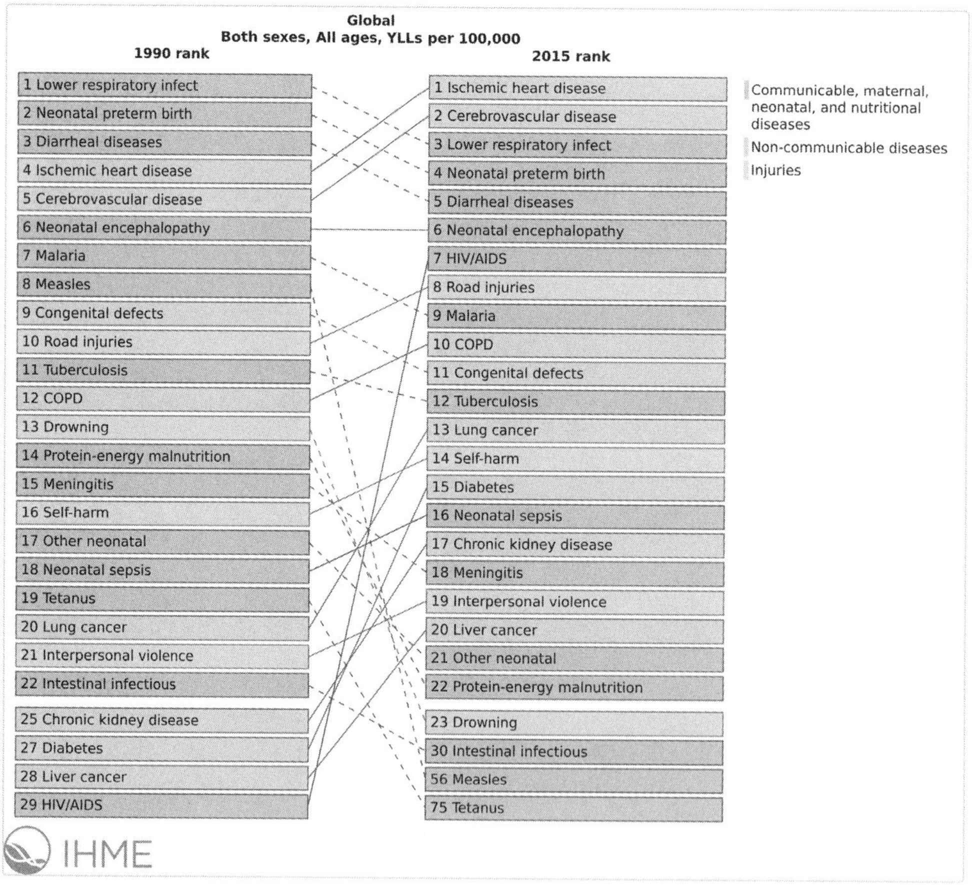

Note: This figure uses GBD 2015 data. This figure comes from IHME's Global Burden of Disease Compare visualization tool, available at http://vizhub.healthdata.org/gbd-compare.

children and mothers, and tend to be associated with young populations in less developed countries.) Such causes of death accounted for 7 of the top 10 causes of YLLs in 2015. Because these health problems tend to impact younger people (unlike NCDs, which are more likely to affect adults), the total amount of lost life they cause is huge.

NCDs remain the most common causes of people's disabilities. The lists of top causes of **years lived with disability** (YLDs) in 1990 and 2015 are considerably more stable than those for YLLs. YLDs are years lived in less than ideal health, and include health loss that may last for only a few days or a lifetime. The top 10 causes of YLDs in each year include only one change over 25 years: oral disorders moved into the 10th spot on the list, and asthma dropped from 10th to 11th (see Figure 5.6). The world made little progress in treating the non-communicable causes of disability from 1990 to 2015.

FIGURE 5.6   Causes of YLDs per 100,000, Global, 1990 and 2015

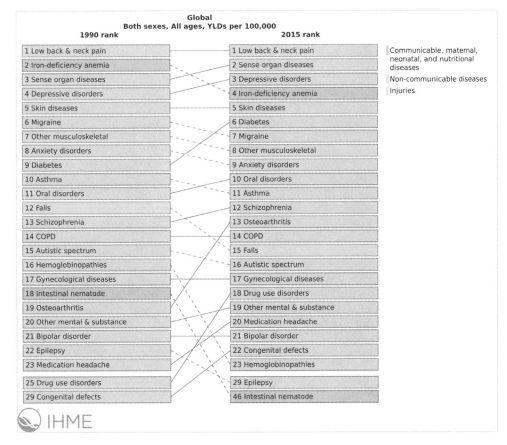

Note: This figure uses GBD 2015 data. This figure comes from IHME's Global Burden of Disease Compare visualization tool, available at http://vizhub.healthdata.org/gbd-compare.

Considering the total burden of global disease, as expressed in disability-adjusted life years (DALYs), also shows the impact of NCDs. As discussed earlier, DALYs are years of healthy life lost to premature death and disability. DALYs are the sum of years of life lost and years lived with disability. The role played by communicable, maternal, neonatal, and nutritional diseases in the top causes of DALYs declined between 1990 and 2015 (see Figure 5.7), with the exception of HIV/AIDS. (DALYs from this cause have declined since 2005, however.) Lower respiratory infections, neonatal preterm births, and diarrheal diseases—the top three causes of DALYs in 1990—fell to causes three, five, and six, respectively, in 2015. Many communicable diseases showed sharper declines. By contrast, NCD and injury DALYs increased from 1990 to 2015, with ischemic heart disease and stroke (cerebrovascular disease) occupying the first and second spots in the 2015 list.

FIGURE 5.7   Causes of DALYs per 100,000, Global, 1990 and 2015

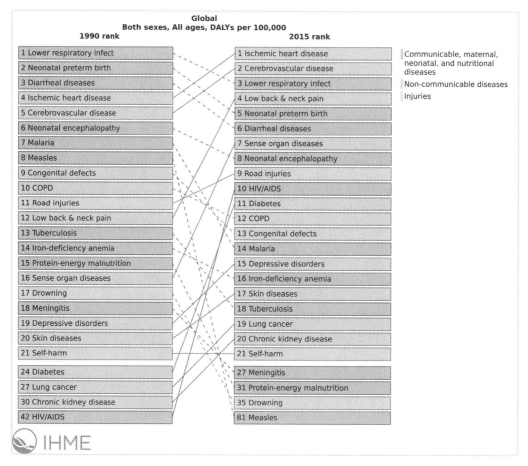

Note: This figure uses GBD 2015 data. This figure comes from IHME's Global Burden of Disease Compare visualization tool, available at http://vizhub.healthdata.org/gbd-compare.

Development Is Driving Changes in the Risk Factors That Cause Disease Burden

When considering how to address disease burden within their societies, policymakers often try to address the risk factors that are likely to increase disease burden in their countries. Risk factors are potentially modifiable causes of disease and injury. By focusing on risk factors, the GBD Study points to the potentially modifiable hazards in our world—levels of indoor air pollution, for instance, or poor diets—that could be reduced to improve human health over the coming decades.

Over the past 25 years, many low-SDI countries have decreased exposure to risk factors such as unsafe sanitation and water, and reduced the burden of disease attributable to these risks. At the same time, exposure to other risk factors tends to increase with development, such as high body mass index, which is an indicator for obesity/overweight; high fasting plasma glucose (also known as high blood sugar); and drug use. One of the big questions for population health during the coming decades is whether middle- to high-SDI countries can succeed in reducing exposure to those risk factors going forward.

From a population health standpoint, the most pressing targets for intervention are those risk factors that cause the largest burden of disease and are increasing rapidly. Those risk factors include high body mass index, high fasting plasma glucose, ambient air pollution, and drug use.

These risk factors appear toward the upper right side of Figure 5.8, which plots risk factors on an axis that combines those risks' overall burden on human health as of 2015 (the *x*-axis) and their change in exposure level from 1990 to 2015 (the *y*-axis). Thus risk factors on the left of the chart have a smaller DALY burden and those on the right a larger one.

Risk factors at the top of the chart have increased markedly in exposure from 1990 to 2015, whereas those on the bottom have declined in exposure during that time. Most of the risk factors in the top half of Figure 5.8 are those associated with older populations living in more developed countries. Their exposure levels and attributable burdens tend to rise as countries move upward in the spectrum of development. Many of the risk factors in the bottom half of the chart are associated with younger populations living in less developed countries, and exposure to them has declined as countries have become more developed.

The risk factors that contribute to the greatest burden of disease are also important priorities for improving population health. For example, even though exposure to tobacco smoking has declined, it is one of the top drivers of burden worldwide. Risks such as high systolic blood pressure (high blood pressure), ambient particulate matter (air pollution), and diets high in sodium continue to cause appreciable disease burdens, even though their exposure levels have not risen nearly as quickly.

Figure 5.8 indicates that public health efforts to combat risk factors linked to NCDs, with the exception of tobacco smoking, have largely failed. It is essential to identify strategies that actually work to reduce these risk factors. Health care—not public health interventions—is likely responsible for global reductions in death rates from NCDs such as ischemic heart disease and stroke.

FIGURE 5.8 Risk Factors by Attributable DALYs, 2015, and Percentage Change in Summary Exposure Value, 1990–2015

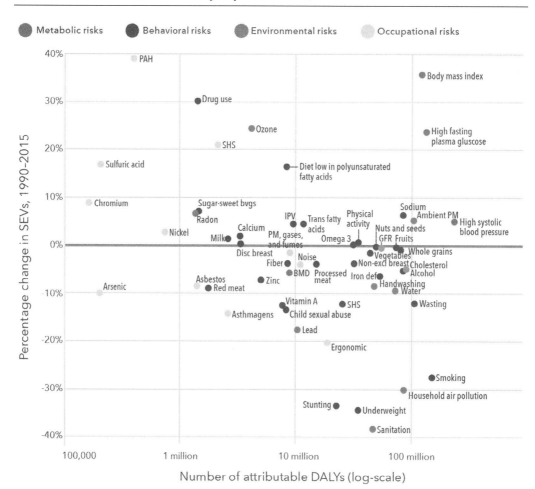

Note: This figure uses GBD 2015 data.

Despite Gains, Health Is Distributed Unequally

The world has made much progress since 1990. Life expectancy has risen in most countries around the world, and mothers and children are dying far less often. Disease burden is shifting toward the problems long associated with wealth. The burdens of a few key environmental risks—in particular those related to sanitation—have declined substantially. But all of this progress leaves us with a world in which geography has an outsized effect on health outcomes.

Figure 5.9 shows the overall burden of disease in the countries of the world in 2015. High levels of DALYs are concentrated in sub-Saharan Africa and a few other countries. People living in the Central African Republic are far less likely to enjoy long, healthy lives than those in Saudi Arabia. Where people live continues to have a huge effect on their health.

FIGURE 5.9   DALYs per 100,000, 2015

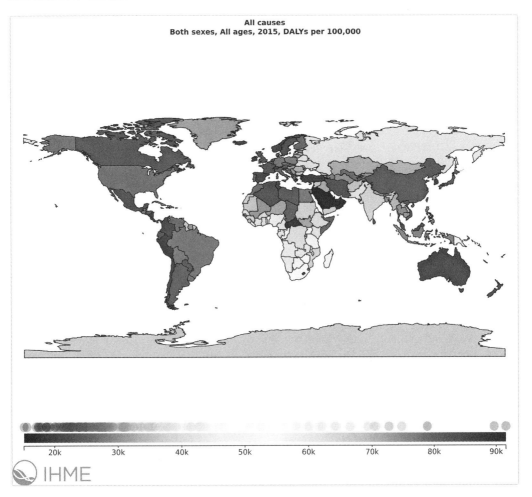

Note: This figure uses GBD 2015 data. This figure comes from IHME's Global Burden of Disease Compare visualization tool, available at visit http://vizhub.healthdata.org/gbd-compare.

GBD Will Help Measure Progress toward the United Nations Sustainable Development Goals

There are many ways—not just using SDI-based comparisons—to judge the performance of health systems. The United Nations, for example, has set benchmark goals for health and development, first in the form of the Millennium Development Goals (MDGs) for 2000 to 2015 and then in the Sustainable Development Goals (SDGs) for 2015 to 2030. Health plays a huge role in the SDGs. Of the 17 SDGs, 11 contain targets related to health. One SDG is focused entirely on health: SDG 3 is to "ensure healthy lives and promote well-being for all at all ages." (For the full list of SDGs, go to http://www. un.org/sustainabledevelopment.) Within each goal are targets and indicators related to health that will be used to judge success, such as "halve the number of global deaths and injuries from road traffic accidents" by 2020 and "by 2030, reduce the global maternal mortality ratio to less than 70 per 100,000 live births." Just measuring the progress made toward meeting the SDGs is an enormous task—one that will require coordinated action across institutions and governments around the world. In this respect, the GBD project offers to the SDG effort independent measurements of health and development indicators that can be used to assess progress toward the goals.

GBD data are available to measure many of the indicators for SDG 3. For instance, as part of the 2015 update of the GBD Study, GBD researchers used data for 33 health indicators to generate a baseline picture against which SDG progress can be measured (GBD 2015 SDG Collaborators, 2016). As of the SDG era's beginning in 2015, there were many targets that have not yet been achieved by any country in the world, such as eliminating new HIV infections or intimate partner violence. The world has made significant progress on a few targets, such as reducing the maternal mortality ratio to 70 per 100,000 live births (achieved by 61% of countries) and reducing the neonatal mortality rate to 12 per 1,000 live births (58%).

As efforts to achieve the SDGs go forward, GBD data will be a valuable resource. Benchmark data on many of the health-related SDG targets will be compared with data collected in the coming years. Countries that make particularly fast progress toward the SDGs—particularly if that progress is faster than expected based on those countries' SDI rankings—could be examined closely to establish best practices that might be replicated in other countries striving toward SDGs.

Using the GBD to Inform Health Policy in the Coming Years

The health estimates generated by GBD serve as benchmarks of world population health covering the last few decades, highlighting progress as well challenges. This study will continue to provide a checkup on the world's health while incorporating the newest data and scientific breakthroughs.

The picture of world health features a few key themes. First and foremost, the world's population is in the midst of an epidemiological transition. Life expectancy is increasing around the world as more children live past the age of five and more mothers survive the childbirth process. Fewer people overall are dying from communicable and nutritional diseases.

That positive picture is complicated, though, by other aspects of the epidemiological transition. Although people are living longer lives, they are still dying early, often from preventable causes, with NCDs claiming an increasing share of deaths around the world. Although progress in treating some of these NCDs, such as many cancers, has been steady, improvements in treatment have mostly succeeded in lengthening the amount of time people live with NCDs instead of eliminating them entirely.

There are a host of NCDs for which we have made very little progress in treatment or prevention. Diseases affecting mental and musculoskeletal health, for example, remain just as widespread and problematic as they were 25 years ago, contributing to increases in disability burden. As years lost to premature death have decreased, much of that time gained has been compromised by disability.

Increases in years lost to disability are especially disconcerting when considered in conjunction with exposure to risk factors. Many of the risk factors that contribute to disability—poor diet, high blood pressure, low physical activity, and alcohol and drug use—are characterized by rising levels of exposure, which will likely increase their health burden in the future. At the same time, concerted efforts have resulted in reductions in exposure to tobacco smoke and infection-spreading sanitation deficiencies around the world; there is no reason to believe that exposure to other risks cannot be reduced as well.

The assessment of global health is further complicated by development and equity. Even though some of the biggest improvements in health outcomes during the recent past have occurred in places with lower SDI rankings, health is still a personal and social good that is distributed unequally. Life expectancy and other health outcomes are markedly higher in higher-SDI countries than in those lower in SDI. Inequitable access to health continues to be, perhaps, the great health-related problem for the whole world.

Work left to be done, and questions left unanswered, will drive efforts on future iterations of the GBD project. Increasing the amount of and access to quality data will be vital to improving health in the coming decades. Ultimately, future GBD work will be directed toward the same goal that has sustained the GBD Study in the past: putting better information into the hands of policymakers in order to improve the quality and equity of world population health.

Chapter Summary

The concept of the global burden of disease starts with a simple premise: everyone, all over the world, deserves to live a long life in full health. The GBD Study seeks to measure everything that prevents countries throughout the world from achieving this goal. It helps decision makers identify the biggest health problems in their countries and tracks more than 300 diseases, injuries, and risk factors in 195 countries and territories; findings from the study are available free of charge on the Institute for Health Metrics and Evaluation's website. Before the GBD Study began, there was no way to make apples-to-apples comparisons between diseases that cause death and diseases that cause disability, and the available studies of how many people died from different diseases overestimated deaths. The latest update of the study found that life expectancy is increasing around the world as more children live past the age of five and more mothers survive the childbirth process. Although people are living longer lives, many are still dying early, often from preventable causes, with NCDs claiming an increasing share of deaths around the world. Public health efforts to combat risk factors linked to NCDs, with the exception of tobacco smoking, have largely failed, and health care is likely responsible for most of the progress made in tackling NCDs to date.

Key Terms

Disability-adjusted life years (DALYs)
Global burden of disease
Non-communicable diseases (NCDs)
Population health
Risk factor
Years lived with disability (YLDs)
Years of life lost (YLLs)

Review Questions

1. Using information from this chapter, explain the purpose of the Global Burden of Disease Study.
2. Name two questions that decision makers can answer using GBD Study data.
3. How does a list of the top causes of disability-adjusted life years in a country differ from a list of the top causes of death?
4. Describe which risk factors pose the greatest threats to population health.

Suggested Reading

GBD 201 5 DALYs and HALE Collaborators. (2016). Global, regional, and national disability-adjusted life years (DALYs) for 315 diseases and injuries and healthy life expectancy (HALE), 1990–2015: A systematic analysis for the Global Burden of Disease Study 2015. *The Lancet, 388*, 1603–1658. doi:10.1016/S0140-6736(16)31460-X

GBD 2015 SDG Collaborators. (2016). Measuring the health-related Sustainable Development Goals in 188 countries: A baseline analysis from the Global Burden of Disease Study 2015. *The Lancet, 388*, 1813–1850. doi:10.1016/S0140-6736(16)31467-2

Smith, J. (2015). *Epic measures*. New York, NY: HarperCollins.

References

GBD 2013 Mortality and Causes of Death Collaborators. (2015). Global, regional, and national age–sex specific all-cause and cause-specific mortality for 240 causes of death, 1990–2013: A systematic analysis for the Global Burden of Disease Study 2013. *The Lancet, 385*, 117–171.

GBD 2015 DALYs and HALE Collaborators. (2016). Global, regional, and national disability-adjusted life years (DALYs) for 315 diseases and injuries and healthy life expectancy (HALE), 1990–2015: A systematic analysis for the Global Burden of Disease Study 2015. *The Lancet, 388*, 1603–1658. doi:10.1016/S0140-6736(16)31460-X

GBD 2015 SDG Collaborators. (2016). Measuring the health-related Sustainable Development Goals in 188 countries: A baseline analysis from the Global Burden of Disease Study 2015. *The Lancet, 388*, 1813–1850. doi:10.1016/S0140-6736(16)31467-2

Kindig, D., & Stoddart, G. (2003). What is population health? *American Journal of Public Health, 93*, 380–383.

Murray, C. J., & Lopez, A. D. (1997). Alternative projections of mortality and disability by cause 1990–2020: Global Burden of Disease Study. *The Lancet, 349*, 1498–1504.

CHAPTER 6

THE RIGHT TO HEALTH AND A FRAMEWORK CONVENTION ON GLOBAL HEALTH

Eric A. Friedman, JD
Fernanda Alonso, LLM, LLB
Ana Ayala, JD, LLM
Andrew Hennessy-Strahs, JD
Sarah Roache, LLM, LLB

Amidst the poverty of Africa, I stand before you because I am able to purchase health and vigour. I am here because I can pay for life itself. To me this seems a shocking and monstrous iniquity of very considerable proportions—that, simply because of relative affluence, I should be living when others have died; that I should remain fit and healthy when illness and death beset millions of others.

—Justice Edwin Cameron of the South African Constitutional Court, at the International AIDS Conference in South Africa, July 10, 2010

LEARNING OBJECTIVES

- Discuss the concept of global health with justice
- Explain the basis for considering health as a human right
- Describe the Framework Convention on Global Health (FCGH) as a promising way to address global health challenges
- Provide examples of where framework conventions and other legal instruments and covenants show promise in responding to global health challenges

Foundations for Global Health Practice, First Edition. Lori DiPrete Brown.
© 2018 John Wiley & Sons, Inc. Published 2018 by John Wiley & Sons, Inc.

What is the state of global health today? This seemingly straightforward question may have deeply divergent answers. One is a tale of triumph of public health and human ingenuity over disease, with growing life expectancies, increasing access to lifesaving medications, and expanding application of basic measures of public health. From 1990, the beginning of the period tracked by the Millennium Development Goals (MDGs, the UN global development targets formulated in 2001), global life expectancy rose from 64 years to 71, with the gains greatest among low-income countries (World Health Organization [WHO], n.d., "Life Expectancy"; 2015e). Maternal deaths fell by more than 40% and child deaths more than 50%, with the latter falling from 12.7 million to fewer than 6 million (WHO, 2015b; United Nations [UN], 2015a). Meanwhile, HIV/AIDS is no longer a death sentence but instead a chronic disease, with more than 15 million people on lifesaving treatment by 2015 (UNAIDS, 2015), and the world has been making progress against a long-standing scourge, malaria (UN, 2015b; WHO, n.d., "Malaria").

A second tale, though, is one of continued avoidable pain, suffering, disability, disease, and death, concentrated among the world's poor and marginalized people, in low-income countries but also in middle- and high-income countries. By one metric, comparing under-five and adult (ages 15–60) mortality rates in low- and middle-income countries to those in high-income countries, inequities in global health and their drivers are responsible from some 20 million deaths every year, an unconscionable toll that stubbornly persists (Garay, 2015). In 2012, the public health spending in wealthy countries was more than 200 times greater than in low-income countries (WHO, 2015c). Deep discrimination—for example, against transgender individuals and people with mental disabilities—within countries persists. In the United States, transgender women of color have been reported to have a life expectancy of 35 years, less than half the national average and far below even the world's poorest country (Vincent, 2015).

Even as maternal and child deaths have fallen considerably, in many countries, dilapidated health systems and other barriers leave women with reason to be in fear for their lives with every pregnancy. Risks are far greater for poorer and less educated women. Globally, a median of 96% of women in the highest wealth quintile were attended by a skilled attendant during birth, compared to 57% of women in the lowest wealth quintile, with some country-level disparities far greater (WHO, 2015c). Although mortality rates for tuberculosis—a disease concentrated among marginalized populations, from migrants to prisoners to people living with HIV/AIDS—fell 47% since 2000, incidence has fallen far more slowly, and the disease killed 1.5 million people in 2014 (WHO, 2015a). The growth of non-communicable diseases (NCDs), such as cardiovascular illnesses, cancers, and diabetes, burdens health systems already weighed down by infectious diseases. Tobacco is moving from richer to poorer countries, and concentrating in poorer populations.

The Right to Health

The **right to health** is, more precisely, "the right of everyone to the enjoyment of the highest attainable standard of physical and mental health." This right was included in the WHO Constitution (1946) and in Article 25 of the Universal Declaration of Human Rights (1948).

BOX 6.1

THE UNIVERSAL DECLARATION OF HUMAN RIGHTS, 1948

Article 25

1. Everyone has the right to a standard of living adequate for the health and well-being of himself and of his family, including food, clothing, housing and medical care and necessary social services, and the right to security in the event of unemployment, sickness, disability, widowhood, old age or other lack of livelihood in circumstances beyond his control.
2. Motherhood and childhood are entitled to special care and assistance. All children, whether born in or out of wedlock, shall enjoy the same social protection.

Source: Universal Declaration of Human Rights, by the United Nations, 1948.

The right to health was further delineated in the **International Covenant on Economic, Social and Cultural Rights (ICESCR)**, which was adopted in 1966 by the United Nations General Assembly and entered into legal force in 1976 (ICESCR, 1966).

The right to health has since been incorporated into numerous international and regional treaties, and is included in more than 100 national constitutions, including 32 of 33 constitutions adopted from 2000 to 2011 (Heymann, Cassola, Raub, & Mishra, 2013). Some obligations in the ICESCR, such as nondiscrimination, are immediately enforceable (Committee on Economic, Social and Cultural Rights [CESCR], 2000). However, in recognition of the resource requirements that the right to health entails, the ICESCR links state obligations to the right to health and other economic, social, and cultural rights to states' resources. In particular, states must "take steps, individually and through international assistance and co-operation, especially economic and technical, to the maximum of [their] available resources, with a view to achieving progressively the full realization of the [rights]" (ICESCR, 1966, art. 2). Notably, this statement of

---

BOX 6.2

INTERNATIONAL COVENANT ON ECONOMIC, SOCIAL AND CULTURAL RIGHTS, 1966

Article 12

1. The States Parties to the present Covenant recognize the right of everyone to the enjoyment of the highest attainable standard of physical and mental health.
2. The steps to be taken by the States Parties to the present Covenant to achieve the full realization of this right shall include those necessary for:
   a. The provision for the reduction of the stillbirth-rate and of infant mortality and for the healthy development of the child;
   b. The improvement of all aspects of environmental and industrial hygiene;
   c. The prevention, treatment and control of epidemic, endemic, occupational and other diseases;
   d. The creation of conditions which would assure to all medical service and medical attention in the event of sickness.

Source: International Covenant on Economic, Social and Cultural Rights, by the United Nations General Assembly, 1966.

---

state responsibility includes a requirement for states to provide international assistance, though states' specific obligations to provide international assistance are vague.

The Committee on Economic, Social and Cultural Rights, which issues authoritative interpretations of the rights in the ICESCR, issued its General Comment 14 on the right to health in 2000 (CESCR, 2000). The committee justified the need for clarifications about the freedoms and entitlements intended in the right to health as follows:

> Since the adoption of the two International Covenants in 1966 the world health situation has changed dramatically and the notion of health has undergone substantial changes and has also widened in scope. More determinants of health are being taken into consideration, such as resource distribution and gender differences. A wider definition of health also takes into account such socially-related concerns as violence and armed conflict. Moreover, formerly unknown diseases, such as human immunodeficiency virus and acquired immunodeficiency syndrome (HIV/AIDS), and others that have become more widespread, such as cancer, as well as the rapid growth of the world population, have created new obstacles for the realization of the right to health which need to be taken into account when interpreting article 12. (CESCR, 2000, para. 10)

This comment goes on to clarify that the right extends beyond health care to include such underlying determinants of health as nutritious food, safe water, and adequate sanitation. It encompasses such principles as nondiscrimination and equity, participation, and accountability. States are required to respect the right themselves, protect against violations from other actors, and to proactively fulfill the right. The CESCR also identifies four "interrelated and essential elements" of the right to health (CESCR, 2000, para. 12). Health goods, facilities, and services must be available, accessible (including economically and geographically), acceptable (including culturally), and of good quality.

In addition, the CESCR has recognized that at a minimum, for the right to have any meaning, states must ensure everyone essential primary health care. The CESCR proceeds to delineate "core obligations" that this minimum encompasses, including not only nondiscrimination but also equitable distribution; food, water, and other underlying determinants of health; a national health strategy and action plan that are developed through participatory processes and "give particular attention to" marginalized groups; and health care elements including essential drugs, immunizations, reproductive health care, preventing and treating endemic and epidemic diseases, health education, and health personnel training, including on health and human rights (CESCR, 2000, paras. 43–44). International health assistance should also prioritize these areas, while international responsibilities extend to respecting the right to health in other countries, protecting the right to health in their participation with international institutes (like the World Bank and International Monetary Fund), and providing humanitarian relief during emergencies.

A Framework Convention on Global Health

In spite of the aspirations and progressive clarifications expressed in the International Covenant on Economic, Social and Cultural Rights and other human rights treaties, the lived experiences of a large portion of the world's population remain at odds with the more encouraging tale of aggregate global health improvements. It is not enough, however, to have a solid framework of standards for and interpretations of the right to health. The greatest task in bringing this legally binding commitment into people's lived realities is to shift power dynamics so that people who are traditionally pushed to society's fringe are instead respected as rights-holders and full partners in the pursuit of their, their community's, and their country's health—respected and equal participants in the decisions that will affect this central aspect of everyone's lives. One proposal to integrate and strengthen the execution of current policy trends, and to help change these dynamics, would be a global treaty, a **Framework Convention on Global Health (FCGH)**. It would bring the benefits of medical and broader public health advances to all people, including the poorest and most marginalized, and endeavor to address—at least as much as one instrument that ultimately requires government support can—the broader social determinants of public health and the unequal power dynamics underlying health disparities.

The FCGH and Global Health Policy

The treaty, conceived shortly after the World Health Organization (WHO) adopted the Framework Convention on Tobacco Control, would build on both the right to health and more recent global health commitments (Gostin, 2008; WHO, 2004). Chief among these are the Sustainable Development Goals (SDGs); universal health coverage, which is the centerpiece of the SDGs' health goal; and a focus on social determinants of health and health in all policies.

The Sustainable Development Goals A stronger legal instrument like the FGHC is critical if the Sustainable Development Goals (SDGs) are to realize their transformative promise. Agreed to by all members of the United Nations in 2015 to follow the Millennium Development Goals (MDGs), at the heart of the SDGs' health goals and targets is the promise of universality: that by 2030, everyone will have safe, nutritious, and sufficient food; safe and affordable drinking water; adequate sanitation and hygiene; and universal health coverage (UN, 2015b).

Universal Health Coverage The focus on universal health coverage represents its own global health trend. In one sense, it returns to the commitment of health for all stated in the 1978 Declaration of Alma-Ata, issued at a WHO and UNICEF conference that included delegations from most countries and calling for "an acceptable level of health for all the people of the world by the year 2000" through primary health care (International Conference on Primary Health Care, 1978, p. 3). Yet shortly after it was issued, the vision of comprehensive health care for everyone had fractured, from an early focus on a narrow set of interventions targeted especially to child health to the MDG focus on infectious diseases, specific diseases, and maternal and child health. This led to fragmented financing and programming, as well as neglect of such major health problems as mental illness and the entire array of NCDs. In the spirit of Alma-Ata, WHO sought to regalvanize the world around primary health care for the 21st century and universal health coverage (WHO, 2008, 2010b). These efforts culminated in a 2012 UN General Assembly resolution calling for universal health coverage, as well as the universal health coverage target in the SDGs (UN, 2012).

WHO has defined universal health coverage as "access to key promotive, preventive, curative and rehabilitative health interventions for all at an affordable cost, thereby achieving equity in access" (World Health Assembly, 2005). It encompasses three dimensions: the proportion of the population covered, the level of health services covered, and the portion of costs covered. As there are different pathways to universal health coverage, to meet its promise of universality and equity, policymakers must choose equitable pathways, such as by extending the same set of benefits to all segments of the population (rather than more benefits for formal sector workers or others who can pay into the system) and by prioritizing coverage and removing user fees for high-priority health services, based on such factors as prevalence and the needs of disadvantaged populations (WHO Consultative Group on Equity and Universal Health Coverage, 2014).

Social Determinants of Health Good health requires more than health care, and even more than the underlying determinants of health incorporated in the right to health. It also requires action on the social determinants of health, the wide-ranging factors spanning "the circumstances in which people are born, grow, live, work, and age"—such as education, employment, and the environment—and disparities rooted in "the inequitable distribution of power, money, and resources" (WHO, Commission on Social Determinants of Health, 2008, p. 2). The understanding of the importance of these social determinants of health has led to the **Health in All Policies** approach. This approach recognizes the potential for policies in all sectors to have a "a profound effect on population health and health equity," and subsequently insists that "public policies across sectors systematically takes into account the health implications of decisions, seeks synergies, and avoids harmful health impacts in order to improve population health and health equity" (WHO, 2013a).

The FCGH Focus on Governance

To better realize the right to health and enable everyone to enjoy the conditions required for good health, the FCGH would focus on four persisting problems of global governance for health: lack of accountability, insufficient funding, persisting social marginalization, and lack of coherence for health across sectors.

Accountability One challenge is lack of accountability. At the most fundamental level, if states do not do as they commit, then commitments to universal health coverage or human rights mean little. States often fail to meet health commitments, from health financing targets unmet to nondiscrimination and other right-to-health commitments unfulfilled. For example, African governments committed in 2001 to spend at least 15% of their budgets on the health sector, yet the vast majority fail to do so (Organisation of African Unity, 2001, para. 26; WHO 2015c). States impose travel and trade restrictions in the face of epidemics like Ebola, beyond those that can be justified by public health protection, violating governments' commitments under the **International Health Regulations (IHR)**, a WHO (2005) treaty protecting against the international spread of disease. People often have limited means to hold their governments accountable—that is, to force the state to explain its actions, acknowledge shortcomings, and take measures to redress them—and even fewer means to hold foundations and other nonstate actors to account. The lack of accountability extends to international organizations, such as the anemic UN response to the cholera outbreak in Haiti for which UN peacekeepers were responsible, or sexual violence by UN peacekeepers (Piarroux, 2016).

The FCGH could establish a global health accountability framework, covering states, international institutions, and nonstate actors such as foundations and even corporations, with such principles as transparency, monitoring and evaluation, and mechanisms for independent oversight and redress. This framework could feed into other accountability mechanisms, such as those developed by human rights treaties and UN human rights special rapporteurs. Meanwhile, at the national level, the FCGH could set standards for inclusive participation, to enable people, including the most marginalized, to participate in the policymaking process, from priority setting to monitoring and evaluation and determining appropriate corrective measures. National health accountability strategies could ensure that avenues of accountability and participation are established and funded from community to national levels, spanning all branches of government and national human rights institutions, and incorporating transparency, disaggregated data, and social empowerment (Friedman, 2016).

Financing A second health governance deficit is in financing. States cannot achieve universal coverage of conditions required for good health without adequate financing. Yet countries often do not meet their human rights obligation to spend the maximum of their available resources to address health and other economic, social, and cultural rights (ICESCR, 1966, art. 2). International assistance, meanwhile, is too little and may be driven by the priorities of funders rather than those of the people of the countries receiving the funds.

In response, the FCGH could establish a national and global health financing framework, for the first time creating clear national and global health financing standards, which would be sufficient to enable comprehensive health coverage and underlying determinants of health, such as clean water and adequate sanitation. The treaty could also include cooperative measures to help states unleash new funding, from improving tax collection and reducing corruption to establishing taxes on unhealthy foods and beverages. The FCGH could also commit countries to equitable funding, ensuring that those with the fewest resources benefit most from public finances.

Social Marginalization Even with sufficient financing at national and global levels, many people might not benefit due to persisting marginalization and discrimination, a third health governance area that the FCGH would help address. Today, populations are marginalized and precluded from the conditions required for health, due to a host of factors. One is simply poverty, preventing people from affording health services and medicines. People who are poor, along with other groups—women, indigenous people, sexual minorities, and people with disabilities, among others—may face discrimination and other mistreatment. Immigrants and certain minority populations may face language barriers. People with physical disabilities may be unable to access health facilities. Undocumented immigrants are frequently legally barred from the benefits of public health services altogether, while customary practices may prevent women from accessing necessary health services. Meanwhile, structural factors well beyond the health system, from polluting industrial sites located near impoverished communities to violence against transgender people, further undermine the health of vulnerable and oppressed populations.

The FCGH would aim to empower marginalized populations and set into motion inclusive policies and prioritized measures to meet their health-related needs. One approach could be national health equity strategies. At their core would be targeted and synergistic plans of action for health equality across the spectrum of marginalized populations, addressing the obstacles to health equality for each population and the policy reforms required to overcome those obstacles, backed by funding and disaggregated data, and ensuring a gendered approach to health and equitable pathways to universal health coverage. Critically, marginalized populations and civil society must be integral to the process of developing these strategies, which would also include analysis and policies to ensure the equitable distribution of resources (Friedman, 2015).

Lack of Coherence for Health across Sectors The best-functioning, fairest health sector will still be unable to fulfill people's right to health if measures taken outside the health sector undermine health policies and operations. Lax pollution regulations can contribute to respiratory, cardiovascular, and other illnesses. Overly protective patent regimes, including through treaty protections, may impede access to medicines. Regulations on narcotics control may severely limit access to morphine and other painkillers (Piana, 2014).

The FCGH could begin to redress this, including by clarifying the obligation of all sectors and of states, including in international agreements and their other actions with extraterritorial effects, to respect the right to health. One specific instrument could be **right to health impact assessments**. Much like environmental impact statements, these would analyze the likely effects of policies, programs, and projects across sectors and legal regimes that may significantly affect the right to health, so that they can be adjusted to prevent harms and maximize synergies with the right to health. People whose right to health may be affected would participate in conducting these assessments to ensure their accuracy and to build accountability into the assessment process (MacNaughton, 2015).

Precedents and Examples of Governance for Global Health

The Framework Convention on Tobacco Control

In 2015, over 1.1 billion people smoked tobacco (WHO, n.d., "Prevalence of Tobacco Smoking"). Although smoking rates have leveled off or declined during the last decades in developed nations, such as the United States and Australia, as tobacco consumption continues to rise in developing nations. More than 80% of all smokers now live in low- and middle-income countries, with prevalence continuing to increase in several regions, including Africa (WHO, n.d., "Prevalence of Tobacco Smoking"). Even in developed countries, the tobacco industry disproportionately targets the most vulnerable populations. Tobacco use is more prevalent among such populations, including racial minorities, people with mental health problems or substance and alcohol abuse, those involved in the criminal justice system, and those who are homeless.

The high rates of tobacco prevalence worldwide have devastating health consequences. Globally, tobacco kills nearly six million people a year and is responsible for one in 10 adult deaths. It has been estimated that if the current trend continues, tobacco use will kill approximately 8 million people per year, mostly in developing countries, by 2030 (Mathers & Loncar, 2006).

Yet tobacco use can largely be prevented. Experience in recent decades has shown that a range of tobacco control measures, such as comprehensive bans on smoking in public places, tobacco taxes, and limits on tobacco advertising, can greatly reduce smoking prevalence. Where implemented, these measures have slowly curtailed the epidemic, despite strong opposition from various sectors led by the tobacco industry.

The **Framework Convention on Tobacco Control (FCTC)** has been a powerful legal instrument to catalyze such measures. Adopted by the World Health Assembly in 2003, the FCTC gives countries the foundation and framework necessary to enact comprehensive, effective tobacco control measures that span all sectors of government. In the words of WHO, "the FCTC is an evidence-based treaty that reaffirms the right of all people to the highest standard of health." To this end, the treaty's provisions include rules that govern smoke-free spaces and the production, sale, distribution, advertisement, labeling, and taxation of tobacco, among others. By ratifying the FCTC, states recognize that the tobacco epidemic is a major public health threat and that the FCTC provides the minimum standards to protect public health.

The FCTC entered into force in 2005. In the decade since, the number of parties has risen to 180 (179 states plus the European Union), covering more than 90% of the world's population and making it one of the most successful and rapidly embraced treaties in history. The FCTC represents a unique breakthrough in global health. Not only was it the first WHO treaty of its kind, but it also marks one of the first multilateral, binding agreements regarding NCDs.

Regardless of whether states have ratified the FCTC, the instrument serves as an international legal standard for interpreting right-to-health obligations regarding the tobacco epidemic. Given the burden of tobacco-related diseases, states have an obligation to intervene to protect the right to health of their citizens regardless of whether they have ratified the FCTC. Moreover, some courts have gone so far as to declare the FCTC a human rights treaty, as it explicitly and directly seeks to protect the right to health.

The process leading to FCTC implementation at the national level has pushed governments and public health groups to better understand the role that law, including tobacco control litigation, can play in protecting the right to health. Because the FCTC provides a minimum standard for domestic tobacco control policies, courts faced with tobacco control litigation can use this treaty to legitimize and guide determinations that would substantively affect national policies. The potential of tobacco control litigation is epitomized by a 2001 case in India where that country's Supreme Court banned smoking in public places throughout the country, including schools, libraries, railway waiting rooms, and public transport, citing the right to health and to life.

Much of the more recent tobacco control litigation comes from Latin America and is based on FCTC standards, which, by providing a legal standard and supported by scientific evidence, defines concrete measures states should take to address the tobacco epidemic, highlighting the importance of substantive international standards in fulfilling the right to health. For example, in 2010, the Constitutional Court of Colombia ruled on the constitutionality of a tobacco control law that, among other policies, prohibited all forms of tobacco advertising. The court stated that this prohibition "is a measure suitable for accomplishing the constitutionally-binding purpose of the State of guaranteeing the health of the inhabitants and the environment ... in this case by discouraging the consumption of tobacco products."

The FCTC is the most salient example of the use of international law to prevent NCDs. Nonbinding legal instruments, including WHO's Global Action Plan for the Prevention and Control of Noncommunicable Diseases (WHO, 2013b) and Global Strategy to Reduce the Harmful Use of Alcohol (WHO, 2010a), provide normative guidance, which can also help reduce NCD risk factors. At the national level, law is an essential tool to address NCDs as part of comprehensive and integrated approaches that also include public education and quality health care. For example, bans on sales of alcohol and tobacco products to minors and taxes on unhealthy products require implementation through law. Laws can also be used to provide access to and ensure affordability of healthier food and beverage options and to promote physical activity through active transport and physical education.

The Convention on the Rights of Persons with Disabilities

People living with mental illness and cognitive or physical disabilities are some of the world's most marginalized. They are often institutionalized, isolated from society and the opportunity to participate in it, and subject to physical and sexual abuse and neglect rather than care and treatment. Extremely inhumane care has been documented in some cases; for example, patients have been put into cages, constrained with duct tape, left in their own excrement, and chained to trees (Abbott et al., 2015; Carey, 2015).

Seeking to change this and reframe global understanding is the **Convention on the Rights of Persons with Disabilities**, a 2006 treaty that took effect in 2008. The convention recognizes that disability is an evolving concept and defines **persons with disabilities** to include "those who have long-term physical, mental, intellectual or sensory impairments which in interaction with various barriers may hinder their full and effective participation in society on an equal basis with others" (Convention on the Protection and Promotion of the Rights and Dignity of Persons with Disabilities, 2006).

The Convention would prohibit all forms of discrimination against people with disabilities; guarantee rights ranging from the rights to health, education, and work to freedom from exploitation, violence, and abuse; support their full inclusion and participation in society; and provide a right to live in the community and have their legal capacity recognized on an equal basis in relation to others.

Alongside these policy efforts for all people with disabilities is a growing international commitment to meeting the health needs of one important subgroup, people with mental illnesses. In 2013, WHO adopted a Mental Health Action Plan (WHO, 2013c). The stakes could hardly be higher, considering that according to one estimate, one in four people will experience a mental disorder at some point in their lives (WHO, 2001). Mental disorders, including substance abuse, collectively account for more years lived with a disability than any other set of health conditions (Baxter et al., 2013). As people live longer, the number of people experiencing dementia, with its enormous human and economic toll, soars. Unlike other major mental illnesses, including depression, bipolar disorder, and schizophrenia, effective treatments for dementia have yet to be developed.

Emerging Infectious Diseases

Globalization has linked different corners of the world in ways never imaginable—individuals can travel from one end of the world to another in a matter of hours, information can be disseminated in seconds across the globe, and products that were once available in only certain parts of the world can now be easily found in others or via online retailers. However, globalization has also brought with it new challenges, such as the (re)emergence and rapid spread of infectious diseases like the flu, Ebola, and Zika.

Diseases know no boundaries, and with increased travel and trade among countries, more recent infectious disease outbreaks have challenged our ability to prevent and even control them. Over the past two decades, we have observed a rise in the number of these public health crises. The Severe Acute Respiratory Syndrome (SARS) outbreak between 2002 and 2003 killed close to 800 people and infected more than 8,000 within the span of eight months (Centers for Disease Control and Prevention [CDC], 2012). The 2009 Influenza A (H1N1) virus rapidly traveled across the globe, killing approximately 576,000 people worldwide within a single year (Cheng et al., 2012). More recently, the 2014 Ebola virus outbreak in West Africa infected close to 30,000 people, more than 11,000 of whom died (CDC, 2016a). Currently, the Zika virus epidemic in the Americas, though not deadly in itself, has caused an increased number of infants born with severe birth defects that can lead to premature death as well as lifelong complications, including seizures, developmental delay, intellectual disability, problems with movement and balance, feeding problems, hearing loss, and vision problems (Gostin & Lucey, 2016; CDC, 2016b).

When it comes to addressing these challenges in a sustainable manner, law can play an important role. WHO's International Health Regulations (IHR) (WHO, 2005) have been designed to create a global network of disease surveillance and response led by WHO with the aim of preventing large-scale public health emergencies. The IHR legally bind 196 countries to build their capacity to monitor and respond to infectious disease outbreaks, as well as communicate effectively with WHO on public health threats that have the potential of becoming "public health emergencies of international concern" (PHEICs). A PHEIC is defined in article 1 as "an extraordinary event which is determined … (i) to constitute a public health risk to other States through the international spread of disease and (ii) to potentially require a coordinated response."

The IHR are critical tools for triggering international action when a PHEIC is declared. PHEIC declarations are issued in exceptional cases, and the decision to do so falls with WHO's director-general, who consults with an emergency committee of experts in making the determination.

Infectious disease outbreaks pose a substantial threat to the health of populations across the world and to the economic well-being of countries, particularly those with weak health systems, as Ebola so devastatingly demonstrated. Once again, the poorest are most vulnerable. Reducing this threat requires a reliable global infrastructure for preventing the spread of infectious diseases before they become large epidemics or pandemics—and, to the extent possible, preventing their emergence.

Chapter Summary

As this brief survey of global health today demonstrates, despite the progress in global health, immense challenges remain, especially that of bringing health justice to the most marginalized among us. The world has forged a consensus around the right to health, yet too often, the commitment is in name only. More effective rights-based rules of the road are needed, with strong accountability. The use of legal approaches, such as the FCGH and international health regulations, can provide the foundation for effective global governance for health and realization of health rights. These approaches build on human rights covenants and complement efforts related to the Sustainable Development Goals.

Key Terms

Convention on the Rights of Persons with Disabilities (CRPD)
Framework Convention on Global Health (FCGH)
Health in All Policies
International Covenant on Economic, Social and Cultural Rights (ICESCR)
International Health Regulations (IHR)
Persons with disabilities
Right to health
Right to health impact assessment

Review Questions

1. What is the right to health? How has the concept developed over time?
2. What are some of the shortcomings of national and global governance? How could the FCGH begin to address them?
3. What is the Framework Convention on Tobacco Control? How does it contribute to reductions in smoking? What implications does this have for other global health challenges?
4. What are the International Health Regulations, and how can they prevent the spread of disease and positively impact global health?

Suggested Reading

Eric A. Friedman and Lawrence O. Gostin, "Imagining Global Health with Justice: In Defense of the Right to Health," *Health Care Analysis* 23, no. 4 (December 2015): 308–329. http://link. springer.com/article/10.1007/s10728-015-0307-x

Lawrence O. Gostin, "Global Health Narratives" (pp. 1–9) and "Global Health Justice" (pp. 13–31) in *Global Health Law* (Cambridge, MA: Harvard University Press, 2014).

References

Abbott, M., Ahern, L., Boychuk, C., Guerrero, H., Rodriguez, P., & Rosenthal, E. (2015, July 22). *No justice: Torture, trafficking and segregation in Mexico.* Disability Rights International. Retrieved from http://www.driadvocacy.org/wp-content/uploads/Sin-Justicia-MexRep_21_Abr_english-1.pdf

Baxter, A. J., Degenhardt, L., Erskine, H. E., Ferrari, A. J., Rehm, J., Whiteford, H. A., . . . Vos, T. (2013). Global burden of disease attributable to mental and substance use disorders: Findings from the Global Burden of Disease Study 2010. *The Lancet, 382,* 1575–1586. doi:10.1016/S0140-6736(13)61611-6

Carey, B. (2015, October 12). The chains of mental illness across West Africa. *New York Times*, p. A1.

Centers for Disease Control and Prevention. (2012). SARS basics factsheet. Retrieved from http://www.cdc.gov/sars/about/fs-sars.html

Centers for Disease Control and Prevention. (2016a). 2014 Ebola outbreak in West Africa—Case counts as of April 13, 2016. Retrieved from https://www.cdc.gov/vhf/ebola/outbreaks/2014 -west-africa/case-counts.html

Centers for Disease Control and Prevention. (2016b). Facts about microcephaly. Retrieved from http://www.cdc.gov/ncbddd/birthdefects/microcephaly.html

Cheng, P., Dawood, F. S., Iuliano, A. D., Meltzer, M. I., Reed, C., Shay, D. K., . . . Widdowson, M. (2012). Estimated global mortality associated with the first 12 months of 2009 pandemic influenza A H1N1 virus circulation: A modelling study. *Lancet Infectious Diseases, 12,* 687–695. doi:10.1016/S1473-3099(12)70121-4

Committee on Economic, Social and Cultural Rights. (2000, August). *General comment 14, the right to the highest attainable standard of health,* U.N. Doc. E/C.12/2000/4. Report on the 22nd session, April 25–May 12, 2000. Retrieved from http://hrlibrary.umn.edu/gencomm/escgencom14.htm

Constitutional Court of Colombia. (2010, October 20). Case C-830/10. Retrieved from http://www.globalhealthrights.org/wp-content/uploads/2013/08/C-830-10-Colombia-2010.pdf

Convention on the Protection and Promotion of the Rights and Dignity of Persons with Disabilities, G.A. Res. 61/106, U.N. Doc. A/RES/61/106. (2006). Retrieved from http://hrlibrary.umn.edu/instree/disability-convention2006.html

Friedman, E. A. (2015, October 5). SDG series: National health equity strategies to implement the global promise of SDGs [Web blog post]. Retrieved from https://www.hhrjournal.org/2015/10/sdg-series-national-health-equity-strategies-to-implement-the-global-promise -of-sdgs/

Friedman, E. A. (2016). An independent review and accountability mechanism for the Sustainable Development Goals: The possibilities of a framework convention on global health. *Health and Human Rights Journal, 18*(1), 129–140. Retrieved from https://www.hhrjournal.org/2016/01/an-independent-review-and-accountability-mechanism-for-the-sustainable -development-goals-the-possibilities-of-a-framework-convention-on-global-health/

Garay, J. (2015). *Health equity: The key to transformational change.* Retrieved from http://isags-unasur.org/uploads/biblioteca/6/bb[245]ling[3]anx[757].pdf

Gostin, L. O. (2008). Meeting basic survival needs of the world's least healthy people: Toward a framework convention on global health. *Georgetown Law Journal, 96,* 331–392. Retrieved from http://georgetownlawjournal.org/files/pdf/96-2/Gostin-Article.PDF

Gostin, L. O., & Lucey, D. R. (2016). The emerging Zika pandemic: Enhancing preparedness. *Journal of the American Medical Association, 315,* 865–866. doi:10.1001/jama.2016.0904

Heymann, J., Cassola, A., Raub, A., & Mishra, L. (2013). Constitutional rights to health, public health and medical care: The status of health protections in 191 countries. *Global Public Health, 8,* 639–653.

International Conference on Primary Health Care. (1978, September). *Declaration of Alma-Alta (1978).* Retrieved from http://www.who.int/publications/almaata_declaration_en.pdf

International Covenant on Economic, Social and Cultural Rights, G.A. Res. 2200A (XXI), U.N . Doc. A/6316. (1966).

MacNaughton, G. (2015, June 11). Human rights impact assessment: A method for healthy policymaking. *Health and Human Rights, 17*(1), 63–75. Retrieved from https://www.hhrjournal.org/2015/04/human-rights-impact-assessment-a-method-for-healthy-policymaking/

Mathers, C. D., & Loncar, D. (2006). Projections of global mortality and burden of disease from 2002 to 2030. *PLoS Medicine, 3*(11). doi:10.1371/journal.pmed.0030442

Organisation of African Unity. (2001, April 17). *Abuja Declaration on HIV/AIDS, Tuberculosis and Other Related Infectious Diseases.* OAU/SPS/ABUJA/3. Retrieved from http://www.un.org/ga/aids/pdf/abuja_declaration.pdf

Piana, R. (2014, October 1). Dying without morphine. *New York Times,* p. A27.

Piarroux, R. (2016, October 8). The U.N.'s responsibility in Haiti's cholera crisis. *New York Times,* p. A8.

UNAIDS. (2015). UNAIDS announces that the goal of 15 million people on life-saving HIV treatment by 2015 has been met nine months ahead of schedule [Press release]. Retrieved from http://www.unaids.org/en/resources/presscentre/pressreleaseandstatementarchive/2015/july/20150714_PR_MDG6report

United Nations. (2012, December 12). *Global health and foreign policy. General Assembly Resolution 67/81.* Retrieved from undocs.org/A/RES/67/81

United Nations. (2015a). *The Millennium Development Goals report 2015.* Retrieved from http://www.un.org/millenniumgoals/2015_MDG_Report/pdf/MDG%202015%20rev%20%28July%201%29.pdf

United Nations. (2015b, September 25). *Transforming our world: The 2030 agenda for sustainable development. General Assembly Resolution 70/1.* Retrieved from undocs.org/A/RES/70/1

Vincent, A. R. (2015, August 13). State of emergency continues for trans women of color [Web blog post]. Retrieved from http://www.huffingtonpost.com/addison-rose-vincent/the-state-of-emergency-co_b_7981580.html

WHO Consultative Group on Equity and Universal Health Coverage. (2014). *Making fair choices on the path to universal health coverage: Final report of the WHO Consultative Group on Equity and Universal Health Coverage.* Retrieved from http://apps.who.int/iris/bitstream/10665/112671/1/9789241507158_eng.pdf?ua=1

World Health Assembly. (2005, May). *Sustainable health financing, universal coverage and social health insurance. WHA 58.33.*

World Health Organization. (n.d.). Global Health Observatory (GHO) data: Life expectancy. Retrieved from http://www.who.int/gho/mortality_burden_disease/life_tables/situation_trends_text/en/

World Health Organization. (n.d.). Global Health Observatory (GHO) data: Malaria. Retrieved from http://www.who.int/gho/malaria/en/

World Health Organization. (n.d.). Global Health Observatory (GHO) data: Prevalence of tobacco smoking. Retrieved from http://www.who.int/gho/tobacco/use/en/

World Health Organization. (2001). World health report: Mental disorders affect one in four people [Press release]. Retrieved from http://www.who.int/whr/2001/media_centre/press_release/en/

World Health Organization. (2004). *WHO framework convention on tobacco control.* Retrieved from http://apps.who.int/iris/bitstream/10665/42811/1/9241591013.pdf

World Health Organization. (2005). *International health regulations.* Retrieved from http://whqlibdoc.who.int/publications/2008/9789241580410_eng.pdf

World Health Organization. (2008). *The world health report 2008—Primary health care (now more than ever).* Retrieved from http://www.who.int/whr/2008/en/

World Health Organization. (2010a). *Global strategy to reduce the harmful use of alcohol 2010.* Retrieved from http://www.who.int/substance_abuse/msbalcstragegy.pdf

World Health Organization. (2010b). *The world health report: Health systems financing: The path to universal coverage.* http://www.who.int/whr/2010/en/

World Health Organization (2013a, June 10–14). *The Helsinki statement on health in all policies.* 8th Global Conference on Health Promotion. Retrieved from http://www.who.int/health promotion/conferences/8gchp/statement_2013/en/

World Health Organization. (2013b). *WHO global action plan for the prevention and control of noncommunicable diseases 2013–2020.* Retrieved from http://apps.who.int/iris/bitstr eam/10665/94384/1/9789241506236_eng.pdf?ua=1

World Health Organization. (2013c). *Mental health action plan 2013–2020.* Retrieved from http://www.who.int/mental_health/action_plan_2013/en/

World Health Organization. (2015a). *Global tuberculosis report 2015.* Retrieved from http://apps.who.int/iris/bitstream/10665/191102/1/9789241565059_eng.pdf

World Health Organization. (2015b). Maternal deaths fell 44% since 1990—UN [Press release]. Retrieved from http://www.who.int/mediacentre/news/releases/2015/maternal-mortality/en/

World Health Organization. (2015c). *World health statistics 2015, part II: Global health indicators.* Retrieved from http://who.int/gho/publications/world_health_statistics/EN_WHS2015_Part2.pdf?ua=1

World Health Organization, Commission on Social Determinants of Health. (2008). *Closing the gap in a generation: Health equity through action on the social determinants of health.* Retrieved from http://apps.who.int/iris/bitstream/10665/43943/1/9789241563703_eng.pdf

CHAPTER 7

GLOBAL MENTAL HEALTH, BEHAVIORAL MEDICINE, AND WELLNESS

Giuseppe Raviola, MD, MPH

The arc of the moral universe is long, but it bends towards justice.
—Dr. Martin Luther King Jr.

LEARNING OBJECTIVES

- Discover the relevance of global mental health, behavioral medicine, and wellness to global health
- Understand the burden of illness and the global treatment gap of mental disorders
- Understand challenges and gaps in national policies, governance, and global systems of care for mental disorders
- Learn about innovative strategies for service delivery and program design of mental health services in low-resource settings
- Understand the components of sustained systems to inform the development of safe, cost-effective, and culturally sound approaches to mental and behavioral health integration
- Appreciate the burdens on health care providers and program implementers in global health with regard to personal wellness
- Consider careers in global health that span service delivery and bidirectional training, program management and design, implementation science and research, and staff wellness.

If global health is a set of interdisciplinary collaborations, transactions, and processes encompassing prevention, treatment, and care, emphasizing principles of promotion of social and economic rights and equitable access to services, and also including the organized social response to health conditions at the global level (the

Foundations for Global Health Practice, First Edition. Lori DiPrete Brown.
© 2018 John Wiley & Sons, Inc. Published 2018 by John Wiley & Sons, Inc.

global health system) and the way in which the system is managed (**governance**), then global mental health offers a fascinating opportunity to learn about how these systems function in the attempt to close the significant ongoing gap in global health care (Koplan, Bond, & Merson, 2009; Frenk & Moon, 2013). Notwithstanding optimism about major advancements in global health financing systems and in delivery for HIV and tuberculosis, as well as more recent developments supporting the non-communicable disease (NCD) agenda, parallel goals for scaling up of mental health services for the world's poorest populations present unique challenges, both conceptual and pragmatic.

Global mental health, behavioral medicine, and wellness comprise a range of endeavors focused on the integration of empathic, safe, evidence-based, culturally sound, well-organized, and efficient approaches to care of mental disorders and stress-related conditions, for patients, providers, and program implementers, living and operating in the context of global health. It also comprises preventive approaches to development and health that touch on mental health—for example, encompassing the function of healthy early child development and, by extension, brain development as a foundation for sustainable development broadly (Daelmans et al., 2017). Global mental health challenges include gaps in policy, funding, and treatment, with a need for new models of care; for these reasons, global mental health is a growing area of interest and focus in global health.

Defining Global Mental Health, Behavioral Medicine, and Wellness

As noted in 1954 by the first director-general of the World Health Organization (WHO), Dr. Brock Chisholm, "Without mental health, there can be no true physical health." Yet the definition of what encompasses "mental health" is itself complex. According to WHO (2014), "mental health is a state of well-being in which every individual realizes his or her own potential, can cope with the normal stresses of life, can work productively and fruitfully, and is able to make a contribution to her or his community." **Global mental health** refers to the international perspective on different aspects of the resource-constrained arena of global health, informed by the protection of the human rights of those living with mental illness (Patel & Prince, 2010). It has been described as the area of study, research, and practice that places a priority on improving mental health and achieving equity in mental health for all people worldwide (Patel & Prince, 2010). **Behavioral medicine** describes an interdisciplinary field that aims to integrate biological and psychosocial perspectives on human behavior and to apply them to the practice of medicine (Feldman & Christensen, 2014). **Wellness** refers to the notion of health as a state of complete physical, mental, and social well-being and not merely the absence of disease or infirmity (WHO, 2014). The scope and lack of clear definition of these terms as a cohesive whole, as well as the fact that they span public health and medicine, and preventive and clinical approaches, have contributed to their remaining a particularly unaddressed area of global health.

This gap has been widened by the fact that the primary measure of the burden of mental disorders is disability (embodied by the DALY, or Disability-Adjusted Life Year metric), rather than mortality (although mental disorders also incur significant mortality). Large, impressive, and sustained gains are being made against the majority of leading causes of death in most countries, but these gains are not being accompanied by commensurate declines in rates of disability, especially from major musculoskeletal disorders, mental and substance use disorders, neurological disorders, and diabetes (GBD 2013 DALYs and HALE Collaborators, 2015). Although the disability metric has had greater difficulty in terms of solidifying the political will necessary to effectively argue for the need, there is increasing expert consensus on the usefulness of disability metrics to define health. Significant and universal gaps therefore exist in how these concerns are integrated within health systems and institutions globally, in low-, middle-, and high-income countries.

The current experience of the global mental health movement bears similarities to that of the HIV/AIDS movement 30 years ago, with regard to the effects of stigma, fear, and denial about the biological underpinnings of certain mental disorders, and the pervasive impacts of mental disorders and stress-related problems. **Stigma** refers to an attribute that is deeply discrediting, often informed by false information, which promotes fear and misunderstanding about the experience of those living with a condition such as mental illness (Goffman, 1963; Centers for Disease Control and Prevention, 2015). A review of global mental health, behavioral medicine, and wellness therefore provides a new opportunity to closely examine core challenges in global health, with regard to burden of illness, vulnerability of populations, the importance of culture and context, priority-setting and governance, opportunities to strengthen health systems, exciting and innovative models of service delivery and program design, and challenges to sustainable career development.

This chapter refers primarily to priority mental disorders, the treatment of which can guide the setting of basic standards of care in low-resource settings. These include depression and stress-related anxiety (common mental disorders), disorders caused by psychosis (severe mental disorders), and epilepsy (a highly treatable and common neurological condition). The term **psychosis** refers to a symptom of mental illness in which thinking and functioning are so impaired that contact with external reality is lost (National Institute of Mental Health [NIMH], 2016b). It can include hallucinations and delusions, and is generally a biological phenomenon with complex genetic causes. The term **depression** refers to a state of sustained feeling of low mood, sadness, and hopelessness that causes a significant decrease in functioning (NIMH, 2016a). There are other critical areas of concern that incur significant disability and for which there is also strong scientific evidence with regard to effective intervention. These include, among others, child development and mental health, adolescent mental health, disability- and development-related problems, alcohol and substance abuse, and domestic violence. All of these have significant implications for global health, mental and behavioral health, and wellness.

Burden of Illness and the Treatment Gap: The Need for Integration

Broadly speaking, mental disorders present a significant burden of illness, and are left largely unaddressed. The treatment gap for people with mental disorders exceeds 50% in all countries of the world (Kohn, Saxena, Levav, & Saraceno, 2004). Although 80% of the world's population live in low- and middle-income countries (LMICs), more than 90% of mental health resources are located in high-income countries (Saxena, Thornicroft, Knapp, & Whiteford, 2007; WHO, 2005). It is estimated that in LMICs, between 76 and 85% of people with severe mental disorders receive no treatment for their mental health conditions (Demyttenaere, Bruffaerts, & Posada-Villa, 2004). Recent estimates suggest that the disease burden of mental illness accounts for approximately 32% of years lived with disability (YLDs) and 13% of DALYs (Vigo, Thornicroft, & Atun, 2016). Mental disorders therefore impose a very significant burden on societies, accounting for almost one in three years lived with disability globally. Depression is the most common mental disorder and the leading cause of disability worldwide. Globally, an estimated 350 million people of all ages suffer from depression, more women being affected than men. At its worst, depression can lead to suicide, with almost one million people per year committing suicide globally; however, there are effective treatments for depression, as well as other mental disorders, and many of these deaths are preventable (WHO, 2016a).

Despite this significant burden of illness caused by mental disorders (psychiatric and neurological), including major depression, anxiety disorders, drug and alcohol use disorders, severe mental disorders such as schizophrenia and bipolar disorder, chronic pain syndrome, self-harm, epilepsy, dementias, and various forms of headache—approximately 15% of the total global burden of disability—governments in LMICs tend to spend less than 1 to 2% of their budgets on mental health, often on restrictive, locked psychiatric facilities that threaten human rights (Vigo et al., 2016; DeSilva, Samele, Saxena, Patel, & Darzi, 2014). A range of problems contribute to the lack of access to safe, effective, evidence-based, and culturally attuned mental health services (see Box 7.1).

Mental disorders also cause a significant economic burden due to lost economic output and the link between mental disorders and costly, potentially fatal conditions including cancer, cardiovascular disease, diabetes, HIV, and obesity. Mental disorders

BOX 7.1

REASONS FOR THE MENTAL HEALTH TREATMENT GAP

- Ministry of health budgets are inadequate.

- Locked hospitals promote stigma, fear, and poor quality care.

- Geographical distance for those living in rural or remote areas limits access.

- For people living with illness and their families, the emotional costs of seeking care can be too high.

- There is a dearth of proven, effective, and sustained community-based care models that can be readily adapted across contexts.

- Families are often unable to pay for medications, and psychiatric medications are frequently excluded from payment plans.

- Few specialists are trained in provision of quality care practices.

- Specialist and nonspecialist health care providers can be afraid of people living with mental illness—stigma is embedded within health systems.

- Adaptation of evidence-based tools to context requires specific technical knowledge and expertise that may not be available.

are incurring greater and greater costs to societies, more than any other NCD, including heart disease; the cost of mental health conditions in 2010 was estimated at $2.5 trillion, with the cost projected to rise to $6 trillion by 2030 (Bloom et al., 2011). However, we now know that in terms of health impact, scaled-up treatments can lead to significant increases in healthy life, as well as a 3:1 economic benefit/cost ratio in terms of return on investment (Chisholm et al., 2016).

We also now have evidence that integration of mental health services into services for other global health priority conditions can have very significant impacts on various health indicators (see Table 7.1). This argument is strengthened by our understanding of the complex mechanisms of comorbidity of mental disorders with NCDs such as cardiovascular, lung, and liver diseases, diabetes, and cancer. There are genetic, environmental (e.g., childhood adversity, stressful life events), toxic (e.g., tobacco or alcohol use), lifestyle (e.g., lack of physical activity), behavioral (e.g., adherence), and structural (e.g., lack of adequate insurance systems or access to care) contributors to comorbid illness (Patel & Chatterji, 2015). In addition, there is a very significant lack of trained specialists in LMICs, to the point that care must be delivered by nonspecialists in most global contexts (Kakuma et al., 2011). Today, nonspecialist providers deliver more than 90% of mental health services worldwide (Jakob & Patel, 2014).

Table 7.1 Evidence for Positive Impacts of Integrated Mental Health Care with Major Global Health Priorities

Global Health Concern	Examples of Evidence	References
Prevention of *maternal deaths in childbirth*	The prevalence and severity of antenatal anxiety and depression may be higher in LMICs than in developed countries.[1] Depressive symptoms in mothers are associated with preeclampsia, preterm birth, intrauterine growth retardation, and low birth weight in infants.[2] However, interpersonal psychotherapy was associated with a reduction in or recovery from depressive symptomatology in a US-based study of outpatient pregnant women meeting *DSM-IV* criteria for major depressive disorder.[3]	1. Verbeek T, et al. Anxiety and depression during pregnancy in Central America: a cross-sectional study among pregnant women in the developing country Nicaragua. *BMC Psychiatry.* 2015; 15(1):292. 2. Kim DR, et al. Elevated risk of adverse obstetric outcomes in pregnant women with depression. *Archives of Women's Mental Health.* 2013; 16(6): 475–482. 3. Spinelli MG, Endicott J. Controlled clinical trial of interpersonal psychotherapy versus parenting education program for depressed pregnant women. *American Journal of Psychiatry.* 2003; 160(3):555–62.
Transmission of *HIV from mother to child*	Psychiatric diagnoses are more common in HIV patient groups than in other populations and are associated with poor antiretroviral treatment (ART) adherence.[1,2] However, antidepressant treatment for depressed HIV patients is associated with an improvement in ART adherence.[2] A review of randomized controlled trials found evidence that psychological interventions for HIV-positive people can lead to improved immune status.[3]	1. Gaynes BN, et al. Prevalence and comorbidity of psychiatric diagnoses based on reference standard in an HIV+ patient population. *Psychosomatic Medicine.* 2008; 70:505–511. 2. Kumar V, Encinosa W. Effects of antidepressant treatment on antiretroviral regimen adherence among depressed HIV-infected patients. *Psychiatric Quarterly.* 2009; 80:131–141. 3. Carrico A, Antoni M. Effects of psychological interventions on neuroendocrine hormone regulation and immune status in HIV-positive persons: A review of randomized controlled trials. *Psychosomatic Medicine.* 2008; 70(5): 575–584.

Global Health Concern	Examples of Evidence	References
Deaths from *under-five malnutrition*	WHO considers exclusive breastfeeding one of the safest and most effective interventions to reduce infant morbidity and mortality. However, mothers with high levels of psychological distress exclusively breastfeed for a shorter duration.[1] A cognitive behavioral counseling intervention delivered in a study in rural Pakistan prolonged the duration of exclusive breastfeeding in mothers receiving the intervention, with double the rate of exclusive breastfeeding as compared to the control group at six months.[2]	1. Wachs TD, et al. Maternal depression: A global threat to children's health. development, and behavior and to human rights. *Child Development Perspectives.* 2009; 3(1):51–59. 2. Sikander S, et al. Cognitive-behavioral counseling for exclusive breastfeeding in rural pediatrics: A cluster RCT. *Pediatrics.* 2015; 135(2): e424–e431.
Deaths from *tuberculosis*	Mental health comorbidities can be a barrier to patient adherence to TB treatment.[1] WHO recommends therapeutic relationships and mutual goal-setting as interventions to reduce psychological stress and improve TB treatment adherence.[2]	1. Pachi A, et al. Psychiatric morbidity and other factors affecting treatment adherence in pulmonary tuberculosis patients. *Tuberculosis Research and Treatment.* 2013; 2013. doi:10.1155/2013/489865 2. World Health Organization. Adherence to long-term therapies: Evidence for action. 2003. http://apps.who.int/ medicinedocs/pdf/s4883e/ s4883e.pdf

Note: Four global health concerns based on Partners In Health Four Zeros Strategic Plan; analysis and references compiled by Alexandra Rose, MSc GMH.

Gaps in Governance, Policies, and Financing: The Need for Systems

Over the past decade, there has been significant progress in thinking about **basic treatment packages** for common mental health conditions, referring to evidence-based bundles of interventions that have been tested in context through the mobilization of nonspecialists. Despite these advances, there has only recently begun to be an increasing commitment by funders in global health and by ministries of health to committing resources to the scaling up of such services. Governance challenges for mental health have included power and resource imbalances between actors, information flows and barriers, poor coordination, and poor shared issue framing. The use of power in global governance around mental health has been limited to building a research knowledge base, making ethical arguments, and displaying expertise.

In seeking to impact public policy, former US Surgeon General Dr. Julius Richmond (Richmond & Kotelchuk, 1983) described three key elements: the analysis and development of a *scientific knowledge base*; the analysis and development of a *social strategy*; and the analysis and development of *political will*. The three must work together if we are to develop and implement public policy. Frenk and Moon (2013) have described good governance among a diverse group of actors operating in the area of global health as related in large part to the demonstration of effectiveness with efficient achievement of demonstrable outcomes, demonstration of credibility and legitimacy in decision-making processes, and attention to equity. Taken together, these concepts are instructive in an analysis of any major global health concern, including mental health, as is an inventory of the global policy landscape. In global mental health, the main actors over the past decade have included the following:

National governments. Governments are ultimately responsible for the development of mental health services, and have generally limited the financial and human resource commitments they have made to management and implementation of such services. Barriers in some contexts have included stigma within political systems, lack of adequate or updated legal protections or parity for people living with mental disorders, lack of expertise and basic knowledge in program design and implementation, and lack of political will across ministries, including finance, to build mental health systems.

The United Nations (UN), WHO, and other UN agencies. The mention of mental health promotion in the 2016 UN Sustainable Development Goals (SDG 3, to ensure healthy lives and promote well-being for all at all ages) has been an important development for raising attention to global mental health (United Nations [UN], 2015). Over the past several decades, WHO has developed norms and standards through technical advice on the establishment of mental health systems, provided a platform for coordination and coherence around key areas, provided scientific advice and guidelines for an evidence base in such areas as essential medicines and care pathways, produced statistical data and global oversight, and offered expertise in coordination of emergency relief (WHO, 2003, 2009). Challenges in governance have included weak accountability mechanisms with national ministries of health around adequate resource allocation to mental health, poor coordination among various actors in the context of disasters and emergencies, and lack of shared global consensus on evidence-based practices that can be adapted to context. In 2007, the WHO-collaborating Interagency Standing Committee (IASC) released Guidelines on Mental Health and Psychosocial

Support in Emergency Settings, to inform improved coordination among actors in the context of disasters and humanitarian response (IASC, 2007). In 2011, WHO released a much-anticipated mental health intervention guide called mhGAP for mental, neurological, and substance use disorders for nonspecialist health settings, a significant innovation that was updated in 2016 (WHO, 2016b). WHO and other actors have also promoted the use of Psychological First Aid, a set of skills for supportive, practical, and human rights–based help to fellow human beings suffering serious crisis events (WHO, War Trauma Foundation, and World Vision International, 2011; Brymer et al., 2006). Additional evidence-based packages offered by WHO include mhGAP-IG (clinical management of mental, neurologic, and substance use disorders in humanitarian emergencies), Problem Management Plus (individual psychological help for adults impaired by distress in communities exposed to adversity), and *Thinking Healthy* (a manual for psychosocial management of perinatal depression).

Advocacy organizations and platforms.   In the arena of global mental health, organizations such as the Movement for Global Mental Health and the World Federation for Mental Health have led coalitions embracing collective action to scale up services for mental disorders (Patel et al., 2011). Disability-oriented organizations have also taken a human rights–based approach informed by the UN Convention on the Rights of Persons with Disabilities (2006). A range of perspectives exist about the degree to which all persons have legal capacity for decision making depending on mental status, the defensibility of involuntary hospitalization and treatment, substitute decision making, and diversion from the criminal justice system (Freeman et al., 2015). Various additional organizations are engaged globally in advocacy for psychosocial and mental health needs of vulnerable groups, and protection of human rights for various populations. The Mental Health and Psychosocial Support (MHPSS) Network (http://mhpss.net) is a global platform for connecting people, networks, and organizations for sharing resources and for building knowledge related to mental health and psychosocial support both in emergency settings and in situations of chronic hardship. The World Psychiatric Association (http://www.wpanet.org) has served as a docking point for collaborations and knowledge sharing across global psychiatry. New initiatives such as the Mental Health Innovation Network (http://www.mhinnovation.net), in collaboration with Grand Challenges Canada, are creating platforms for information sharing with regard to effective models of practice, implementation, and scale-up.

International nongovernmental organizations (NGOs).   NGOs such as Basic Needs, Doctors without Borders, Healthnet TPO, International Medical Corps, Partners In Health, and Sangath in India have taken an increasingly important role in advancing services, science, and advocacy around mental health in postdisaster or postconflict situations and in low-resource settings.

Development innovation funds.   In 2008, the government of Canada announced the creation of a development innovation fund called Grand Challenges Canada, to support the search for "breakthroughs in global health and other areas that have the potential to bring about enduring changes in the lives of the millions of people in poor countries" (Grand Challenges Canada, 2011).

Academic institutions, experts (academic, scientific).   In the United States in 2010, the National Institutes of Health opened an Office on Research on Disparities and Global Mental Health, a promising development for research in global mental health. Universities such as Columbia University (US), University of Glasgow (UK), Harvard Medical School (US), Johns Hopkins (US), and London School of Hygiene and Tropical Medicine have developed various training programs in global mental health spanning undergraduate and graduate levels. Mixed qualitative and quantitative research methods have contributed to our understanding of how to develop interventions more appropriate to local conceptions of mental health and illness. There is an awareness of the need for greater evidence around intervention models, with new funding sources emerging, as well as new platforms for dissemination of innovations. Over the past decade, two rounds of a landmark *Lancet* Series on Global Mental Health have been published, as well as a series by *PLoS Medicine* (Horton, 2007; Patel et al., 2012).

"Global health initiatives" (multistakeholder partnerships).   The Clinton Global Initiative and others have increasingly supported global mental health initiatives, usually for special populations. The Human Resources for Health program—a program that represents a new model for health education and the delivery of foreign aid by building health care education infrastructure and workforce in low-income countries such as Rwanda—has integrated psychiatry training in its funded programs (Cancedda et al., 2017).

Media (professional journalists, social media).   The media has presented only a limited number (however increasing) of balanced stories on mental health and global health. The portrayal of the relationship of mental health to other public health concerns, such as gun violence, has served to cloud public perceptions of those living with mental illness.

Transnational corporations, including the pharmaceutical industry.   Concerns about diagnostic colonialism and the imposition of the biomedical approach from the field of psychiatry, and that the psychopharmaceutical industry will use the global mental health movement to increase profits, have also raised concerns about the movement for global mental health (Watters, 2010; Mills, 2014). Some pharmaceutical companies have emerged to promote global access to health care for patients with mental disorders in low-income countries, such as the One Mind Initiative (https://www.onemindinstitute.org), supported by Johnson & Johnson/Janssen.

Multilateral donors.   The World Bank has engaged with issues in global mental health, although in a limited way; however, in 2016. the bank convened a major meeting on global mental health, inviting finance ministers from around the world to begin to coalesce evidence and momentum for greater funding for global mental health care (World Bank, 2016).

Private philanthropy.   The Wellcome Trust (https://wellcome.ac.uk/) in the United Kingdom is one of several private philanthropies supporting global mental health initiatives.

NCD Advocates.   Organizations such as the NCD Alliance are increasingly inclusive of mental and neurological disorders as contributory to the burden of other priority NCDs with shared risk factors, including cardiovascular disease, respiratory illness, diabetes, and cancer.

■ ■ ■

Basic governance functions critical to mental health include the following:

Generating resources for public goods such as knowledge production through research focusing on implementation of interventions in low-resource contexts (such as is being done by Grand Challenges Canada and NIMH)

Norm-setting of expectations for governments in providing basic packages of care and ensuring human rights and dignity for those with mental disorders (such as is being promoted by WHO and some NGOs)

Improved coordination for effective collective action among various actors, including other NCD actors

Policy coherence, including the institution of national mental health policies and plans that meet WHO standards

Efforts to strengthen governance around global mental health can include enhancing access to evidence-based packages of care—for example, by widely implementing the WHO mhGAP guidelines, necessitating task-shifting and integration of mental health care within primary health care systems and other sectors such as education and social welfare; strengthening the human rights commitment enshrined in the Convention on the Rights of Persons with Disabilities in order to ensure that people with mental disorders live a life with dignity; and taking actions to expand knowledge relating to treatment of mental disorders, including establishment of a specific fund akin to the Drugs for Neglected Diseases Initiative (Bass et al., 2012; UN, 2006; DNDi, http://www.dndi.org). Ultimately, through the generation of political will, these efforts have as their aim the mobilization of financial resources to support the human resource, management, and data collection capacities to integrate mental health services into existing health care systems.

Strategies for Program Design and Sustained Service Delivery: The Need to Strengthen Existing Health Systems

Current evidence argues for integrated approaches to delivering mental health services within health systems that include **collaborative, team-based care** in which there is effective communication, and **task-shifting** of care delivery functions across disciplines in contexts where there are few specialists. This method has been employed in delivery of HIV services globally, through the use of community health workers (CHWs) and other providers, to ensure that people are supported in taking antiretroviral medicines. It led, through the development of services for HIV/AIDS in resource-poor contexts, to the strengthening of primary care systems in various parts of the world and to the reduction of HIV rates in many countries. Team members may include community health workers, health coaches, social workers, psychologists, nurse care managers, nurse practitioners, physician assistants, primary care physicians, and/or psychiatrists (Lee, Kolappa, & Raviola, 2014). Evidence also suggests that it is helpful to consider packages of care, bundling of care pathways for priority conditions such as depression or schizophrenia, based on best practices and existing evidence in context, as well as integration of mental health care into primary care (Patel, Simon, Chowdhary, Kaaya, & Araya, 2009; WHO & World Organization of Family Doctors, 2008). Such care locates services closer to people's homes, improving access and reducing costs associated with seeking specialist care in distant locations (Lee et al., 2014). Through research over the past decade, focused interventions have been found to be effective. For example, randomized control trials in Pakistan have shown that CHWs can be effectively mobilized to use cognitive behavioral therapy to treat mothers with depression, with positive health impacts on their children (Rahman, Malik, Sikander, Roberts, & Creed, 2008). A greater challenge, however, involves the scaling up of such interventions within existing public health and primary care health systems, and their sustained integration within government-run services to eventually strengthen those systems.

Key elements to optimizing impact from emerging programs that implement these effective practices will include building the capacity within governments to meaningfully consider context and culture in adaptation of practices, sustaining effective training and supervision of larger numbers of nonspecialist providers, meaningfully measuring outcomes and managing data with technology, providing effective training in tried-and-true quality improvement practices and using those practices with fidelity, concurrent commitment to training of specialists such as psychologists and psychiatrists, and ongoing commitment to also addressing the social determinants of health that create and compound the burden of mental disorders. At the front end of program implementation "on the ground," this includes working to develop and test innovative care delivery models as evidence for the feasibility and cost-effectiveness of developing functional mental health systems of care and long-term services that integrate strong traditional perceptions and beliefs, local community networks and religious influences, and contemporary biopsychosocial approaches (Raviola et al., 2013).

Global Health Worker Wellness: The Need for Professional and Personal Development

As health care systems globally are increasing their focus on efficiency and effectiveness, in part through the mobilization of less specialized providers who are accountable for seeing more patients, there is a risk of burnout and compassion fatigue for both specialist and nonspecialist providers. This is also notable given that many providers operate in areas significantly affected by the impacts of poverty, natural disasters, and societal violence where there is a major lack of mental health services within the biomedical care system, and where there exists a high disease burden, a shortage of specialists, and a lack of integration between primary health care and traditional belief and care systems. Often, providers and program implementers have themselves been significantly impacted at a personal level by these forces. For these reasons, there exists a need for a shift in ethos around the relevance and importance of health worker training and professional development, emotional support, and wellness. This need extends from health care providers to program implementers, managers, and administrators, who as health care workers all bear a high degree of burden from the challenge of a feeling of perpetual need from those suffering and seeking care, and a sense of endlessness to the various aspects of their work. Maintaining an empathic stance vis-à-vis the recipients of (and partners in) our services and care, promoting internal curiosity and deep engagement with regard to the work, nurturing a core ethics of practice, and fostering a sense of partnership and collaboration with colleagues as members of teams—all require a commitment to a personal practice of introspection, the pursuit of balance, and greater attention to **self-care**. This greatly enhances the chances of success for a sustained, long-term career in global health.

The fostering of bidirectional relationships between cross-national teams can also bolster the capacity of teams and individuals to bear these challenges. Creative ways of supporting teams and colleagues in supervising clinical work through mentorship, implementation of programs, and application of tools for safety, quality, outcomes measurement, and performance improvement are needed, and can be improved through effective use of technology. Targeted academic work and research support can also build research capacity within local teams, strengthening engagement as team members make effective intellectual linkages to the work that have relevance to professional development.

There exist many ways to innovate in global health. Academic work in global health includes more than formal research; it can span a continuum from service delivery science and use of quality improvement methods, to implementation science and mixed-methods (qualitative and/or quantitative approaches) research, to formal randomized-control trials or anthropological research. **Implementation science** refers to the scientific study of methods to promote the systematic uptake of proven clinical treatments, practices, and organizational and management interventions into routine practice, and hence to improve health. (For more information, see https://implementationscience.biomedcentral.com/.) Finally, supporting the emotional health and well-being of health care workers and global health implementers in various ways so as to enhance resilience and prevent burnout through self-care require greater attention by organizations, institutions, and individuals truly committed to the endeavor of global health.

Conclusion

Global mental health, behavioral medicine, and wellness are areas of increasing attention in global health. Mental disorders constitute the greatest illness burden to global societies, in terms of disability over the life course and economic burden, with 50% of these problems developing prior to the age of 15. Global mental health, however, includes gaps in policy, funding, and treatment, with a need for new models of care and systems of financing for scaling up of services. The integration of public health and behavioral medicine approaches addressing mental health that are collaborative across provider roles and government sectors in the context of communities and health systems offers the opportunity to strengthen existing health systems and global societies, writ large. This will require an appreciation of the impact of these problems on societies, and of the role of stigma and fear in impeding progress within societies and health systems with regard to care for people living with mental illness. Progress will require ongoing attention and commitment to Richmond's model for impacting public policy—building a scientific knowledge base, a social strategy, and political will—and an appreciation for the concept of governance in global health in order to leverage change at local and global scales. The work required by practitioners in this area, as in all areas of global health, requires not only technical knowledge and experience but also commitment to professional and personal development for oneself and others at emotional, physical, spiritual, ethical, and interpersonal levels. For these reasons, a review of global mental health, behavioral medicine, and wellness offers an instructive study of key issues and concerns in contemporary global health.

Chapter Summary

In this chapter, we described the relevance of global mental health, behavioral medicine, and wellness to global health. This includes a description of the burden of illness and the global treatment gap of mental disorders; an overview of challenges and gaps in national policies; governance and global systems for care for mental disorders; and the concept of global health governance. We also looked at strategies both for policy change and for innovative care delivery in low-resource settings, building on previous work done in the field of HIV/AIDS in engaging communities and community health workers in mobilizing care. The potential burdens on health care providers and program implementers in global health with regard to personal wellness are also described. The reader is encouraged to consider that careers in global health can span service delivery and bidirectional training, program management and design, implementation science and research, and staff wellness.

Review Questions

1. What are some ways to define or consider mental health in the context of global health?
2. What are the elements of Richmond's model for impacting public policy?
3. Describe innovative strategies being used in low-resource settings to increase access to mental health services.
4. Describe some ways to consider personal and professional wellness in global health practice.

Key Terms

Basic treatment packages
Behavioral medicine
Collaborative, team-based care
Depression
Disability
Global mental health

Governance

Implementation science

Psychosis

Self-care

Stigma

Task-shifting

Wellness

References

Bass, J. K., Bornemann, T. H., Burkey, M., Chehil, S., Chen, L., Copeland, J.R.M., . . . Patel, V. (2012). A United Nations General Assembly special session for mental, neurological, and substance use disorders: The time has come. *PLoS Medicine, 9*(1), e1001159. doi:10.1371/journal.pmed.1001159

Bloom, D. E., Caero, E. T., Jané-Llopis, E., Abrahams-Gessel, S., Bloom, L. R., Fathima, S., . . . Weinstein C. (2011). *The global economic burden of non-communicable diseases.* Geneva: World Economic Forum. Retrieved from http://www3.weforum.org/docs/WEF_Harvard_HE_GlobalEconomicBurdenNonCommunicableDiseases_2011.pdf

Brymer, M., Jacobs, A., Layne, C., Pynoos, R., Ruzek, J., Steinberg, A., . . . Watson, P. (2006). *Psychological first aid: Field operations guide* (2nd ed.). Retrieved from www.nctsn.org

Cancedda, C., Riviello, R., Wilson, K., Scott, K. W., Tuteja, M., Barrow, J. R., . . . Golan, D. E. (2017). Building capacity in a low-income country while strengthening global health programs at home: Participation of seven Harvard-affiliated academic institutions in a health professional training initiative in Rwanda. *Academic Medicine, 92,* 649–658. doi:10.1097/ACM.0000000000001638

Centers for Disease Control and Prevention. (2015). Stigma and mental illness. Retrieved from https://www.cdc.gov/mentalhealth/basics/stigma-illness.htm

Chisholm, D., Sweeney, K., Sheehan, P., Rasmussen, B., Smit, F., Cuijpers, P., & Saxena, S. (2016). Scaling-up treatment of depression and anxiety: A global return on investment analysis. *The Lancet, 3,* 415–424. doi:10.1016/ S2215-0366(16)30024-4

Daelmans, B., Darmstadt, G. L., Lombardi, J., Black, M. M., Britto, P. R., Lye, S., . . . *Lancet* Early Childhood Development Series Steering Committee. (2017). Early childhood development: The foundation of sustainable development. *The Lancet, 389,* 9–11. doi:10.1016/S0140-6736(16)31659-2

Demyttenaere, K., Bruffaerts, R., & Posada-Villa, J. (2004). Prevalence, severity, and unmet need for treatment of mental disorders in the World Health Organization World Mental Health Surveys. *Journal of the American Medical Association, 291,* 2581–2590. doi:10.1001/jama.291.21.2581

DeSilva, M., Samele, C., Saxena, S., Patel, V., & Darzi, A. (2014). Policy actions to achieve integrated community-based mental health services. *Health Affairs, 33,* 1595–1602. doi:10.1377/hlthaff.2014.0365

Feldman, M., & Christensen J. (2014). Preface. In M. Feldman & J. Christensen (Eds.), *Behavioral medicine: A guide for clinical practice* (4th ed., pp. xvii–xviii). New York, NY: McGraw Hill.

Freeman, M. C., Kolappa, K., Caldas de Almeida, J. M., Kleinman, A., Makhashvili, N., Phakathi, S, . . . Thornicroft, G. (2015). Reversing hard won victories in the name of human rights: A critique of the General Comment on Article 12 of the UN Convention on the Rights of Persons with Disabilities. *Lancet Psychiatry, 2,* 844–850. doi:10.1016/S2215-0366(15)00218-7

Frenk, J., & Moon, S. (2013). Governance challenges in global health. *New England Journal of Medicine, 368*, 936–942. doi:10.1056/NEJMra1109339

GBD 2013 DALYs and HALE Collaborators. (2015). Global, regional, and national disability-adjusted life years (DALYs) for 306 diseases and injuries and healthy life expectancy (HALE) for 188 countries, 1990–2013: Quantifying the epidemiological transition. *The Lancet, 386*, 2145–2191. doi:10.1016/S0140-6736(15)61340-X

Goffman, E. (1963). *Stigma: Notes on the management of spoiled identity.* Upper Saddle River, NJ: Prentice Hall.

Grand Challenges Canada/Grand Défis Canada. (2011, January). The Grand Challenges approach. Retrieved from http://www.grandchallenges.ca/wp-content/uploads/2011/02/thegrandchallengesapproach.pdf

Horton, R. (2007). Launching a new movement for global health. *The Lancet, 370*, 806–808. doi:10.1016/S0140-6736(07)61243-4

Interagency Standing Committee. (2007). Interagency Standing Committee guidelines on mental health and psychosocial support in emergency settings. Retrieved from http://www.who.int/mental_health/emergencies/guidelines_iasc_mental_health_psychosocial_june_2007.pdf

Jakob, K. S., & Patel, V. (2014). Classification of mental disorders: A global mental health perspective. *The Lancet, 383*, 1433–1435. doi:10.1016/S0140-6736(13)62382-X

Kakuma, R., Minas, H., van Ginneken, N., Dal Poz, M. R., Desiraju, K., Morris, J. E., . . . Scheffler, R. M. (2011). Human resources for mental health care: Current situation and strategies for action. *The Lancet, 378*, 1654–1663. doi:10.1016/S0140-6736(11)61093-3

Kohn, R., Saxena, S., Levav, I., & Saraceno, B. (2004). The treatment gap in mental health care. *Bulletin of the World Health Organization, 82*, 858–866. doi:10.1590/S0042-96862004001100011

Koplan, J., Bond, T. C., & Merson, M. H. (2009). Towards a common definition of global health. *The Lancet, 373*, 1993–1995. doi:10.1016/S0140-6736(09)60332-9.

Lee, P., Kolappa, K., & Raviola, G. (2014). Global health and behavioral medicine. In M. Feldman & J. Christensen (Eds.), *Behavioral medicine: A guide for clinical practice* (4th ed., pp. 65–76). New York, NY: McGraw Hill.

Mills, C. (2014). *Decolonizing mental health: The psychiatrization of the majority world.* London, United Kingdom: Routledge.

National Institute of Mental Health. (2016a). Depression. Retrieved from https://www.nimh.nih.gov/health/topics/depression/index.shtml

National Institute of Mental Health. (2016b). Schizophrenia. Retrieved from https://www.nimh.nih.gov/health/topics/schizophrenia/index.shtml

Patel, V., & Chatterji, S. (2015). Integrating mental health in care for noncommunicable diseases: An imperative for person-centered care. *Health Affairs, 34*, 1498–1505. doi:10.1377/hlthaff.2015.0791

Patel, V., Collins, P., Copeland, J., Kakuma, R., Katontoka, S., Lamichhane, J., . . . Skeen, S. (2011). The movement for global mental health. *British Journal of Psychiatry, 198*(2), 88–90. doi:10.1192/bjp.bp.109.074518

Patel, V., Jenkins, R., Lund, C., & the *PLoS Medicine* Editors. (2012). Putting evidence into practice: The *PLoS Medicine* series on global mental health practice. *PLoS Medicine, 9*(5), e1001226. doi:10.1371/journal.pmed.1001226

Patel, V., Simon, G., Chowdhary, N., Kaaya, S., & Araya, R. (2009). Packages of care for depression in low- and middle-income countries. *PLoS Medicine, 6*(10), e1000159. doi:10.1371/journal.pmed.1000159

Patel, V., & Prince, M. (2010). Global mental health—A new global health field comes of age. *Journal of the American Medical Association, 303*, 1976–1977. doi:10.1001/jama.2010.616

Rahman, A., Malik, A., Sikander, S., Roberts, C., & Creed, F. (2008). Cognitive behaviour therapy-based intervention by community health workers for mothers with depression and their infants in rural Pakistan: A cluster-randomised controlled trial. *The Lancet, 372*, 902–909. doi:10.1016/S0140-6736(08)61400-2

Raviola, G., Severe, J., Therosme, T., Oswald, C., Belkin, G., & Eustache, E. (2013). The 2010 Haiti earthquake response. *Psychiatric Clinics of North America, 36*, 431–450. doi:10.1016/j.psc.2013.05.006

Richmond, J. B., & Kotelchuk, M. (1983). Political influences: Rethinking national health policy. In C. McGuire, R. Foley, A. Gorr, & R. Richards (Eds.), *Handbook of health professionals and education* (pp. 386–404). San Francisco, CA: Jossey-Bass.

Saxena, S., Thornicroft, G., Knapp, M., & Whiteford, H. (2007). Resources for mental health: Scarcity, inequity, and inefficiency. *The Lancet, 370*, 878–889. doi:10.1016/S0140-6736(07)61239-2

United Nations. (2006). *Convention on the rights of persons with disabilities and optional protocol.* Retrieved from http://www.un.org/disabilities/documents/convention/convoptprot-e.pdf

United Nations Development Program. (2015). *Transforming our world: The 2030 agenda for sustainable development.* Retrieved from https://sustainabledevelopment.un.org/content/documents/21252030%20Agenda%20for%20Sustainable%20Development%20web.pdf

Vigo, D., Thornicroft, G., & Atun, R. (2016). Estimating the true global burden of mental illness. *Lancet Psychiatry, 3*(2), 171–178. doi:10.1016/S2215-0366(15)00505-2.

Watters, E. (2010). *Crazy like US: The globalization of the American psyche.* New York, NY: Free Press.

World Bank. (2016, June). *Out of the shadows: Making mental health a global development priority. Report of proceedings of event.* Retrieved from http://pubdocs.worldbank.org/en/391171465393131073/0602-SummaryReport-GMH-event-June-3-2016.pdf

World Health Organization. (2003). *Organization of services for mental health.* Retrieved from http://www.who.int/mental_health/policy/services/4_organisation%20services_WEB_07.pdf

World Health Organization. (2005). Mental health atlas. Retrieved from http://www.who.int/mental_health/evidence/atlas/global_results.pdf

World Health Organization. (2009). *Mental health and development: Targeting people with mental health conditions as a vulnerable group.* Retrieved from http://apps.who.int/iris/bitstream/10665/44257/1/9789241563949_eng.pdf

World Health Organization. (2014). Mental health: A state of well-being. Retrieved from http://www.who.int/features/factfiles/mental_health/en/

World Health Organization. (2016a). Depression fact sheet. Retrieved from http://www.who.int/mediacentre/factsheets/fs369/en/

World Health Organization. (2016b). *mhGAP intervention guide for mental, neurological and substance use disorders in non-specialized health settings: Mental Health Gap Action Programme (mhGAP). Version 2.0.* Retrieved from http://apps.who.int/iris/bitstream/10665/250239/1/9789241549790-eng.pdf

World Health Organization, War Trauma Foundation, and World Vision International. (2011). *Psychological first aid: Guide for field workers.* Retrieved from http://www.searo.who.int/srilanka/documents/psychological_first_aid_guide_for_field_workers.pdf

World Health Organization and World Organization of Family Doctors. (2008). *Integrating mental health into primary care: A global perspective.* Retrieved from http://www.who.int/mental_health/policy/Mental%20health%20+%20primary%20care-%20final%20low-res%20140908.pdf

CHAPTER 8

WATER, SANITATION, HYGIENE, AND HEALTH

Eric Hettler, PE

We are called to assist the Earth to heal her wounds and in the process heal our own—indeed, to embrace the whole creation in all its diversity, beauty and wonder.

—Wangari Maathai, winner of the 2004 Nobel Peace Prize

LEARNING OBJECTIVES

- Describe the key aspects of water and sanitation from a global health perspective
- Understand the basic causes of and types of diseases associated with water and sanitation
- Summarize the historic and current efforts surrounding global water and sanitation
- Evaluate the current challenges facing water and sanitation

Access to clean water and adequate sanitation and hygiene are vital to the health of populations. To appreciate the importance of water, imagine your daily routine. When you wake up, perhaps you shower, brush your teeth, brew yourself a cup of coffee, and prepare breakfast. Throughout the day, you may use the restroom, wash your hands, drink from a water fountain, and water your garden. In the evenings, you may cook dinner, wash the dirty dishes in the sink or in a dishwasher, wash your face, and once again brush your teeth. All of these relatively simple activities require immediate and reliable access to water, and it is easy to take that access for granted. In the wealthy and well-developed areas of large cities throughout the world, including Nairobi, Shanghai, Mumbai, and San Salvador, your daily routine and relationship with water would not look all that different. For hundreds of millions of people in both rural and peri-urban areas throughout the world, however, the convenience of simply obtaining water from a tap does not exist.

Foundations for Global Health Practice, First Edition. Lori DiPrete Brown.
© 2018 John Wiley & Sons, Inc. Published 2018 by John Wiley & Sons, Inc.

The World Health Organization (WHO, 2015) estimates that approximately 700 million people throughout the world lack access to clean water. Such a large number is difficult to visualize, but it is approximately equivalent to the entire population of the United States and Western Europe combined. If the number of people lacking access to water were grouped into a single country, it would be the third most populous nation in the world behind China and India. Even more significant is the number of individuals in the world lacking access to adequate sanitation. Current estimates approximate that 2.4 billion individuals living in the world do not have access to adequate sanitation as it is defined by WHO (2015). That staggering number means that one out of every three people in the world lacks access to what we would consider a safe, hygienic toilet facility. It is equivalent to eight times the population of the United States.

The realties associated with the lack of access to water and sanitation have a very important impact on the overall health of populations throughout the world. Diarrheal disease, which is routinely caused by unsafe water and inadequate sanitation and hygiene, is a major cause of morbidity and mortality in global populations (WHO, 2015). Water and sanitation are wide-ranging, multifaceted issues that require complex and multidisciplinary approaches. Although national governments, multinational organizations, and nongovernmental organizations have undertaken work to address the problem, much effort and financing are still required to ensure clean water and adequate sanitation for every person worldwide.

Water, Sanitation, and Hygiene: Contextual Considerations

To understand the complex issues of water, sanitation, and hygiene, we must establish a few foundational concepts. First, a broad understanding of what characterizes effective water, sanitation, and hygiene is required to adequately meet the needs of populations. Second, knowledge of the specific diseases associated with inadequate water and sanitation is needed to develop appropriate solutions. Third, insights into the historic and current efforts associated with global water and sanitation are needed to appreciate what has already been accomplished. Finally, a thoughtful assessment of the gendered, political, economic, and environmental challenges related to water and sanitation is required so that future policies, programs, and activities can be properly implemented.

Four Components of Effective Water, Sanitation, and Hygiene Systems

Although as already noted, water and sanitation are complex issues that require multidisciplinary approaches, the subject can be summarized by four main components (Figure 8.1): accessibility of safe and clean water, availability of sufficient water quantity, protection of water resources, and access to adequate hygiene and sanitation.

FIGURE 8.1   Four Critical Components of Water- and Sanitation-Related Health

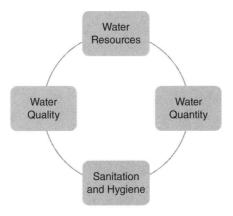

Accessibility to Safe and Clean Water When one thinks of water in a global health context, the picture of a child fetching water from a dirty water source may come to mind (Figure 8.2). Unfortunately, this situation is a reality for many people throughout the world. When water infrastructure is not in place, individuals must rely on whatever sources of water are available. Poor water quality extends beyond just aesthetic characteristics, however. Even water that appears clean can contain pathogens and other contaminants that are detrimental to human health. The most significant concern for water quality is pathogens that cause acute illness. Water containing harmful metals or chemicals, such as arsenic or pesticides, also cause illness, but the impact of this contamination can be less apparent, as it usually accumulates over a long period of time. To avoid these negative health impacts, access to clean, uncontaminated water sources is vital to ensuring the well-being of global populations.

Availability of Sufficient Water Quantity The availability of sufficient water quantity is also a major concern. In some areas, water sources may not be located in close proximity to households that rely on them. As a result, individuals and community members must travel long distances to collect water for drinking, cooking, washing, and other household needs. The burden of collecting water falls primarily on women, but children are also sometimes assigned the task of collecting water (United Nations Children's Fund [UNICEF] & WHO, 2015). The time spent collecting water can consume many hours in any given day, restricting the ability of women to work or of children to attend school. The lack of sufficient water quantity poses significant challenges to many communities around the world.

Protection of Water Resources A common threat to both water quality and water availability is poor management of existing water resources. **Water resources** are commonly

FIGURE 8.2   Surface Water Source in Rural Uganda

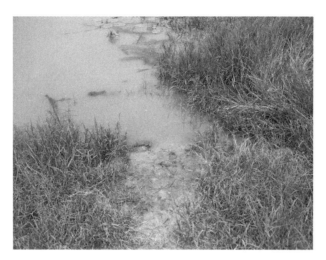

Photo: Eric Hettler

defined as sources of water that are useful or potentially useful to humans. The definition encompasses both the quality and the quantity of water available. For example, if water becomes excessively polluted such that it no longer can be utilized by humans, it amounts to a reduction in the available water resources. Further, if water is used for agricultural or industrial purposes and cannot be recovered, the water resources of an area are decreased. The protection of water resources by ensuring that water does not become contaminated and by responsibly managing the amount of water used is an important consideration for all communities in the world. The need is especially great for those who already live in areas where access to water is limited.

Accessibility of Adequate Sanitation and Hygiene   Finally, access to adequate sanitation and hygiene is vital to the overall health and well-being of individuals. The most visible example of adequate sanitation is improved sanitation facilities. UNICEF/WHO (2015) define an **improved sanitation facility** as one that "hygienically separates human excreta from human contact." Improved sanitation facilities in the United States are typically toilets that are connected to sanitary sewers or septic systems. In very rural settings, properly maintained household latrines with permanent slabs are classified as improved sanitation facilities. Later sections of this chapter provide a more in-depth discussion of sanitation facilities. Related to sanitation, **hygiene** is defined as referring to "conditions and practices that help to maintain health and prevent the spread of disease" (WHO, 2016). Face, body, and hand washing are all critical elements of proper hygiene, and they all require a sufficient supply of water to be done properly.

Summary of Components of Water and Sanitation Although the components of water, sanitation, and hygiene can be broken into four distinct categories, they are all intimately linked. If any of these four components is missing from a community, the burden of disease on individuals will increase. Improving only one aspect without addressing the others will have limited benefit for an individual's health. Therefore, any project or program being implemented should include a holistic focus that incorporates all four components.

Diseases Associated with Water, Sanitation, and Hygiene

The four components of water and sanitation are important to understand, but a more in-depth understanding of disease is required when relating water and sanitation to health and wellness. In a global health context, water-related diseases are typically grouped into four functional categories: water-borne, water-washed, water-based, and water-related insect vectors (Choffnes & Mack, 2009).

Water-Borne Diseases **Water-borne diseases** are "diseases caused by the ingestion of water contaminated by human or animal feces or urine containing pathogens" (UNICEF, 2008). A number of debilitating diseases are related to poor water quality. Water-borne diseases include pathogenic viruses, bacteria, and protozoa. Examples include rotavirus, pathogenic *E. coli*, cholera, typhoid, dysentery, hepatitis A, and hepatitis E. Individual water-borne diseases all present unique symptoms, but they are almost always accompanied by vomiting and diarrhea. The major concern with vomiting and diarrhea is dehydration, which is especially dangerous for young children, persons with compromised immune systems, and the elderly. Dehydration is the main mechanism of death associated with water-borne diseases (UNICEF & WHO, 2015).

Many options are available for improving the quality of water, and they vary tremendously in their scope. The variation in water treatment options is demonstrated in Figure 8.3. In large, well-developed areas, water is typically treated at a centralized water treatment plant. Although the water leaving the treatment plant may be safe for human consumption, it can become contaminated as it is distributed to different areas. Contamination of once-treated water is especially prevalent in peri-urban areas, where poorly constructed connections or illicit connections are common. These poor connections allow once-clean water to become compromised with polluted surface water.

Where wide distribution of centralized water is not available, improved water sources can be utilized to provide clean drinking water. An **improved water source** is defined as a water collection point that "adequately protects the source from outside contamination, particularly fecal matter" (WHO, 2015). Examples of improved water sources in rural areas include protected springs (Figure 8.3), protected wells, and rainwater.

FIGURE 8.3   Variation in Water Treatment Systems

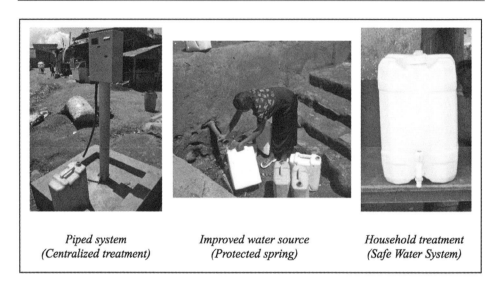

| Piped system (Centralized treatment) | Improved water source (Protected spring) | Household treatment (Safe Water System) |

Photos: Eric Hettler

Even if clean water sources are available, water must be transported to the household when direct household water connections are not available. The act of transporting water provides opportunities for the water to become contaminated either by contaminated transport vessels, contaminated storage vessels, or dirty hands or utensils being introduced to the water. To overcome the challenges associated with water transportation, point-of-use water treatment can be utilized. Point-of-use water treatment refers to any form of water treatment that occurs where the water is being consumed or used. Examples include household chemical disinfection (chlorine), household water filters, and boiling.

Water-Washed Diseases Water-borne diseases typically receive the most attention in international programs addressing clean water, but water-washed diseases are also very common in areas with undeveloped or underdeveloped water supplies. **Water-washed diseases** are "diseases caused by inadequate use of water for domestic and personal hygiene" (UNICEF, 2008). Lack of sufficient water quantity has a negative impact on hygiene and sanitation. Water-washed diseases differ from water-borne diseases because they refer directly to the diseases resulting from a lack of adequate water for washing and sanitation purposes rather than diseases caused by the consumption of unsafe water. Water-washed diseases include skin and eye infections. One example of an eye infection transmitted by poor hygiene conditions is trachoma, a chronic bacterial infection of the cornea and conjunctiva (Choffnes & Mack, 2009). If left untreated, trachoma can cause blindness. Although skin or eye infections may not cause as much mortality as water-borne diseases, they are a significant source of morbidity (UNICEF, 2008). They can cause infections that could ultimately lead to loss of limb, loss of sight, or loss of life.

Water-washed diseases can be prevented by increasing the availability of water for hygiene. In urbanized areas, increasing availability of water can be achieved by extending the reach of the piped distribution system. In more rural areas without piped water distribution, water quantity can be increased by strategically drilling boreholes or digging wells in areas where groundwater is known to exist. Pumps can also be used to transmit water from far-away areas to a more centralized location, although the energy and maintenance costs of high-powered pumps can make this solution unavailable for communities that lack adequate financial resources.

Water-Based Diseases Other diseases related to the lack of availability of water are water-based diseases. **Water-based diseases** are "infections caused by parasitic pathogens found in aquatic host organisms" (UNICEF, 2008). One example of a water-based disease is schistosomiasis, caused by a parasitic worm that affects the human liver. The parasitic worms that infect humans live in freshwater snails, and the disease is typically contracted when humans enter water bodies in which the snails live. Another example of a water-based disease is Guinea worm. Guinea worm is transmitted when water containing tiny water fleas is consumed. The water fleas contain Guinea worm larvae, and the larvae are released when the fleas are digested. The larvae enter the body through the lining of the stomach and the intestine, where they reproduce. As the larvae grow and reproduce, they spread through the body. The worms eventually seek to leave the body through the skin through very painful and debilitating blisters.

The best way for a person to prevent infection by schistosomiasis is avoiding water bodies that are home to the freshwater snails containing the parasitic worms. Unfortunately, for many, avoiding contact with their water source is not an option. If infection occurs, medication can kill the parasitic worms once they infect the body. Medication is only a temporary solution, however. In the absence of improved sanitation and hygiene practices, an outbreak of parasitic worms can be perpetual, especially when medication is discontinued (Campbell et al., 2014).

The reduction in cases of Guinea worm is one of the major success stories in disease eradication. Led by the Carter Center, the eradication efforts focus on ensuring that people do not consume water contaminated with the fleas that carry the larvae and by preventing people who are infected with the worms from entering water sources. Largely due to the efforts of the Carter Center and other organizations, cases of Guinea worm infection have decreased from approximately 3.5 million people per year in 1986 to just 22 cases recorded in 2015 (Carter Center, 2016).

Water-Related Insect Vectors The final functional category of water-related diseases is water-related insect vectors. **Water-related insect vector diseases** are diseases "caused by insect vectors which either breed in water or bite near water" (UNICEF, 2008). The most common water-related insect vectors are mosquitoes, which carry an array of diseases that are detrimental to human health. Examples of mosquito-borne diseases include dengue fever, malaria, chikungunya, and Zika. Flies that rely on water for breeding are also capable of transmitting diseases to humans. The tsetse fly in sub-Saharan Africa transmits trypanosomiasis, more commonly referred to as "sleeping sickness," to humans.

Control of water-related insect vectors requires coordinated efforts. The easiest mechanism for controlling water-related insect vectors is reducing the amount of standing water around populated areas. It is not possible to eliminate all standing water, however, so additional measures are required to reduce the burden of disease caused by the vectors. These measures include spraying insecticides to kill the insects and introducing fish or other aquatic wildlife to feed on the larvae of the insect vectors. Spraying insecticides must be done carefully, however, because these chemicals can damage water resources and have negative impacts on human health and the environment.

Historic and Current Efforts Surrounding Global Water, Sanitation, and Hygiene

The causes of water-related diseases have been understood for many years, and these diseases have been minimized in the United States and Western Europe over the last century and a half. Many people throughout the world, however, still lack basic access to the water and sanitation facilities required to alleviate the burden of disease. Many programs implemented by national governments, international organizations, and nongovernmental organizations have attempted to reduce the burden of water-related diseases in populations that still lack clean water and adequate sanitation.

Brief History of Water and Sanitation To understand the current efforts being undertaken to address water and sanitation around the world, we need to review a general history of water and sanitation coverage in Europe and the United States. During the Industrial Revolution, a large number of people started to migrate to large cities. As people increasingly lived in relatively close proximity to one another, diseases associated with poor water and sanitation became more apparent. For a time, the exact nature of how water and sanitation caused negative health outcomes was not understood. One of the early theories about the relation of poor sanitation to human health came from the idea of the miasma. The theory of miasma essentially hypothesized that many diseases arising in large urban centers were caused by the foul odors that were ever present in the densely populated areas. Although it is now known that unpleasant smells are not the direct cause of disease, the idea did lead to some important public health interventions.

During this period, cities were focused on decreasing the odors by clearing waste and sewage away from populated areas. Although the theory behind the intervention was flawed, the act of clearing waste did decrease the burden of disease by reducing the presence of pathogens that were in sewage.

Not everyone was convinced that foul odors were causing disease. John Snow, a physician in London, suspected that contaminated water supplies were causing the outbreaks of disease that were so common in London. During a cholera outbreak in London, Snow deduced that water from a public water pump at Broad Street was the main cause of the outbreak. He convinced the local leaders to disable the pump, and the outbreak came to an end. This well-known event contributed to research into a new theory called the **germ theory of disease**, which states that disease can be caused by specific microorganisms. This theory has since been expanded, and it is the basis of most water and sanitation programs today.

Current Practices for Treating Water and Wastewater Once the idea that pathogens and sewage in water were causing disease, cities in the United States and in Europe began to treat the water they distributed to households and the sewage they deposited in rivers. Today, most communities in the United States are equipped with water treatment plants and wastewater treatment plants. Although the exact treatment mechanisms vary by location, water treatment focuses on the removal or deactivation of harmful pathogens from water before the water is distributed to households. Pathogens are generally removed by filtering out impurities and treating the water with a chemical agent or ultraviolet light. The water is distributed through pipes at a high pressure so that no outside contaminants can enter the water distribution system.

Sewage and wastewater are typically treated by essentially speeding up the natural processes that break down sewage in nature. Sewage treatment plants create an environment that encourages good bacteria to consume and break down the organic matter and pathogens in water. Occasionally, the processed sewage is treated with chemicals or with ultraviolet light to make it even safer before it is introduced back into the environment.

Millennium Development Goals One of the recent efforts to alleviate the burden of disease worldwide was the Millennium Development Goals (MDGs), which were established at the United Nations in 2000. The goals were developed to address the major issues facing many nations around the world. Each goal had corresponding targets, which allowed the progress of the goals to be tracked. The seventh goal of the MDGs was ensuring environmental sustainability. This goal focused on sustainable development, biodiversity loss, water and sanitation access, and slum-dweller livelihoods. The specific target related to water and sanitation, Target 7.C. aimed to "halve, by 2015, the proportion of the population without sustainable access to safe drinking water and basic sanitation" (UN, 2015a). The goals of the MGD target related to water and sanitation were relative to the baseline condition established in 1990 through the Joint Monitoring Programme for Water Supply and Sanitation (JMP). The JMP is a collaborative effort between UNICEF and WHO to monitor and track the progress of developments related to water and sanitation.

The JMP uses specific definitions for improved water sources and improved sanitation facilities in its monitoring efforts. As described previously, improved water sources are those that adequately protect the water source from contamination. Unimproved water sources include surface water, unprotected wells, and unprotected springs. Improved water sources include taps, tube wells, protected springs, protected wells, and rainwater (UNICEF & WHO, 2015). The major difference between protected and unprotected wells and springs is the installation of the facilities. Unprotected wells do not have any casing within the well to prevent fecal matter or other contaminants from entering the well after construction. Similarly, unprotected springs are those that do not have any protective barrier at the outlet to prevent contamination.

Improved sanitation facilities are defined slightly differently than improved water sources. As previously noted, improved sanitation facilities are those that separate human excreta from human contact. Examples of unimproved sanitation are open defecation, pit latrines lacking a slab, and sanitation facilities shared by two or more households. Improved sanitation facilities are those that utilize flushing or pouring to wash the excreta into a sewer or a latrine, pit latrines with slabs, and composting toilets (UNICEF & WHO, 2015). The definitions of improved water sources and improved sanitation sources are important when evaluating the success of the MDG target for water and sanitation.

The MDG target for halving the number of people utilizing unimproved water sources was declared as met in 2010. Between 1990 and 2015, the percentage of the world population using improved water sources increased from 74 percent to 91 percent (UNICEF & WHO, 2015). When evaluating the MDGs, however, it is important to take a closer look at the regional successes. The majority of the improvement in access to improved water sources during this time period occurred in Eastern Asia, especially in China. Although the global targets were met, sub-Saharan Africa and Oceana did not meet the targets. Despite not meeting the goals, these two regions have seen a notable increase in access to improved water sources.

The MDG target for sanitation has not been nearly as successful as the target for water. Between 1990 and 2015, the percentage of the world population with access to improved sanitation facilities increased from 54 percent to 68 percent (UNICEF & WHO, 2015). The increase is significant and indicates that a large number of individuals now have access to improved sanitation facilities, but the explicit MDG target has not been met. More than 2.4 billion people worldwide still lack access to adequate sanitation facilities, and nearly 1 billion of those people are still practicing open defecation.

The claimed MDG successes did not come without some controversy, which is well summarized by Fehling, Nelson, and Venkatapuram (2013). First, the MDGs were established with relatively little input from the countries at the focus of the goals (sometimes referred to as "developing countries"). Second, the regional variation in successes indicated earlier may paint a more optimistic picture than the reality in certain parts of the world. Third, the establishment of eight separate goals ignores the important interconnectedness among goals. Fourth, the goal related to environmental challenges, which includes water and sanitation, was seen as not being robust enough to encompass the importance of the topic. Many other criticisms have been levied on the MDGs, and the UN has attempted to address the concerns in their post-2015 agenda.

Sustainable Development Goals To continue with the successes of the MDGs and to address their shortcomings, new goals and targets for water and sanitation were established in 2015 in the form of the Sustainable Development Goals (SDGs). Whereas the MDGs included only eight main goals, the SDGs established 17 goals with 169 targets. The sixth SDG is specifically related to water and water resources, and the goal is to "ensure availability and sustainable management of water and sanitation for all." SDG 6 includes six main targets and two subtargets, which are listed here (UN, 2015b).

Target 6.1: "By 2030, achieve universal and equitable access to safe and affordable drinking water for all"

Target 6.2: "By 2030, achieve access to adequate and equitable sanitation and hygiene for all and end open defecation, paying special attention to the needs of women and girls and those in vulnerable situations"

Target 6.3: "By 2030, improve water quality by reducing pollution, eliminating dumping and minimizing release of hazardous chemicals and materials, halving the proportion of untreated wastewater and increasing recycling and safe reuse globally"

Target 6.4: "By 2030, substantially increase water-use efficiency across all sectors and ensure sustainable withdrawals and supply of freshwater to address water scarcity and substantially reduce the number of people suffering from water scarcity"

Target 6.5: "By 2030, implement integrated water resources management at all levels, including through transboundary cooperation as appropriate"

Target 6.6: "By 2020, protect and restore water-related ecosystems, including mountains, forests, wetlands, rivers, aquifers and lakes"

Target 6.a: "By 2030, expand international cooperation and capacity-building support to developing countries in water- and sanitation-related activities and programs, including water harvesting, desalination, water efficiency, wastewater treatment, recycling and reuse technologies"

Target 6.b: "Support and strengthen the participation of local communities in improving water and sanitation management"

Target 6.1 and Target 6.2 are continuations of the MDGs. The other targets, however, are more specifically focused on the protection and appropriate use of existing water resources. As discussed earlier, this update is more consistent with the holistic approach of managing water for the protection of human health. More information about the SDGs can be found on at UN Water's website, www.unwater.org.

Current Challenges Facing Water and Sanitation

Despite the successes of recent initiatives to address the water and sanitation shortcomings around the world, many challenges still exist. The challenges include the gender disparities associated with water and sanitation, the inadequacy of studies related to water and sanitation, the gap in applicability of current water technologies, forced migration, rapid urbanization, and climate change. These challenges will define the future of the work required to improve global health related to water and sanitation.

Gender Disparities in Water and Sanitation The first major challenge that has been and continues to be an issue for the improvement of global health associated with water and sanitation is the gender disparity that exists within the water and sanitation realm. The most visible example, noted earlier, is the disproportionate burden placed on women in collecting water for household use. Households need water, and women are more likely to be tasked with collecting it. Carrying large volumes of water over long distances for long periods of time can cause musculoskeletal issues. Further, the time and energy spent collecting water (and firewood for boiling water) is time taken away from other tasks, such as education or work.

The less visible challenges that disproportionately affect women are related to sanitation, hygiene, and water access. Insufficient access to hygiene resources and facilities for young women during menstruation can lead to increased absenteeism in school (Jewitt & Ryley, 2014). Missing many days of school can cause young women to fall behind in their studies, which can have significant negative impacts on their future educational and occupational opportunities. In addition, when the water and sanitation facilities are located far from school or home, women are exposed to sexual harassment and assault. These factors can cause psychosocial distress for women who lack access to sufficient water resources (Stevenson et al., 2012), and the social factors associated with water and sanitation as they specifically relate to women must be considered in all future efforts.

Applicability of Current Technologies Another major challenge related to water and sanitation is the gap in applicability of current water technologies. In US communities and in some cities around the world, water and sanitation coverage is typically addressed by using large, piped infrastructure to serve individuals at the household level. Although the systems are extremely effective, they present many challenges. First, the initial investment associated with large water and sanitation infrastructure is extremely high. Second, the maintenance of the systems is costly and complex. Third, the funding and operation of large infrastructure projects rely on federal, state, and community organizational and taxing structures to ensure the continued operation of the infrastructure.

The large, centralized systems work well in areas with a broad and prosperous tax base, but the high implementation and maintenance costs are not currently practical for lower-income communities throughout the world. Also, the large infrastructure is not as applicable to rural areas with dispersed populations. Because the majority of the individuals living without adequate access to water and sanitation reside in rural areas, an alternative model for water supply, treatment, and distribution must be developed. A description of the water supply issues facing rural communities is provided in case study 1 (Box 8.1).

BOX 8.1

CASE STUDY 1: WATER SYSTEM IN CALABAZAL, PANAMA

KEVIN ORNER

It was 8 a.m. when I pulled open my wooden bamboo door and greeted the chickens and roosters who had been making noise for the past hour. My morning routine consisted of getting water from the tap and cooking oatmeal on my propane stove. I rotated the red water faucet outside at the tap counterclockwise, but nothing came out. There must not be a lot of water at the spring. This was often the case during the dry season from January to April in Panama, as the heavy rains of October and November were long gone, replaced in the dry summer months by weeks of sun.

The water system in Calabazal, an indigenous community in western Panama, consisted of a spring box to capture water leaving a small spring on the edge of the community and PVC pipe that transported the water from the spring to a collection tank and then to the thirty household taps spread throughout the community. After a fifteen-minute hike to the spring, I figured out why the tap had no water. The water was exiting from a spring 11 meters uphill from where a concrete spring box was constructed years ago. It is likely that the spring box was constructed during the rainy season, when water fell abundantly, and small streams of water covered most of the hill. Now, the water fell slowly from the trickling spring down the hill, around the existing spring box, and into the nearby river, while the pipe running to the community for their water supply lay empty.

I walked down the hill past the grassy soccer area in the center of the community to the tin-roofed house of the current water committee president, Jose. Each small community usually has its own small water system; the system was maintained through the water committee. The committee voted each year for a president, vice president, treasurer, secretary, and two spokespeople. The committee was in charge of hosting regular meetings to collect the monthly water quota of $0.50 per family for maintenance of the system, roughly a tenth of a day's wage. During these meetings, the committee organized workdays to perform upkeep on the system and updated the community of any other news.

I found Jose behind the wall at the store attached to his house, where he sold beans, rice, coffee, sugar, and candy. I told him about the issue with the spring, and after making a trip together to the spring, we plotted our next move. There were a few options to fix the spring, but the most promising one was to contact the local Ministry of Environmental Health (MINSA). This would help the community build a relationship with the ministry and tap into their technical knowledge. A relationship with MINSA would serve the community long after my return home to the States. We decided the next step would be making a visit to the MINSA office in the nearby town of San Felix to see if someone there could fix the springbox.

MINSA in this region was severely understaffed: fewer than 10 workers were in charge of working with indigenous communities spread over both sides of the Cordillera mountain range. Accessing some communities would often mean a hike of over four hours or a long boat ride. Because of the inability of the workers to adequately serve all the communities in their region, the best way to receive help would be to contact MINSA directly and see when a worker would have an open date in his schedule.

To go to the MINSA office in San Felix, Jose and I hiked our normal 20-minute route over two rivers and two streams to the bus stop, where we hopped in the back of a pickup truck and traveled to San Felix. After discussing our spring box issue, the MINSA worker made an offer: if the community could provide sand and rock from the nearby river and raise $75 for the other supplies, MINSA would provide transportation for the materials and a MINSA worker to help for the two days of construction.

It is not easy to raise $75 when families often have several children who rely on the sporadic employment of the father, who could work at a nearby farm for around $6 a day. A creative solution emerged to raise the money: a party. A temporary wood and bamboo structure was built, speakers were borrowed, and caseloads of beer and chicha fuerte, a fermented corn drink, were bought. After the party, the committee had enough money for the supplies.

The water committee scheduled a workday and organized the community members. Three men hiked early in the morning 45 minutes down to the river, where they collected the sand and the rock. Two other members and I met the MINSA technical worker at his office in San Felix and drove with the worker to the members gathering sand and rock by the river. The sand and rock were loaded into the truck, and we piled in and drove back to Calabazal. However, the farthest point the truck could go was a

30-minute hike from the spring. We loaded horses' and men's backs with the heavy bags of sand and rock and hauled them to the spring.

The construction of the spring box took place over the following two days. Wood forms were placed, concrete was poured, the PVC pipe was placed, and the new spring box was created that would now provide a permanent collection of water for the community in both the wet and dry seasons.

The opposite of the large-scale infrastructure model of water and wastewater treatment is small-scale groundwater wells, point-of-use water treatment, and disconnected household-level sanitation facilities. Small-scale groundwater wells are currently found throughout rural areas in the United States, and they typically provide safe and adequate water to many millions of people. The strategy can be implemented throughout the world, although care must be taken to ensure that the water originating from the groundwater wells is safe for human contact and consumption. **Point-of-use treatment systems** are technologies that treat small amounts of water for use in the home. They are very advantageous in situations where only polluted surface or groundwater is available. Disconnected household-level sanitation facilities are facilities that serve a single household and are not connected to a formal sewer system. If properly designed and constructed, the systems can safely serve a household's sanitation needs.

In recent years, implementation of these technologies has become more common. The goal of the point-of-use and household-level models is to address the water and sanitation needs of individuals who do not have access to the large, centralized systems described previously. The technologies have limitations, however. First, a large number of these technologies are developed in Western counties without direct consultation with the individuals who will actually be using the technologies. Examples of these types of technologies include complex household water filtration technologies and complicated biogas-generating composting toilets. As a result, the technologies tend to be poorly understood, expensive, and difficult to use. Second, many point-of-use technologies require perfect adherence for every single use in order to be effective. The technologies therefore require a high level of education and training upon implementation to ensure proper use. Third, many of the point-of-use systems have components that must be replaced on a semiregular basis. Replaceable parts require an ability and willingness to pay, a thorough understanding of the replacement procedure, and a well-organized supply chain to ensure that the consumable parts are available at all times. Although these challenges to point-of-use water and household-level sanitation efforts can be overcome, they present significant barriers that have led to the poor long-term success of many projects. Therefore, the point-of-use treatment systems need to be applied with caution, and they are unlikely to be a long-term solution to the water and sanitation needs.

Forced Migration Another major issue that confronts water and sanitation coverage is the forced migration of individuals. Forced migration occurs when people are forced to flee their homes to "escape persecution, conflict, repression, natural and human-made disasters, ecological degradation, or other situations that endanger their lives, freedom, or livelihood" (International Organization for Migration, 2000). In 2015, the United Nations High Commissioner for Refugees (2015) estimated that over 65 million people in the world were forcibly displaced from their homes. As a whole, that represents approximately 1 out of every 113 people in the world who are currently displaced.

When people are forced to leave their established communities, they must seek out refuge in other areas. The rapid influx of individuals to a new area places extreme strain on water, sanitation, and health care infrastructure. The construction of new infrastructure requires time, money, and coordinated efforts. In the interim period before adequate water and sanitation provisions can be provided, water-related diseases among refugee populations are likely to increase. Case study 2 (Box 8.2) examines the water supply situation at the Nyarugusu refugee camp, Tanzania.

BOX 8.2

CASE STUDY 2: NYARUGUSU REFUGEE CAMP—THE CHALLENGES AND COMPLEXITIES OF ENGINEERING IN AN UNFAMILIAR SETTING

ERIC HETTLER

When I was living in Tanzania, I was asked to provide technical training and technical assistance to a group of engineers working at the Nyarugusu refugee camp in the western part of the country. The camp was initially established in the late 1990s to accommodate refugees fleeing from civil war in the Democratic Republic of Congo (DRC). In the early 2000s, the camp also began to receive refugees fleeing from unrest in Burundi.

When I arrived at the camp in early 2014, its population had momentarily stabilized. Many of the remaining refugees were from the DRC and had lost everything in their home countries during the constant unrest. For many, returning to their country was not an option, and they essentially had become permanent residents of the camp. The long-term settlement of populations is not a goal of refugee camps, but it can become a reality when conflicts are protracted. In fact, a number of the younger teenagers I met in the camp were born and raised entirely within the confines of the camp.

The population of the camp when I arrived was approximately 70,000, and access to water was a major consideration and challenge. Water was distributed throughout the camp from large water storage tanks that received pumped water from nearby surface water sources. Given the high demand for water, the water available from the taps was intermittent, irregular, and often insufficient to meet the needs of the population. As a result, individuals waited in long queues for water, and they often were not able to collect enough water to serve the needs of their family.

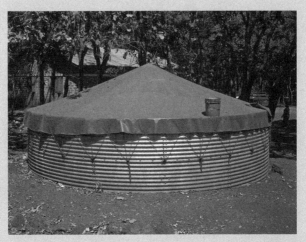

The primary goal of my involvement was to determine improvements that could be made to the system to alleviate the challenges with water quantity and water availability. When I first started working on the task, I was confident that I had the technical training and experience necessary to provide meaningful assistance. Further, I was collaborating with a team of very skilled local engineers who fully understood the water distribution system in the camp.

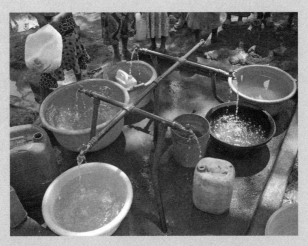

Before a five-day site visit to the camp, I prepared materials for a multiday workshop to train the local engineers in the use of a freely available water distribution modeling software. I figured that if we could model the details of the water distribution system, we could see where the improvements needed to be made. When I first arrived at the field office located just outside the camp, one of the engineers made a very direct statement. He said, "I really hope this is not like the last group of technical experts who came. They came for a week, talked about all these grand ideas, left, and we never heard from them again." Having lived in East Africa for almost two years at that point, I was well aware of this problematic dynamic. I was sure my workshop would be different.

Within the first few hours of my presentation, it became pretty clear that I had misjudged the complexity of the issues in the camp. Similar to many engineers, I have a tendency to latch on to the interesting technical aspects of a project and fail to see the larger picture. I was sure the fancy software would help identify the issues. What I failed to realize, however, was that these local engineers who worked in the camp every day already knew where the key issues in the system were located; they just lacked the approval and resources to make the changes needed. In addition, the computer model I was proposing requires very precise information about the system layout, pipe sizes, water demand, elevation, and so on. This information was not readily available, so my efforts to create a computer model of the system were doomed from the start.

After recognizing my shortcomings, I shifted my focus away from the computer modeling and toward visiting the camp and assessing the system. I attended a few fairly productive meetings, but ultimately the engineers were pulled away from their regular and important tasks to essentially babysit me and walk me through the system. I assured them that I would build the computer model for them if I received the appropriate information. After I returned to Dar es Salaam after the trip, however, the communication slowly fizzled. The team of engineers in the field saw what I failed to see: spending the time to build a computer model was not the most pressing issue they faced. In the end, I had become another "technical expert" who showed up for a week, presented some big ambitious ideas, left, and was never heard from again.

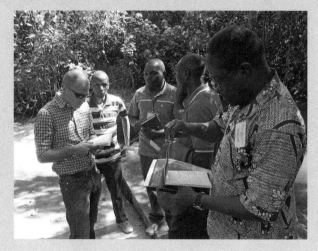

One of the key principles of engineering is to first do no harm. It could be argued that I technically did not do any material harm because I provided some suggestions on how to improve the system, and I did not recommend anything that would cause major water shortages or water contamination issues. The reality is, though, I did do harm. By arriving relatively unprepared with ideas that were not necessary or realistic, I was unable to meet the ultimate goals of my participation. In addition to that, my involvement provided false hopes that something would change. Everyone was initially very excited about what I might offer, but that excitement quickly dwindled. My travels, which were funded by the organization, used precious resources that could have been better spent elsewhere. Further, I had reinforced the idea that outside experts are unreliable, self-serving, and unhelpful.

Although my efforts were unsuccessful, I still feel that the lessons I learned through this experience were valuable. What could I have done differently? Here is a short, albeit incomplete, list of ideas:

1. From the outset, I should have coordinated directly with the engineers already living at or near the camp. Most of my communication was through the field office in Dar es Salaam, so I did not fully understand the extent of the problem and the potential solutions.
2. I should not have been so focused on using the latest and greatest technologies to characterize the issues of the camp. A fancy computer model with nice graphics would have been an interesting tool, but it was not entirely necessary. The resident engineers already had a good grasp of the key issues facing the water distribution system, and they did not need the model to confirm those ideas.
3. I should have spent my time at the camp observing and learning from the residents and the resident engineers rather than trying to lead a workshop. It is clear that I was not qualified to be leading a workshop for engineers who understood the system better than I did.
4. I should have considered the wider picture rather than solely focus on the technical and engineering details. The politics and funding at a refugee camp are extremely complex, and those complexities must be factored into any proposed engineering design.

After I left Tanzania, civil unrest in Burundi forced hundreds of thousands of people to flee their homes, and the population of the camp swelled to over 150,000 individuals. The water resource challenges were already difficult when the camp was at a relatively stable population of 70,000, and the conditions they must have faced during that time are unimaginable. Although it is unlikely that any amount of engineering expertise alone would fully alleviate those challenges in an emergency situation, I still look back at my inability to provide meaningful insights as the greatest failure of my engineering career.

Rapid Urbanization Another major challenge facing water and sanitation in the world is the large and rapid movement of individuals from rural to urban areas. As cities continue to grow, their existing water and sanitation infrastructure can become stressed. When infrastructure is stressed beyond its capacity, water shortages and untreated sewage discharges become more frequent. Also, when individuals from rural areas move to urban areas, it is not uncommon for them to settle in informal settlements on the outskirts of cities. These settlements generally lack well-planned and well-organized water and sanitation infrastructure.

The cost of establishing a formal and legal connection to the municipal water system in informal settlements can be prohibitively high for a household, so access to water is often controlled by only a few individuals. As a result, water is typically more expensive in lower-income informal settlements than it is in more wealthy developed sectors of the cities—an example of what economists call a "poverty tax." This high cost of water can have an impact on the amount of water available for sanitation and hygiene practices, which can increase the burden of disease. Similarly, extending sanitation coverage to informal settlements is commonly cost-prohibitive, so sewage and wastewater are not generally properly disposed. As cities continue to grow, the challenges facing inadequate water and sanitation supply will continue to intensify.

Climate Change Finally, one of the most daunting and unpredictable challenges related to water and sanitation is climate change. Climate change can have dramatically different effects on different parts of the world. The biggest threat associated with climate change and water and sanitation is an increased frequency both of droughts and of extreme weather events.

When an area experiences more frequent droughts, the availability of water ultimately decreases. As described in previous sections, adequate access to water quantity is extremely important for health because it facilitates adequate hygiene and sanitation. Also, as water sources dry up, individuals must travel farther to access the same amount of water. The increased time and effort required to collect water can negatively impact the economic development of a community.

More frequent extreme rainfall events causing flooding are also a major cause for concern. The acute consequences of extreme rainfall events and flooding include drowning and the destruction of infrastructure. Destruction of infrastructure requires communities to reinvest in rebuilding; as a result, money focused on improving water and sanitation facilities is decreased. In addition, critical water infrastructure, such as pipes, boreholes, and protected springs, can be destroyed during massive flooding events.

Flooding also causes lingering issues related to health. Water-related diseases have been shown to drastically increase after major flooding events. First, water-borne diseases may become more common when sewage and other contaminants are washed into water sources. Second, water-washed diseases may increase when critical water infrastructure is destroyed and water supply after the flood decreases. Third, water-based diseases may increase when water sources that were once free of the insects causing water-based diseases are contaminated from other water sources. Finally, lingering pools of water provide additional breeding habitat for water-related insect vectors. The increase of these water-based diseases after floods can have significant negative health impacts for the affected communities.

Chapter Summary

Water, sanitation, and hygiene are all critical to global health. These complex issues encompass a variety of challenges that require thoughtful and multidisciplinary approaches. Programs and initiatives in the past few decades have made considerable progress in reducing the number of individuals living without access to adequate water and sanitation. Nonetheless, many challenges related to water technology, forced migration, rapid urbanization, and climate change still remain. A concerted global effort that focuses on the needs and desires of communities must be continued to ensure that every person in the world has access to adequate water, sanitation, and hygiene.

Key Terms

Germ theory of disease
Hygiene
Improved sanitation facility
Improved water source
Point-of-use treatment system
Water-based disease
Water-borne disease
Water-related insect vector diseases
Water resources
Water-washed disease

Review Questions

1. Explain how the four components of water, sanitation, and hygiene are related to one another.
2. Summarize the four functional categories of water-related diseases. Using a rural area lacking access to water and sanitation coverage as an example, brainstorm some potential solutions that could address all four functional categories of water-related diseases.

3. The Millennium Development Goal (MDG) target for water supply was achieved, but the target for sanitation has still not been met. Why do you think the increase in access to improved sanitation facilities has lagged behind the increase in access to improved water sources?

4. The Sustainable Development Goals (SDGs) expanded on the successes of the MDGs, and the goals and targets for the SDGs are more numerous than the goals and targets for the MDGs. What are some advantages of the increased number of targets and goals, especially related to water and sanitation? What are some of the disadvantages?

5. Describe policies that are not directly related to water and sanitation coverage that would have an impact on water, sanitation, hygiene, and health.

Suggested Reading

Evaluating Household Water Treatment Options: Health-based Targets and Microbiological Performance Specifications, distributed by WHO. Free download available at http://www.who.int/water_sanitation_health/publications/2011/evaluating_water_treatment.pdf

Field Guide to Environmental Engineering for Development Workers, by J. R. Mihelcic, L. M. Fry, E. A Myre, L. D. Phillips, and B. Barkdoll. Distributed by ASCE Press.

Global Issues in Water, Sanitation, and Health: Workshop Summary, by E. R. Choffnes and A. Mack. Free download available at http://www.nap.edu/catalog/12658/global-issues-in-water-sanitation-and-health-workshop-summary

Progress on Sanitation and Drinking Water—2015 Update and MDG Assessment, distributed by UNICEF and WHO. Free download available at http://www.wssinfo.org

Unbowed: A Memoir, by W. Maathai. Knopf, 2006.

UNICEF Handbook on Water Quality, distributed by UNICEF. Free download available at http://www.unicef.org/wash/files/WQ_Handbook_final_signed_16_April_2008.pdf

References

Campbell, S. J., Savage, G. B., Gray, D. J., Atkinson, J. M., Soares Magahaes, R. J., Nery, S. V., . . . Clements, A.C.A. (2014). Water, sanitation, and hygiene (WASH): A critical component for sustainable soil-transmitted helminth and schistosomiasis control. *PLoS Neglected Tropical Diseases, 8*(4), e2651.

Carter Center. (2016). Guinea Worm Eradication Program. https://www.cartercenter.org/health/guinea_worm/

Choffnes, E. R., & Mack, A. (2009). *Global issues in water, sanitation, and health: Workshop summary.* Washington, DC: National Academies Press.

Fehling, M., Nelson, B. D., & Venkatapuram, S. (2013). Limitations of the Millennium Development Goals: A literature review. *Global Public Health, 8,* 1109–1122.

International Organization for Migration. (2000). *World migration report 2000.* New York, NY: United Nations.

Jewitt, S., & Ryley, H. (2014). It's a girl thing: Menstruation, school attendance, spatial mobility and wider gender inequalities in Kenya. *Geoforum, 56,* 137–147.

Stevenson, E. G., Greene, L. E, Maes, K. C., Ambelu, A., Tesfaye, Y. A., Rheingans, R., & Hadley, C. (2012). Water insecurity in 3 dimensions: An anthropological perspective on water and women's psychosocial distress in Ethiopia. *Social Science & Medicine, 75,* 392–400.

United Nations. (2015a). *The Millennium Development Goals report: 2015.* New York, NY: Author.

United Nations. (2015b). *Transforming our world: The 2030 Agenda for Sustainable Development.* New York, NY: Author.

United Nations Children's Fund. (2008). *UNICEF handbook on water quality.* New York, NY.

United Nations Children's Fund & World Health Organization. (2015). *Progress on sanitation and drinking water—2015 update and MDG assessment.* Retrieved from http://www.wssinfo.org/

United Nations High Commissioner for Refugees. (2015). *Global trends: Forced displacement in 2015.* Retrieved from http://www.unhcr.org/576408cd7

World Health Organization. (2015). *World health statistics 2015.* Retrieved from http://www.who.int/gho/publications/world_health_statistics/2015/en/

World Health Organization. (2016). Hygiene. Retrieved from http://www.who.int/topics/hygiene/en/

CHAPTER 9

FOOD, AGRICULTURE, AND NUTRITION

Michele Joseph Aquino, MS

A sustainable agriculture does not deplete soils or people.
—Wendell Berry

LEARNING OBJECTIVES

- Establish basic understanding of food system considerations
- Build core vocabulary related to human nutrition and agriculture
- Evaluate the current state of food scarcity
- Define the dimensions of food security

Chī le ma? Have you eaten yet? This is a common informal greeting, at least among some generations of Chinese. The phrase is rooted in days past, when food scarcity may have been more top of mind for some than it is today. It is a very relevant greeting to begin this chapter, in which we will explore foundational topics on food systems. By **food system**, we simply mean a collection of interconnected resources that produce and bring food to people. Most of us eat multiple times each day, so your response to this opening question may very well have been yes. If so, why did you eat, what did you consume, and where did that nourishment come from?

Thinking critically about questions like these can help build fluency for a future problem solver in this field. We must be able to connect the dots between physiological need for food, cultural norms surrounding diet, and the journey food takes from field to market. Of course, many people around the world would still respond to this opening question with *no*. Hunger and food scarcity remain a problem, even in relatively wealthy societies. This emphasizes the importance of continuing to work on food issues and

Foundations for Global Health Practice, First Edition. Lori DiPrete Brown.
© 2018 John Wiley & Sons, Inc. Published 2018 by John Wiley & Sons, Inc.

why we are discussing food security in the context of global health and development. **Food security** is defined as reliable access to a sufficient quantity of affordable, nutritious food. We will briefly explore our capacity to grow enough food and challenges to equitable distribution of that food, such as food waste. This chapter will also build some basic agricultural literacy while exploring how food and nutrition are interconnected with the health topics discussed throughout the rest of this book. The ideas presented here aim to help prepare global health professionals to (1) analyze food policies and (2) make culturally appropriate decisions about potential food security interventions in the communities they serve.

Global Food System, Local Solutions

Massive quantities of foods are grown, traded, and wasted around the world. In 2016, the Food and Agriculture Organization of the United Nations (FAO) forecast total cereal production at approximately 5.6 trillion pounds, which would equal just over two pounds per day for each of the world's 7.4 billion people—and that is just cereal crops (Food and Agriculture Organization of the United Nations [FAO], 2016b; United Nations [UN], 2015b). With so much food production, why is there still hunger? Of course, not all of that food is available at once (there are crop seasons), nor are those grains equally distributed around the globe. Before discussing nutrition and food security, let's first look upstream at the agricultural origins of our globe's diet. Going back to the farm level, we will see a myriad of crops, growing practices, and outcomes. Not surprisingly, the combination of those three factors (crops, growing practices, and outcomes) will be connected to geography and locally available resources. A small **subsistence farm** may aim to produce enough food for the same family that works the land. In contrast, a commercial farmer may choose to grow different crops that are valuable in the marketplace, perhaps because such cash crops cannot be grown efficiently in the geography where demand is strong (e.g., bananas grown for export to North America). For the former, the success of harvest will directly affect the amount of food available for the household. Harvest success or failure for a **commercial farm** will likely impact the farmers' available income for purchasing food in the marketplace.

Agricultural solutions should be implemented with consideration of such local realities as land availability, soil type and quality, seed availability, appropriate seed varieties, water, weather, labor, traditions, technology, and other economic factors. When designing and implementing sustainable development interventions related to agriculture, we must acknowledge the unique characteristics of the target region and market dynamics (i.e., trade), or we will increase the risk of unintended consequences and unsustainable programming. It cannot be emphasized enough that grassroots, bottom-up planning for food and nutrition interventions are often more responsible and sustainable because of the aforementioned cultural ties associated with farming and diet. Families plan many household routines around meals, and agrarian communities will have many traditions that can be difficult for a development professional, especially one from a different culture, to immediately comprehend. Something that adds value to one culture's food might be completely unappealing to another culture. Consider the example of introducing a new lettuce into a kitchen in a culture different from your own. Depending on the context, one cook in the kitchen may prefer to eat the leaves fresh, another may want to sauté. If it is not a cultural norm to eat such a plant, someone in the kitchen might think the food is better suited for farm animals. Collaboration and coplanning alongside all community stakeholders should be considered a prerequisite for success with food security interventions, especially when adaptation is necessary to encourage new practices or new foods. Let's now consider the diverse set of growing practices in the world and then think critically about how farming styles might influence health through the different dimensions of food security.

The Farm Spectrum

It is helpful to think about **agriculture** as a spectrum of practices that produce food, fiber, and fuel. **Food** refers to the agricultural products that people and animals eat (to differentiate, we refer to food for livestock as feed). **Fiber** can be thought of as the inedible agricultural commodities that become items such as cotton clothing or the paper used to print a book. **Fuel** refers to products that we burn for energy outside of our bodies, such as biomass for electricity or corn ethanol to power a vehicle.

On the far left of the agriculture spectrum (see Figure 9.1) we have small, low-to-no synthetic input, **extensive agriculture**. On the far right are large, high-input, **intensive agricultural** practices. The connotation around various farming methods may be interpreted differently by region and culture. "Small and local" in the United States might produce farmers' market vegetables for relatively wealthy urban consumers, but the small end of the spectrum might also describe a **smallholder** farming family in rural Central America attempting to grow sufficient maize (corn) and beans to eat throughout the year. The large-scale systems will more often be associated with **monocultures** (the planting of one or few crop types); high **productivity** (the amount of food or food energy/calories produced per area of land); and heavier use of agricultural technology, including chemical inputs, improved seed varieties, precision irrigation, and machinery. Dr. Paul B. Thompson of Michigan State University has described these contrasting farming styles in terms of two philosophies, "agrarian" and "industrial" (Thompson, 2010; National Research Council, 2010).

At both ends of the spectrum, we can find both beneficial and problematic examples of growing practices for food, fiber, and fuel. There are also farming techniques

FIGURE 9.1   The Agricultural Spectrum, a Generalized View of Farming Systems

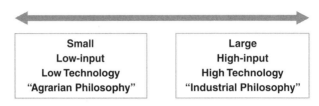

| Small
Low-input
Low Technology
"Agrarian Philosophy" | Large
High-input
High Technology
"Industrial Philosophy" |

Note: Agrarian and industrial philosophies adapted from Thompson, 2010.

that fall all along the middle of the spectrum. It is likely that some viable solutions to the world's agricultural dilemmas exist in this middle ground; however, good outcomes are rarely achieved without some trade-offs. The techniques implemented across the agriculture spectrum should not be thought of as good or bad at face value. It is not always clear what type of system is "best."

The purpose of including a primer on agriculture in a global public health text is to link the growing of food with human livelihoods. With that in mind, it is worth noting two specific concepts that fall along the farming spectrum and offer unique benefits to people and planet. First, "kitchen scale" home gardening should be mentioned because of its potential to positively affect household food supply. Numerous food security and international development organizations have embraced this means of increasing self-reliance and diversified food production. (One such organization is highlighted later in this chapter.) In his book *Square Foot Gardening*, gardener Mel Bartholomew describes the potential: in a single 16-square-foot area, with proper technique and adequate resources, a family could harvest around 12 different varieties of healthful vegetables over a two-month period. Another alternative concept found along the agricultural spectrum is soil management through intensive, rotational grazing. In this context, *intensive* refers not to heavy use of synthetic inputs but to systematic use of livestock to cycle nutrients into the soil. We recommend reading further on this topic. (See the book by Allan Savory in the recommended reading section.)

BOX 9.1
THE FARM AS A SYSTEM

Advancing sustainability in agriculture may be achieved, in part, by considering each farm system that depends heavily on various ecological services. Donella Meadows (2008), author of *Thinking in Systems*, defines a system as "an interconnected set of elements that is coherently organized in a way that achieves something" (p. 11). For a farm, that "something" to be achieved could be a crop harvest that meets expectations of feeding the people or livestock reliant on that farm's output. When one is designing projects aimed at increasing the success rate of achieving that outcome, consideration should be given to each of the farm's interconnected elements, including the crops selected, soil, soil microbial life, insect populations, and water. Changing the farm's management practices or using a new tool (such as a chemical pesticide) might achieve a desired outcome, but at some cost (and/or benefit) to other parts of the system.

For a practical systems example, consider the dung beetle (Bertone et al., 2016; Hammer et al., 2016). In some grazing cattle herds, a farmer may observe signs of worms in the cattle and opt for a parasiticide deworming treatment. However, such treatments may also decrease dung beetle populations in the pastures. This scenario is an example of an effective pesticide possibly damaging beneficial living organisms in addition to reducing the target pest. In this case, dung beetles are helpful in the grazed livestock system; they help control the spread of parasite larvae that become the worms that the medicine aims to treat. The beetles also promote nutrient cycling by facilitating the decomposition of the manure left behind by cows. The faster the manure decomposes, the less time there is for manure to breed flies, which cause stress to the livestock.

The dung beetle example illustrates that the addition of a new element to a farm system is often not achieved without affecting other parts of the system. Some farmers might focus more on preventive measures or separation of an infected animal from the herd rather than sacrificing the dung beetle

Historical Context

Understanding how we arrived at the agricultural spectrum described earlier would certainly be a story for a book of its own. However, some introductory knowledge related to the use of agricultural inputs (e.g., fertilizer) and **the Green Revolution** provides helpful context for exploring the current state of farming.

As various fields of physical science progressed through the 19th century, we gained a better understanding of how plants grow and how to control growth. Just as our bodies need nutrition, so do the plants grown to feed us. As described by Vaclav Smil (2001) in *Enriching the Earth*, cultivating food depends on plants' assimilating key nutrients, such as nitrogen, found in the soil where they grow. Smil describes how increasingly dense populations led to intensification of agriculture, or growing more food per area of land. Traditional methods of replenishing soil nutrition, such as application of manures and returning plant materials to the earth, were eventually replaced or supplemented with new forms of fertilizer, thus ushering in an era of newfound agricultural scale.

In the latter half of the 20th century, improved agricultural practices went global—bringing improved crop varieties, fertilizer, pesticide, and irrigation to many parts of the developing world. This Green Revolution is widely associated with the improved varieties of wheat and rice introduced by 1970 Nobel Peace Prize laureate Norman Borlaug. Spreading from research programs in Mexico to many parts of Asia (but not as successfully in Africa), the Green Revolution techniques greatly increased crops yields and food self-sufficiency for struggling regions (Smil, 2001; "Norman Borlaug—facts," 2016). Economist Jeffrey Sachs (2008) explains that such improved agricultural productivity for a nation whose "core livelihood" is farming can be an integral step in pulling that nation out of a "poverty trap." However, history has shown that, in some communities and geographies, Green Revolution practices were not as sustainable by today's standards as they were beneficial from a production standpoint (Sachs, 2008). Heavy reliance on chemical inputs, mechanized farming, and rapid extraction of water for irrigating crops certainly cannot be sustained in some agricultural communities.

Moving forward, the need to tackle agricultural production constraints remains as the population continues to grow. The call to action after the 2012 UN Conference on Sustainable Development in Rio (Rio+20) was, "End hunger and make the transition to sustainable agricultural and food systems" (Food and Agriculture Organization [FAO], 2012). The tools of the "new" Green Revolution include more precise use of water to achieve what Sachs (2008) calls "more crop per drop," more judicious use of agricultural chemicals, and more focus on environmental resiliency (FAO, 1996). We will also see that, in light of two worldwide problems, obesity and food waste, some organizations are promoting initiatives to influence food consumption behaviors in parallel with the ongoing efforts to grow more food.

Our Bodies Need Food: Nutrition Basics

We all share a basic reason for eating: our body's need to extract nutrients and calories from foods. A calorie is a unit of heat measurement that is used to quantify the energy derived from foods. Food energy may also be expressed using the International System of Units, or SI units, as joules (J). It is generally accepted that in the context of nutrition, the food calorie is understood to represent one kilocalorie (kcal). This represents a relatively straightforward physiological connection between food and health—a mix of macro- and micronutrients is necessary to thrive in daily life. **Macronutrients** are the fats, proteins, and carbohydrates that provide the energy that our bodies require. Proteins, which serve a variety of invaluable metabolic functions in the body, are worth noting because of how they vary in quality by dietary source and because diets worldwide are shifting toward more animal-based protein sources (meat and dairy) (WRI, 2016; Smil, 2013). Proteins are made of smaller building blocks called **amino acids**, some of which are not produced by the body and therefore must be consumed in our diets; these are classified as the *essential* amino acids (Gropper, Smith, & Groff, 2005). Plant and animal protein sources vary in composition based on amino acid profiles. Animal food diets and traditional diets based on legumes, rice, and corn will typically provide more balanced proteins compared to diets based on crops such as wheat and some root crops (Smil, 2001; Lappé & Collins, 1977). **Micronutrients** refer to the vitamins and minerals that facilitate the body's metabolic processes, in some cases aiding the transfer of energy from macronutrients to a form that is biologically available to help the body function.

There are two primary types of malnutrition, described by the FAO (2014) as undernourishment and undernutrition. **Undernourishment** is summarized as a calorie problem—the inability to secure enough food to derive sufficient energy from the diet. **Undernutrition** should be thought of as a micronutrient deficiency. Rather than not enough food, the root-cause issue is likely either consumption of the wrong types of foods (usually a lack of access to diversity of foods), or disease preventing the body's utilization of the nutrients contained in the foods. Sometimes referred to as *hidden hunger,* undernutrition can be present even in regions where food access does not appear to be challenging. For example, food deserts—areas in which access to healthy, fresh foods is limited—are a common problem in urban areas of the United States. Multiple socio-economic factors have led to food deserts, often characterized by lower income, lower transportation access, and corner-store food shopping with disproportionate availability of processed foods relative to fresh offerings. These conditions also lead to another of today's global health challenges, **overnutrition**, which is leading to a growing number of people around the world who are overweight or obese, or carrying excess body fat. This nutritional imbalance can lead to poor health outcomes and can increase risk for chronic diseases such as diabetes and heart disease (World Health Organization [WHO], 2016b). This problem was once considered a "developed world" issue, but now the FAO reports that occurrence of overnutrition is on the rise worldwide. In the next section, we will discuss food scarcity and briefly revisit obesity with regard to shifting diets. As you read, consider the societal and community-level factors that shape diet and influence the nutrition outcomes described here.

Introduction to Food Security

Food Security Defined

As a framework for understanding and evaluating how food systems impact nutrition, we will now outline the dimensions of food security. Recently, the United Nations (UN) reaffirmed the call to action to solve the world's problems of food security. As of January 2016, the UN continued its international development efforts under the Sustainable Development Goals (SDGs), which set development targets for the next 15 years. The SDGs generally aim to tackle poverty alleviation and ensure well-being of both people and planet. Hunger and food security are covered by SDG 22: "End hunger, achieve food security and improved nutrition and promote sustainable agriculture" (UN, 2015a). Echoing this multilateral call to action, the US Global Food Security Act of 2016 authorizes a robust strategy for continued foreign food security assistance through such programs as the US Agency for International Development's Feed the Future program.

Various definitions of food security have been put forth by different development organizations through the years (FAO, 2003). The World Food Programme (WFP, 2016) defines people as food secure "when they have available access at all times to sufficient, safe, nutritious food to maintain a healthy and active life." The food security of an individual, family, or community is typically discussed in the context of stable food availability, access, and utilization (FAO, 2008). Frequently, food security is part of the broader topic of poverty alleviation because poverty is often associated with malnutrition. Consider a landless family that may experience low food availability because they cannot grow enough food. They may also lack steady income to access food grown by others. However, financial instability is not the only driver of food insecurity. Some people lack food because of political conflicts, weather events, and price volatility; of which the latter two are interconnected to problems of climate change (FAO, 2014, 2016a).

Availability. Food availability refers to the physical quantity present in an area, whether the area in question is an individual village, a country, or a region. Assessment of availability involves determining the area's capacity to procure and store sufficient stocks of foods, whether procurement involves growing locally, trading, food assistance, or some combination of the three. Availability is most connected to the evaluation of whether or not agriculture is producing enough food, but it also encompasses the quality or types of food produced (FAO, 2014).

Access. Just because food may be available for the population in question, it does not mean that everyone will be able to access sufficient quantities of that food. Does a family have the economic means to purchase or trade to bring that food home? Access is often synonymous with purchasing power (CIRAD, 2016). Access may also involve physical infrastructure constraints that impede food from reaching groups of people in need (FAO, 2014).

Utilization. Once food is acquired, a household must process (cook), store, and consume it in a fashion that allows the nutrients within the food to be absorbed by the body. Does a household have the knowledge to prepare the available food in a healthy way before it spoils? Is the food that has come into the household safe—free of contamination or pathogens? Public health organizations must not only concern themselves with whether or not sufficient quantities of food exist but also work on community health factors which ensure that a person is healthy enough for their body to properly receive food when it is available.

An underlying factor in the utilization of nutritionally balanced food is the requirement for food (and water) to be clean and free of pathogens. Food-borne illness can cause both acute discomfort and chronic malabsorption of nutrients, as is the case for many of the 760,000 children under five years old who die each year from diarrhea (WHO, 2016a). Therefore, in tackling food security through the lens of public health, one must consider not only the agricultural origin but also the entire **value chain**, which includes storage and processing steps that could contaminate foods before consumption.

Elusive Food Stability

Do we produce enough food? The question is not a new one, and policymakers have been pondering the root causes of food scarcity for many years. There are countless reasons for the persistence of hunger, and we will not be able in this chapter to sufficiently answer the question of *why* food scarcity still exists. Frances Moore Lappé and Joseph Collins (authors of food policy books including *Food First*, 1977) have written about unjust distribution of "productive assets"—the tools and land needed to produce. Countless organizations have identified insufficient productivity as a root cause. It is true that **yield gaps**, or disparities in the amount harvested on any given area of land versus what could potentially be harvested, remain between some developing and developed nations. Researchers have found a relevant example of this cause by looking at women in agriculture. In some developing nations, up to one fifth of the agricultural landowners may be women, but they use markedly less synthetic fertilizer (and have lower yields). One reason for this may be disparate access to agricultural extension resources (education) and financial tools (credit)(FAO, 2011b; OECD, 2012). This example also demonstrates the complexity of food scarcity—root causes may be biological, economic, political, cultural, or any combination of such factors. We challenge you to become an innovative systems thinker in this field so that, project by project, new advances in food systems work can enrich lives through improved access to nutritious diets. Often such solutions need to be tailored to local conditions rather than based on one-size-fits-all thinking.

According to the FAO, over 800 million people worldwide were estimated to have experienced chronic undernourishment between 2012 and 2014. Although the undernourished portion of our population has fallen by over 200 million since the 1990s, the problem persists as global population continues to grow (FAO, 2013, 2014). In a business-as-usual projection, assuming no major changes to current policies and food security programs, the FAO (2015) estimates that over 650 million people will still be undernourished in 2030. The World Resources Institute (WRI, 2016) projects a need for 70% more calories to be grown between 2006 levels and anticipated caloric needs in 2050—and by that time, around two thirds of the 10 billion people projected to be living on the planet will live in cities. This projection implies that (1) even fewer people will be involved in producing food, and (2) diets will continue to shift. "As nations urbanize and citizens become wealthier, people generally increase their calorie intake and the share of resource-intensive foods—such as meats and dairy—in their diets" (p. 1).

We should consider how socioeconomic shifts and agricultural trade policies affect how nations eat. For example, Turkey is a country with a growing GDP and an urbanizing populace. Increased wealth, changing lifestyles, and more women working outside the home appear to be influencing eating behaviors. The US Department of Agriculture (USDA) Foreign Agricultural Service notes increased consumption of food outside the home and more purchases of processed convenience foods (Atalaysun, 2016). Mexico has been identified by some as an example of how trade policy creates side effects. In their article "Exporting Obesity," Sarah Clark and colleagues (2012) propose that commodity and processed food exports from the United States to Mexico under the North American Free Trade Agreement (NAFTA) provide data relevant to how policy can influence food systems and health outcomes, such as obesity.

BOX 9.2

AGRICULTURAL TRADE: WHAT'S AHEAD FOR CUBA?

As critics will point out, the United States has an unsavory history related to some rice exports as food aid. Maura O'Connor (2013) highlights this in her article "Subsidizing Starvation," in which she describes how imports of rice from a subsidized production system (the United States) to a nation like Haiti can have the unintended consequence of pricing Haitian rice farmers out of the marketplace. In recent years, former president Bill Clinton has acknowledged that such well-intended policy actions were indeed detrimental and that food self-sufficiency in developing countries should have been emphasized more ("We Made a Devil's Bargain," 2010). In recent years, we have seen softening of US policies against Cuba, and, in the summer of 2016, the state of Missouri donated 20 tons of rice to the island nation. Is such a donation setting a good precedent? As diplomatic relations continue to evolve between the two countries, Cuban policymakers should consider the long-run implications of such aid for the island's food system.

After the nation's revolution in the 1950s, Cuba experienced growing pains of land reform (redistribution of productive resources). The state took control of the majority of farmland, and the country shifted away from sugar to a more diversified portfolio of food crops (Lappé & Collins, 1977). Between US embargoes and trade benefits that ended along with the Cold War, Cuba has largely operated on low-input agriculture for decades (Severson, 2016). With changing policies toward Cuba under the Obama administration, the island nation appears to be nearing a crossroads: should they allow big agribusiness to enter, or should they go organic? Which style of agriculture would benefit the people, the economy, and the land the most? Leading proponents of the organic movement in the United States see an opportunity to leverage Cuban land for production of certified organic crops. Philosophically, those leaders would argue that Cuba should open up its agriculture marketplace in a way that promotes organic growing practices. Of course, some conventional agribusiness companies also see opportunity. Perhaps farmers and policymakers will soon need to make decisions that influence what mix of growing practices exist in the country to balance economic, environmental, and food security benefits.

Now consider the following 10 Principles for Responsible Investment in Agriculture and Food Systems, published by the FAO's Committee on World Food Security (CFS, 2014). Think about how these principles relate to the Cuban situation we've described.

Principle 1: Contribute to food security and nutrition

Principle 2: Contribute to sustainable and inclusive economic development and the eradication of poverty

Principle 3: Foster gender equality and women's empowerment

Principle 4: Engage and empower youth

Principle 5: Respect tenure of land, fisheries, and forests, and access to water

Principle 6: Conserve and sustainably manage natural resources, increase resilience, and reduce disaster risks

Principle 7: Respect cultural heritage and traditional knowledge, and support diversity and innovation

Principle 8: Promote safe and healthy agriculture and food systems

Principle 9: Incorporate inclusive and transparent governance structures, processes, and grievance mechanisms

Principle 10: Assess and address impacts and promote accountability

The USDA National Organic Program (7 CFR §205.2, n.d.) defines organic production as an approach that accounts for local "conditions by integrating cultural, biological, and mechanical practices that foster cycling of resources, promote ecological balance, and conserve biodiversity." The USDA (2015) also estimates that Cuba imports the majority of its food. Moving into the future, it is worth evaluating: Would the Cuban government and trade partners be champions of the CFS principles if they promoted a system of widespread organic agriculture? Does conventional agriculture, using modern techniques and precision technology, have a place? Perhaps the solution is a mix of these two farming methodologies.

Historically, the conversation has emphasized agricultural production shortfalls, noting sizable yield gaps between developed and developing economies. As mentioned, the technologies transferred during the Green Revolution succeeded in boosting yields (not without some environmental trade-offs), but this did not eliminate hunger. However, as mentioned at the beginning of this chapter, data show that we *do* grow enough food to feed the population. We *have* been able to grow food faster than our population has grown as we entered the 21st century (FAO, 2012). For decades, the world has produced sufficient amounts of food, despite some regions still failing to realize potential crop yields (Lappé & Collins, 1977; FAO, 2013). "For the world as a whole, per capita food supply rose from about 2,200 kcal/day in the early 1960s to more than 2,800 kcal/day by 2009" (FAO, 2013). The FAO sets the worldwide average daily energy requirement at 2,353 kcal.

As discussed, there is seemingly enough food on the planet, and research continues to explore how best to grow more. As well, disparities remain in how that food is distributed around the globe. If we accept the premise that there are limited agricultural resources (i.e., land) and those resources remain unevenly distributed, then looking at better utilization of what we do produce seems logical. For this reason, numerous multilateral government organizations and nongovernmental organizations (NGOs) are working on efficiencies in food chains downstream of the farm. *How can we waste less?*

Waste and Wealth

Excluding severe weather events and political conflicts, if hunger persists despite sufficient caloric production, targeting waste appears ripe with opportunity. The National Resource Defense Council reports that the United States wastes approximately 40% of its food, along with the productive resources used to bring that food to market (Gunders, 2012). Worldwide, the FAO estimates that one third, or 1.3 billion tons, of all food for human consumption are wasted. These organizations have looked at where the losses occur from "farm to fork," and the contrast between the developed and the developing world in terms of loss distribution provides insight into how to tailor food waste initiatives to local needs (see Figure 9.2). Speaking generally, the more developed economies tend to waste food once it reaches the consumer (such as extra vegetables expiring in the fridge). In the less developed regions of the world, the food waste is more prevalent closer to the farm; for example, grain may be exposed to the elements or pests in unimproved postharvest storage situations (Lipinski et al., 2013; FAO, 2011a). The waste problem has no easy solution. (One Acre Fund work in this area is mentioned later in the chapter, however.) Crops in most systems have a finite number of harvests in any given year. Following harvest, there is inevitably a large available supply that people will need to consume all throughout the time until the next harvest. Global trade, financial markets, food packaging, transportation infrastructure, and sophisticated storage techniques all serve a purpose in managing the postharvest supply glut, but disparate access to food and inefficiencies along supply chains remain.

Another proposal to address waste is to look at waste as (1) calories that people consume but do not *need* to thrive (i.e., overnutrition) and (2) calories that are

FIGURE 9.2   A Visualization of Food Losses throughout an Agricultural Value Chain

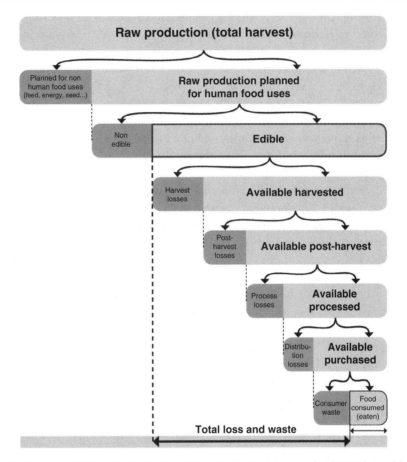

Source: *Food Losses and Waste in the Context of Sustainable Food Systems,* by the High Level Panel of Experts on Food Security and Nutrition, June 2014. http://www.fao.org/3/a-i3901e.pdf

produced less efficiently, in terms of environmental resources, such as meat and dairy. When one is evaluating food production and distribution, the amount of grains necessary to grow animal proteins (i.e., meat) should be considered—and not all animal production is created equal. Typically, smaller livestock (e.g., chickens and pigs) convert feed to edible protein more efficiently than do cattle (Smil, 2001). WRI has proposed promoting consumption shifts including reducing consumer waste, reducing overconsumption of calories, and promoting plant-based diets (i.e., eating less meat).

Agricultural Technology and Public Health

Farming is a gamble. Even with meticulous planning and textbook use of available resources (farming inputs and tools), weather can ultimately decide the fate of a harvest. We cannot control rainfall and weather disasters. Aside from financial tools that may be in place to manage risk, such as subsidies and crop insurance, farm technology helps some farmers achieve the harvests they seek. A farmer may rely on the increased certainty provided by genetically engineered (GE) seeds, or they may focus less on purchased inputs and more on farm system self-sufficiency, with hopes that self-sufficiency builds resiliency. This section is intended to give an overview of how agricultural technology should be evaluated from a global health perspective. Even the phrase "increased certainty" could be debated at length. The certainty provided by a GE crop could be only temporary when we consider a changing climate and the reality that new crop pests and diseases can emerge in new regions.

One widespread agricultural tool that helps farmers manage risk is improved seed varieties. Hybrid seeds from traditional selective plant breeding offer farmers a seed with better chances of succeeding in the local geography and growing conditions. GE seeds are also available—commonly known as **genetically modified organisms (GMOs)**. Such seeds have been developed for various purposes, including but not limited to drought tolerance and herbicide resistance. Some GE crops feature one major selling point, such as herbicide resistance, whereas an emerging class of GE crops have the potential to "stack" or combine multiple genetic characteristics in a single seed variety. GEs are developed through different methods. Genetic alterations may be the product of inserting one species' genetic material into a different species. Methods also exist to modify genes without going to another species or organism. (For further study, read about CRISPR technology.) Production methods and classification of GE products will continue to evolve, so it is important that food and health professionals develop an understanding of the details of farming with GE technology. First, let's observe that the current (2016) scientific consensus on GE crop varieties in the marketplace is that such crops are safe for consumption. The World Health Organization (WHO), the FAO, and numerous governmental regulatory agencies have ruled that these products are safe. However, many groups oppose or encourage continued research of these crops for precautionary, philosophical, environmental, and health reasons (Landrigan & Benbrook, 2015). We will not address the arguments for and against GE crops in this chapter. However, we propose that the biotechnology toolbox used for GE may have many benefits beyond agriculture. GE technology should not be written off completely, even if one does not believe in the use of such technology in food production. We encourage readers to think critically about how use of a GE crop variety fits into each specific farm system, and then to ask *why* the GE technology is being utilized (or not) in each case. In industrialized agriculture, many proponents of GE technology are also advocates of sustainability—which leads to the need to examine the motivations, sustainability metrics, and criteria for success when evaluating agriculture and food yield. For example, do certain seeds typically require fewer pesticide applications, saving money and preventing farmworker exposure to pesticides? Do some farmers have more stability from one season to the next if they are self-sufficient in producing seed for themselves? Perhaps a smallholder lacks access to credit and would find it risky to rely heavily on GMO seed purchases, even if the GMO seed offers yield benefits. There are numerous sociological and biological perspectives to be explored as GE science and GE crops continue to evolve in the marketplace.

As mentioned, GE technology, though debated, is currently thought to be safe. However, glyphosate-based herbicides often associated with GMO crops are causing concern as water contaminants and potential carcinogens (Myers et al., 2016; Landrigan & Benbrook, 2015). Even before these chemicals contaminate the environment or reach a consumer on food or via drinking water, farm laborers are at high risk of exposure in fields during and after chemical applications. Although widespread use of some agricultural chemicals provide farmers with more certainty and high yields, such use should be of concern to public health authorities. For example, the Florida tomato industry has been exposed as a particularly heavy user of pesticides with particularly poor policies for worker protection. Unfortunately, similar to many farm laborers around the world, residents of Immokalee, Florida, in the heart of the tomato growing region have high rates of both acute and chronic health outcomes associated with pesticide exposure (Estabrook, 2011). Furthermore, if industrialized farming moves away from GMO crops in the future, will other chemicals replace glyphosate? If so, will they be more dangerous?

Some farming philosophies draw from different toolboxes, avoiding genetically engineered seeds and many synthetic agrichemicals. Organic and related methodologies (e.g., biodynamic) aim to build resiliency to manage risk instead of using GMO crop technology. It is worth noting that USDA organic legislation does not allow GMO seed or animal feed. Organic agriculture is a good example of a holistic systems approach to growing, one that considers the environmental impact of food production. In part, this means understanding the farm's place in the surrounding ecosystem, strategically rotating crops, and building rich topsoil. The idea of building on the soil's nutrition aligns with a broader methodology referred to as **regenerative agriculture**, which aims not only to avoid negative environmental impacts but also to build soil health and biodiversity in a farm system (Francis, Harwood, & Parr, 1986). A multi-stakeholder group led by the Regenerative Agriculture Initiative at California State University, Chico, and the Carbon Underground recently drafted a formal definition of regenerative agriculture. The definition speaks of farming and grazing practices that reverse climate change by rebuilding soil organic matter. To read further and watch this definition evolve, visit http://regenerationinternational.org/2017/02/24/what-is-regenerative-agriculture/.

We mention these farming philosophies to encourage food system professionals to evaluate whether or not regenerative and/or organic growing practices should be used as a means of building long-term food security for community beneficiaries. Regardless of the crop or farm type, we must strive to promote balance between farm productivity and risks to the environment and human health.

BOX 9.3

THE INTERNATIONAL 4-H PROGRAM

MARY CRAVE

At first glance, learning how to raise a bumper crop of corn, give a demonstration in front of one's classmates, or preserve tomatoes for the off-season doesn't seem like a life-changing event. But it is when it is part of a youth development program like 4-H. 4-H does change lives, especially for women and girls, according to former members.

Ending her studies because her parents did not have the means to pay her school fees was not what Stella of northeast Tanzania had planned as a young girl. Fortunately, she had joined her school's 4-H club while in fifth grade, giving her some of the skills and confidence she needed to become a successful businesswoman in her rural community. She learned such basic skills as record-keeping and how to manage a bank account. She learned how to set goals, get along with others, and be a leader. Now in her mid-20s, she sells, as she has for several years, fruit, juice, and other food to schoolchildren outside a secondary school. She is active in another 4-H club for out-of-school girls as a volunteer peer counselor in sexual and reproductive health and serves as a role model for other girls who are not able to continue formal schooling.

Ana used the skills and profits from her primary school 4-H vegetable gardening project to open a restaurant. Samai owns a dress shop. Like their friend Stella, these women credit 4-H with helping them identify safe and promising opportunities in their communities through life and vocational skills training, including how to manage money, open a bank account, apply for and pay back a small loan, and identify business opportunities. Equally important are the confidence, self-esteem, and creativity that the program builds in participants.

4-H—the H's stand for *head, heart, hands,* and *health,* originated in the United States in the early 1900s under the auspices of the US Department of Agriculture and the state land-grant institutions. Now in more than 70 countries, 4-H might be in-school or after-school, a nonprofit or a group guided by the ministry of agriculture, for boys or girls only or for any gender. Members may be in primary or secondary school, or even in colleges and universities. They may have dropped out of school. Leaders may be parents, teachers, or older youth. In Africa alone, 4-H programs involve more than 300,000 members in nine countries, about half of whom are female. In many countries, especially those where food insecurity is a persistent threat, 4-H programs focus on agriculture and other income-generating practices. Some youth learn cultural arts, technology, and science; others, health and wellness.

What clubs have in common is that they provide a safe space for children to learn and grow. 4-H clubs are based on the positive youth development model. By providing positive, age-appropriate learning opportunities under the guidance of a caring adult, members develop skills critical to a healthy transition to adulthood, to be ready for work and ready for life. These life skills may range from decision making to leadership, record-keeping to problem solving, communication to cooperation. These boil down to "the Six Cs": confidence, competence, connection, character, compassion, and contribution—skills necessary for any walk of life.

Throughout the world, 4-H programs use innovative partnerships to connect youth with positive mentors, healthy living practices, and their communities. Community service and citizenship are important in 4-H programs. In the United States, 4-H members are nearly four times more likely than their peers to make contributions to their communities.

> When we are given leadership training, we all benefit because the boys learn the importance of women becoming leaders.
>
> —Tanzania 4-H member

Research in a couple of African countries has found that culture, tradition, or unconscious bias sometimes keeps some girls from flourishing as much as they might, even in 4-H. The 4-H club in Ghana has addressed this by implementing the Fifth H—Her training program, providing gender awareness and sensitivity training to hundreds of 4-H clubs, reaching tens of thousands of youth. Topics such as gender-based violence, sexual and reproductive health, and rights of the girl-child are taught alongside gardening and poultry production. Boys and girls learn to be advocates for each other. In Tanzania, 4-H clubs for young women who've left school build small business skills while weaving in health and child nutrition. In Kenya 4-K (4-H in Swahili) boys and girls have a policy of alternating club responsibilities and offices between the sexes so that both can develop confidence and other life skills from these experiences. A gender tool kit for club members, leaders, and parents provides strategies for helping girls succeed in school and 4-H across Africa.

Whether located in a rural or urban area, in Africa, Asia, or North America, in or out of school, 4-H is helping boys and girls develop confidence to lead a community project or pursue higher education, build vocational skills to help them succeed in a business, and gain skills that help them contribute to their community. 4-H has a long history in positive youth development, and continues to make sure that a fifth H—*her*—is part of the program.

Sources: Adapted from "4-H Changes the Lives of Girls in Tanzania," by Mary Crave, 2011, in *Girls Grow: A Vital Force in Rural Economies,* Chicago, IL: Chicago Council on Global Affairs. Also cited: *The Positive Development of Youth: Comprehensive Findings from the 4-H Study of Positive Youth Development,* by Tufts University, 2013, Chevy Chase, MD: National 4-H Council; *Preliminary Report: Assessment of Gender in Tanzania 4-H Clubs,* by National 4-H Council, 2011, Chevy Chase, MD: Author.

Sustainability and Equity: Highlights from Successful Programs

To close this chapter, we highlight some successful, progressive programs that are relevant for the field of sustainable agriculture and food security as we work toward a world with sufficient, equitable distribution of health-promoting foods.

4R Nutrient Stewardship and Field to Market

The 4R Nutrient Stewardship (4R) and Field to Market (FTM) programs are examples of industry-led progress in the realm of monitoring sustainability metrics in agriculture, with the goal of maintaining high productivity while also caring for the environment. Some aspects of these programs are adaptable to both small- and large-scale farming operations.

The 4R program teaches best practices for application of agricultural inputs, mainly fertilizer. The 4R techniques promote more judicious use of agrichemicals so that farmers maximize the benefit from each dollar spent on input costs while also minimizing environmental impact, such as excessive runoff. The 4R program is based on applying fertilizer of the right type, using the proper dose, applying it at the right time in the crop's life cycle, and applying it in the right place to ensure optimal uptake of nutrients by the plants. The 4R program provides farmer training (e.g., online video training modules) and funding for progressive agricultural research.

Field to Market (FTM) is a program based on the concept that we must be able to measure the various details of farming practices in order to effectively manage farm operations. FTM is connecting stakeholders across agricultural supply chains to collect agronomic data. By partnering with various technology and precision agriculture companies, FTM is helping characterize on-farm practices for specific crops in specific growing regions. Over time, FTM should facilitate meaningful dialogue in the farming community to help farmers make informed management choices to promote long-term sustainability of their farmland.

Read more online at http://www.nutrientstewardship.com/4rs/4r-principles and https://www.fieldtomarket.org/.

One Acre Fund

One Acre Fund supplies smallholder farmers with the financing and training they need to grow their way out of hunger and poverty. Instead of giving handouts, we invest in farmers to generate a permanent gain in farm income. We provide a complete service bundle of seeds and fertilizer, financing, training, and market facilitation—and we deliver these services within walking distance of the 400,000 rural farmers we serve in Kenya, Rwanda, Burundi, Tanzania, Uganda and Malawi. (One Acre Fund, 2016)

Read more online at www.oneacrefund.org.

World Food Program/Brazilian National School Feeding Program

Brazil has the oldest and most successful school feeding program, known as the Brazilian National School Feeding program. This program provides meals to over 43 million children across the country. In 1963, the World Food Programme collaborated with the Brazilian government to provide technical assistance and support for free meals in schools in the northeast of the country where many children lived in poverty. WFP provided these meals for the first 12 years of the program, until the Brazilian government was able to take it over. This school meals program has proven to be an incentive to attend school, but also has had great impact on malnutrition and hunger outcomes. Hunger has decreased from 22.8 million people in 1992 to 13.6 million in 2012. In addition child malnutrition rates have decreased by 73 percent and child deaths by 45 percent—this as a direct result of school meals, support for small farmers, community kitchens and food banks. More information can be found at the Centre of Excellence. (World Food Programme, 2014)

Gardens for Health International (GFI)

Gardens for Health is aiming to change the way that malnutrition is treated by moving away from short-term handouts and towards equipping families with the knowledge and resources to grow their own nutritious food and improve their health. Their ultimate objective is to integrate agriculture into the clinical care of malnutrition in Rwanda, and throughout the region, so that nutrition focused home gardens become a key strategy for addressing, and ultimately eradicating, chronic malnutrition among vulnerable families. Their community-led development approach includes partnerships with health centers, advocacy for agricultural solutions to malnutrition, and a curriculum and training methodology designed in partnership with mothers that they serve. Their agriculture innovation team works cross-culturally to design interventions that are effective and culturally adaptable. To date, GFI has helped to ensure that approximately 15,700 people have the healthy food they need to grow and thrive. (Gardens for Health International, 2016)

Read more online at http://www.gardensforhealth.org/our-story/.

Chapter Summary

The goal of this chapter was to leave you with some foundational knowledge about agriculture so that you can think critically about the social, environmental, and economic characteristics of food systems. By thinking about farms as complex agricultural systems that exist within ecosystems, including communities of people, you will begin to see that the modern practitioner of global health must consider how any intervention will affect the larger system. Even though food is grown and traded worldwide, consider that the most impactful food security initiatives may be localized and culturally appropriate piecemeal solutions (Easterly, 2006).

Food systems and farming practices around the world are shaped and influenced by countless variables, including access to productive resources (e.g., land), agricultural economic policy, geography, and social traditions. We looked at agricultural practices on a spectrum to demonstrate that food can be grown using a combination of many different tools, with varied guiding philosophies, at virtually any scale.

When evaluating any food system in the context of how it affects community health, we must consider that highly efficient farming operations may not always be the most sustainable and that food's connection to health extends beyond caloric needs (and by what metrics *efficiency* is defined). Consider that agricultural chemicals present risks to environmental health. Sustainability is relative and will be defined by the needs and concerns of a given farming community. Following the widely cited definition for sustainable development from the Brundtland Commission, we should promote programs that consider both immediate needs and the ability for future generations to meet their needs (World Commission on Environment and Development, 1987). We can use the dimensions of food security as a standard tool kit to evaluate how capable a food system is of consistently providing ample food availability, access, and utilization.

The literature indicates that enough food is grown on the planet to feed the current population; however, that food is not equally available to all people at all times. Much of the food supply is wasted before it reaches our mouths, so reducing food waste is seen as a major opportunity in the fight against food scarcity. Continued attention must be paid to agricultural productivity, though not without a focus on good stewardship of our existing farmlands. The Intergovernmental Panel on Climate Change (2014) reports that over 20% of global greenhouse gas emissions are the result of agriculture. If we do not proactively manage the environmental impact of how we grow our food, the resulting changes in weather and climate may exacerbate the food insecurity that already exists. There will not always be additional acres of fertile land (with available water) on the horizon. Going forward, food security practitioners must take a holistic view of food systems. We must increase financial stability by building resilient supply chains and creating progressive agricultural and trade policies that promote diversified farming and food self-sufficiency.

Key Terms

Agriculture
Amino acids
Commercial farm
Extensive agriculture
Fiber
Food
Food security
Food system
Fuel
Genetically modified organisms (GMOs)
The Green Revolution
Intensive agriculture
Macronutrients
Micronutrients
Monoculture
Organic production
Overnutrition
Productivity (yield)
Regenerative agriculture
Smallholder
Subsistence farm
Undernourishment
Undernutrition (hidden hunger)
Value chain
Yield gap

Review Questions

1. The National Research Council Committee on Twenty-First Century Systems Agriculture (2010) states:

   Sustainability in agriculture is a complex and dynamic concept that includes a wide range of environmental, resource-based, economic, and social issues. The committee's definition of sustainable farming does not accept a sharp dichotomy between unsustainable or sustainable farming systems because all types of farming can potentially contribute to achieving different sustainability goals and objectives.

   What is an example of a farming practice for which the concept of sustainability appears relative or debatable?

2. Briefly explain food availability, access, and utilization.
3. Brainstorm: What levers might be pulled to maintain economic viability when converting a farm from GE crops to non-GE crops?
4. List three pros and three cons about increasing food self-sufficiency in Cuba. Should planners promote modernization of Cuba's agriculture sector to grow more food at home, or advocate for preservation of post–Cold War low-input farming practices?
5. For discussion: Why hasn't the international community been able to completely eradicate hunger?

Exercise: Thinking Critically about Genetically Engineered Crops

Golden Rice is a genetically engineered (GE) variety of rice that has been developed with humanitarian intentions over recent decades. The rice has the potential to deliver more vitamin A–producing beta-carotene to the body (International Rice Research Institute, 2005). This offers a potential solution to combat vitamin A deficiency (VAD), which is a leading cause of preventable blindness around the world. VAD is the result of a micronutrient-poor diet and/or chronic diseases causing malabsorption (Gropper et al., 2005). VAD causes a variety of poor health outcomes, notably night blindness in young children and pregnant women. WHO (2016c) estimates that approximately 250 million preschool-age children experience VAD, and many of these children are at risk of blindness and increased mortality.

We mention Golden Rice not to decide whether it is good or bad but to present the questions that may be applied to many agriculture-related issues:

*   Is the GE solution necessary if other interventions (e.g., supplements) already exist?
*   Do the target beneficiaries of the technology want this solution? (In other words, are there barriers to cultural acceptance of eating a different colored staple food?)
*   Generally, how does adoption (or elimination) of GE crops change other farming practices?
*   Would local solutions to grow a more diverse mixture of crops, some of which naturally contain beta-carotene, be a preferred long-term solution compared to introduction of a GE crop? How would we determine the path with the best outcomes?

Suggested Reading

Climate Impacts on Food Security and Nutrition [Review]. World Food Programme, 2012. Available online at https://www.wfp.org/content/climate-impacts-food-security-and-nutrition-review-existing-knowledge

Food First, by Francis Moore Lappé and Joseph Collins, 1977.

"GMOs, Herbicides, and Public Health, by Philip J. Landrigan and Charles Benbrook, 2015. *New England Journal of Medicine, 373,* 693–695. doi:10.1056/NEJMp1505660

Holistic Management (3rd ed.), by Allan Savory, 2016.

The Omnivore's Dilemma, by Michael Pollan, 2006.

Organic 3.0, for Truly Sustainable Farming & Consumption [Report], by IFOAM Organics International, 2015. Available online at http://www.ifoam.bio/en/organic-policy-guarantee/organic-30-next-phase-organic-development

Principles for Responsible Investment in Agriculture and Food Systems [Report]. Committee on World Food Security, 2014. Available online at http://www.fao.org/3/a-au866e.pdf

Shifting Diets [Report]. World Resources Institute, 2016. Available online at http://www.wri.org/publication/shifting-diets

Toward Sustainable Agricultural Systems, by the Committee on Twenty-First Century Systems Agriculture, 2010. Available online at http://www.nap.edu/catalog/12832/toward-sustainable-agricultural-systems-in-the-21st-century

References

Atalaysun, M. (2016, August). *Turkey food processing ingredients report.* GAIN Report No. TR6035. USDA Foreign Agricultural Service. Retrieved from http://gain.fas.usda.gov/Recent%20GAIN%20Publications/Food%20Processing%20Ingredients_Ankara_Turkey_8-15-2016.pdf

Bertone, M., Watson, W., Stringham, M., Green, J., Washburn, S., Poore, M., & Hucks, M. (2016, August). *Dung beetles of central and eastern North Carolina cattle pastures.* North Carolina Cooperative Extension. Retrieved from https://www.ces.ncsu.edu/depts/ent/notes/forage/guidetoncdungbeetles.pdf

CIRAD. (2016). Food security. Retrieved from http://www.cirad.fr/en/research-operations/research-topics/food-security/what-s-cirad-doing

Clark, S. E., Hawkes, C., Murphy, S. M., Hansen-Kuhn, K. A., & Wallinga, D. (2012). Exporting obesity: US farm and trade policy and the transformation of the Mexican consumer food environment. *International Journal of Occupational and Environmental Health, 18*(1), 53–65.

Committee on World Food Security. (2014). *Principles for responsible investment in agriculture and food systems.* Rome: Food and Agriculture Organization of the United Nations.

Easterly, W. (2006). *The white man's burden.* New York, NY: Penguin.

Estabrook, B. (2011). *Tomatoland.* Kansas City, MO: Andrews McMeel.

Food and Agriculture Organization of the United Nations. (1996). *Towards a New Green Revolution.* Rome: Author. Retrieved from http://www.fao.org/docrep/x0262e/x0262e06.htm

Food and Agriculture Organization of the United Nations. (2003). *Trade reforms and food security.* Rome: Author. Retrieved from http://www.fao.org/docrep/005/y4671e/y4671e06.htm

Food and Agriculture Organization of the United Nations. (2008). An introduction to the basic concepts of food security. *Food security information for action: Practical guides.* Rome: EC–FAO Food Security Programme. Retrieved from http://www.fao.org/docrep/013/al936e/al936e00.pdf

Food and Agriculture Organization of the United Nations. (2011a). *Global food losses and food waste: Extent, causes and prevention.* Rome: Author. Retrieved from www.fao.org/docrep/014/mb060e/mb060e00.pdf

Food and Agriculture Organization of the United Nations. (2011b). *The state of food and agriculture: Women in agriculture.* Rome: Author. Retrieved from http://www.fao.org/docrep/013/i2050e/i2050e.pdf

Food and Agriculture Organization of the United Nations. (2012). *Towards the future we want.* Rome: Author.

Food and Agriculture Organization of the United Nations. (2013). *Statistical yearbook.* Rome: Author. Retrieved from http://www.fao.org/docrep/018/i3107e/i3107e00.htm

Food and Agriculture Organization of the United Nations. (2014). *Food and nutrition in numbers.* Rome: Author.

Food and Agriculture Organization of the United Nations. (2015). *Achieving zero hunger.* Rome: Author. Retrieved from http://www.fao.org/3/a-i4951e.pdf

Food and Agriculture Organization of the United Nations. (2016a). *Climate change and food security: Risks and responses.* Rome: Author. Retrieved from http://www.fao.org/3/a-i5188e.pdf

Food and Agriculture Organization of the United Nations. (2016b). *FAO cereal supply and demand brief.* Rome: Author. Retrieved from http://www.fao.org/worldfoodsituation/csdb/en/

Francis, C. A., Harwood, R. R., & Parr, J. F. (1986). The potential for regenerative agriculture in the developing world. *American Journal of Alternative Agriculture, 1*(2), 65–74. doi:10.1017/S0889189300000904

Gardens for Health International. (2016). Our story. Retrieved from http://www.gardensforhealth.org/our-story/

Gropper, S., Smith, J., & Groff, J. (2005). *Advanced nutrition and human metabolism* (4th ed.). Belmont, CA: Thomson Wadsworth.

Gunders, D. (2012). *Wasted.* New York, NY: National Resources Defense Council.

Hammer, T. J., Fierer, N., Hardwick, B., Simojoki, A., Slade, E., Taponen, J., . . . Roslin, T. (2016, May). Treating cattle with antibiotics affects greenhouse gas emissions, and microbiota in dung and dung beetles. *Proceedings of the Royal Society B: Biological Sciences, 283.* doi:10.1098/rspb.2016.0150

Intergovernmental Panel on Climate Change. (2014). *Climate change 2014: Impacts, adaptation, and vulnerability. Contribution of Working Group II to the Fifth Assessment Report of the Intergovernmental Panel on Climate Change.* C. B. Field, V. R. Barros, D. J. Dokken, K. J. Mach, M. D. Mastrandrea, T. E. Bilir . . . L. L. White (Eds.). New York, NY: Cambridge University Press.

International Rice Research Institute. (2005). Golden Rice fact sheet. Retrieved from http://www.goldenrice.org/PDFs/fs_GR_IRRI_2005.pdf

Landrigan, P. J., & Benbrook, C. (2015). GMOs, herbicides, and public health. *New England Journal of Medicine, 373,* 693–695. doi:10.1056/NEJMp1505660

Lappé, F. M., & Collins, J. (1977). *Food first.* New York, NY: Ballantine Books.

Lipinski, B., Hanson, C., Lomax, J., Kitinoja, L. Waite, R., & Searchinger, T. (2013). *Reducing food loss and waste.* Working paper. World Resources Institute. Retrieved from http://www.wri.org/sites/default/files/reducing_food_loss_and_waste.pdf

Meadows, D. H. (2008). *Thinking in systems.* White River Junction, VT: Chelsea Green Publishing.

Myers, J. P., Antoniou, M. N., Blumberg, B., Carroll, L. Colborn, T., Everett, L. G., . . . Benbrook, C. M. (2016). Concerns over use of glyphosate-based herbicides and risks associated with exposures: A consensus statement. *Environmental Health, 15*(19). doi:10.1186/s12940-016-0117-0

National Organic Program, 7 CFR §205.2. (n.d.). *Code of federal regulation.* Retrieved from http://www.ecfr.gov/

National Research Council. (2010). *Toward sustainable agricultural systems in the 21st century.* Washington, DC: National Academies Press. doi:10.17226/12832

Norman Borlaug—facts. (2016, August 15). Nobelprize.org. Retrieved from http://www.nobelprize.org/nobel_prizes/peace/laureates/1970/borlaug-facts.html

O'Connor, M. (2013, January 11). Subsidizing starvation. *Foreign Policy.* Retrieved from http://foreignpolicy.com/2013/01/11/subsidizing-starvation/

OECD. (2012). Achieving sustainable agricultural productivity growth. *In OECD-FAO agricultural outlook 2012* (pp. 49–85). Paris, France: OECD Publishing. Retrieved from http://www.oecd-ilibrary.org/agriculture-and-food/oecd-fao-agricultural-outlook-2012/achieving-sustainable-agricultural-productivity-growth_agr_outlook-2012-5-en

One Acre Fund. (2016). Program model. Retrieved from https://www.oneacrefund.org/our-approach/program-model

Sachs, J. D. (2008). *Common wealth.* New York, NY: Penguin Press.

Severson, K. (2016, June 20). A rush of Americans, seeking gold in Cuban soil. *New York Times.* Retrieved from http://nyti.ms/28LRpw9

Smil, V. (2001). *Enriching the earth.* Cambridge, MA: MIT Press.

Smil, V. (2013). *Should we eat meat?* West Sussex, England: Wiley-Blackwell.

Thompson, P. B. (2010). *The agrarian vision: Sustainability and environmental ethics.* Lexington: University of Kentucky Press.

United Nations. (2015a). Goal 2: End hunger, achieve food security and improved nutrition and promote sustainable agriculture. *Sustainable Development Goals.* Retrieved from http://www.un.org/sustainabledevelopment/hunger/

United Nations. (2015b). *World population prospects.* Retrieved from https://esa.un.org/unpd/wpp/publications/Files/WPP2015_DataBooklet.pdf

US Department of Agriculture. (2015, June 22). *U.S. agricultural exports to Cuba have substantial room for growth.* USDA Foreign Agriculture Service. Retrieved from http://www.fas.usda.gov/data/us-agricultural-exports-cuba-have-substantial-room-growth

"We made a devil's bargain": Fmr. President Clinton apologizes for trade policies that destroyed Haitian rice farming. (2010, April 1). [Transcript]. *Democracy Now.* Retrieved from http://www.democracynow.org/2010/4/1/clinton_rice

World Commission on Environment and Development. (1987). *Our common future.* Oxford, United Kingdom: Oxford University Press.

World Food Programme. (2014, June 24). *Brazil—A champion in the fight against hunger.* Retrieved from http://www.wfp.org/stories/brazil-champions-fight-against-hunger

World Food Programme. (2016). What is food security? Retrieved from https://www.wfp.org/node/359289

World Health Organization. (2016a). Diarrhoeal disease. Retrieved from http://www.who.int/mediacentre/factsheets/fs330/en/

World Health Organization. (2016b). Obesity. Retrieved from http://www.who.int/topics/obesity/en/

World Health Organization. (2016c). Micronutrient deficiencies. Retrieved from http://www.who.int/nutrition/topics/vad/en/

World Resources Institute. (2016). *Shifting diets for a sustainable food future.* Washington, DC: Author.

CHAPTER 10

CLIMATE AND HEALTH

Jonathan Patz, MD, MPH
Evan DiPrete Brown

As human beings, we are vulnerable to confusing the unprecedented
with the improbable.

—Al Gore

LEARNING OBJECTIVES

- Define climate change, explain its basic mechanisms, and consider the impact of human behavior and lifestyles
- Explain the direct and indirect ways in which climate change threatens global public health
- Describe the effects and health cobenefits of cross-sector responses to climate change
- Identify major actors and initiatives in the current climate change policy landscape

What do droughts in sub-Saharan Africa have in common with heavy rainfall in Brazil? Or shellfish poisoning in Alaska with air pollution in Beijing? What about heat waves in Europe and the nutritional value of crops in South Asia? Although it is difficult to pinpoint the cause of any one event, all of these occurrences—and the health problems that result—could be related to the consequences of global climate change.

The health of the environment in which we live has tremendous influence on our own health. Our impact on the world around us has ramifications not just for ourselves and the billions with whom we share this earth but also for the generations that will follow. And although many think of the effects of climate change on agriculture or biodiversity, impacts of climate variability and change on human health are profound and diverse. Indeed, public health concerns are central to this problem. Policies and

Foundations for Global Health Practice, First Edition. Lori DiPrete Brown.
© 2018 John Wiley & Sons, Inc. Published 2018 by John Wiley & Sons, Inc.

actions that grapple with the root causes of climate change could yield large health benefits. Both the health risks of climate change and the potential benefits of addressing it, therefore, are covered in this chapter.

What Is Climate Change?

Human activity alters the world in which we live. **Climate change** refers to changes in climate beyond natural variability that stem directly or indirectly from human activities and their impact on the global atmosphere. It is important to note that climate is distinct from weather. The term *weather* refers to conditions in a particular time and place, whereas *climate* reflects the average weather conditions over a longer period of time. Climate scientists often use a period of 30 years to distinguish between climate and weather.

The earth's surface temperature depends on the balance between incoming solar radiation and outgoing infrared radiation. The balance of radiation entering and exiting is determined by the composition of the atmosphere. Gases such as carbon dioxide (CO_2), methane (CH_4), and nitrous oxide (N_2O) absorb outgoing radiation and redirect it back toward the earth's surface. The presence of these **greenhouse gases** impacts climate as they trap heat in the atmosphere—much like a greenhouse allows sunlight to enter but prevents the heated air from rising. An atmosphere with higher levels of greenhouse gases will retain more heat and result in higher average surface temperatures than will an atmosphere with lower levels of these gases.

Since the preindustrial era, the levels of greenhouse gases present in the atmosphere have changed dramatically. In fact, the increase in atmospheric levels of greenhouse gases since the middle of the 19th century far exceeds any of the changes that occurred in the previous 10,000 years. Historical levels of greenhouse gases can be determined from the analysis of air bubbles found in Antarctic ice cores, making comparisons to modern conditions possible (Etheridge, Steele, Francey, & Langenfelds, 1998; Gulluk, Slemr, & Stauffer, 1998). The concentrations of carbon dioxide, methane, and nitrous oxide in the atmosphere now surpass the highest concentrations recorded over the past 800,000 years. Further, the average rates of increase of these three greenhouse gases over the past century are higher than at any time in the past 22,000 years (IPCC, 2013). In particular, the concentration of carbon dioxide has risen by approximately 35%, from about 280 parts per million by volume (ppmv) in the late 18th century to about 400 ppmv at present. These elevated concentrations of greenhouse gases have contributed to warming the earth and in doing so have altered its climate.

As the atmosphere retains more heat from greenhouse gases, average surface temperatures increase. Between 1880 and 2012, the average surface temperature of the earth increased 0.85°C (Intergovernmental Panel on Climate Change [IPCC], 2014). An assessment of historical climate data is necessary to distinguish such changes from the natural background of climate variability. Analyses of the various sources of this information—instrument records, documentary evidence, and paleoclimatic records—have shown that average North American temperatures in the mid- to late twentieth century appear to have been warmer than during any similar period in the last five centuries and were likely the highest in at least the past 1,300 years (IPCC, 2007). As such, the IPCC has determined that warming of the earth since the 1950s has been "unequivocal" and "unprecedented."

This warming correlates with a number of Earth system changes and environmental consequences. Melting ice from land-based glaciers releases vast amounts of water into the oceans and, combined with thermo-expansion of warmer oceans, has caused sea levels to rise. Since 1961, sea levels have risen approximately two millimeters per year on average (IPCC, 2007), while snow cover and glaciers have diminished in both hemispheres. As with temperatures, these trends are accelerating: Arctic ice caps have melted rapidly in the last 30 years, and according to the IPCC, the sea level will rise between 18 and 59 centimeters over the next 90 years. Earth system changes do not only manifest on this longer time scale: rising temperatures also make "hydrologic extremes" such as floods and droughts more likely to occur. The weather patterns that result from Earth system changes vary greatly from place to place and over short periods of time. For these reasons, the term *climate change* is more accurate than *global warming* when describing these changes.

Although climatologists have been cautious in attributing single extreme weather events (such as a heat wave or flood) to the process of climate change, according to the National Academy of Sciences (NAS, 2016), it is now possible to attach some level of attribution given the advancement in the science of "event attribution." According to this report, "Confidence in attribution findings of anthropogenic influence is greatest for those extreme events that are related to an aspect of temperature, such as the observed long-term warming of the regional or global climate, where there is little doubt that human activities have caused an observed change." The report further describes some confidence in attributing hydrological events (floods and drought), but little or no confidence yet in attributing convective storms and cyclones to climate change.

Climate change entails a number of environmental consequences relevant to public health. Some of these are direct and readily apparent: high temperatures leading to heat-related deaths, or rising sea levels flooding low-lying coastal areas. Others require a deeper understanding of the manifold ramifications of shifts in climate, but pose similarly urgent health risks. These impacts range from food production and the spread of disease to mental health and workforce productivity. The picture that emerges illustrates both the specific threat of climate change and the broader connection between environmental conditions and public health.

Public Health Risks of Climate Change

Climate change has become increasingly relevant to public health as its various impacts have been identified and researched. The following examples of areas in which the consequences of climate change create or amplify public health risks not only highlight specific problems to be addressed but also illustrate the wide variety of pathways through which changes in climate can impact health.

Temperature Extremes

The rise in global temperatures associated with climate change has led to more temperature extremes. Severe temperatures are associated with higher morbidity and mortality compared to the intermediate, or comfortable, temperature range (Kilbourne, 2008). In the United States, an average of 658 deaths are certified as heat related each year, and represent more fatalities than all other weather events combined (Centers for Disease Control and Prevention, 2013; Luber & McGeehin, 2008). More accurate risk estimates compare observed versus expected mortality during heat events. For example, 70,000 excess deaths were estimated for a European heat wave in 2003, and 15,000 for a 2010 heat wave in Russia (Robine et al., 2008; Matsueda, 2011). One estimate, focusing on a set of 12 US cities, projected over 200,000 excess heat-related deaths during the 21st century (Petkova et al., 2014). By midcentury, many US cities could experience more frequent extreme heat days; for example, New York and Milwaukee can expect three times their current average number of days hotter than 32°C (90°F) (Patz, Frumkin, Holloway, Vimont, & Haines, 2014).

Heat waves have been growing more frequent, more intense, and longer in duration over recent decades (Habeeb, Vargo, & Stone, 2015), and this trend is expected to continue, especially in the high latitudes of North America and Europe (Goodess, 2013). In Africa, extreme heat waves that are considered unusual today are projected to become commonplace by the end of the century (Russo, Marchese, Sillmann, & Immè, 2016).

Growing urbanization magnifies this threat due to the **heat island** effect. As a result of human and industrial activities, buildings, and other factors (such as the lack of trees), urban areas tend to generate and retain more heat. This puts those living in cities—an increasing portion of the global population—at special risk of suffering from heat extremes. Heat also disproportionately affects the poor, the elderly, those who are socially isolated, those who lack air conditioning, and those with medical conditions that impair the ability to dissipate heat.

One interesting case that illustrates some of the consequences of heat is its impact on people at work. Outdoor workers (such as farmworkers and construction workers) and those in non-air-conditioned facilities (such as factory workers in developing countries) are most directly affected by heat. Under such conditions, rising temperatures pose a serious threat to the health of these individuals. In addition, the heat can substantially reduce their ability to work. One study estimates that ambient heat stress has reduced global labor capacity by 10% at the peak of summer over the past few decades (Dunne, Stouffer, & John, 2013). By the middle of the 21st century, work days lost due to heat could reach 15%–18% in Southeast Asia, West and Central Africa, and Central America (Kjellstrom, Holmer, & Lemke, 2009). These regions contain some fragile economies that might be particularly susceptible to reduced productivity. Given that the risk burden of heat already falls on the economically disadvantaged, further economic difficulties may exacerbate the health consequences of extreme temperatures.

Rising Seas

As with the increase in global temperatures, the rise in sea level is not merely a signal of climate change but a public health threat in its own right. One expected effect of sea level rise is an increase in flooding and coastal erosion in low-lying areas. This will endanger large numbers of people: 14 of the world's 19 current megacities are situated at sea level. Coastal regions at risk of storm surges will expand, and the population at risk will increase from the current 75 million to 200 million (IPCC, 2001). In addition to directly impacting public health through flooding and storm surges, sea levels may have indirect consequences. As rising seas intrude on coastal areas, salt water could enter aquifers or disrupt storm drainage and sewage disposal. Several kinds of areas are especially vulnerable to this risk. Some countries, such as Vietnam and Bangladesh, have heavily populated, low-lying deltas along their coasts. In the Maldives, 50% of all human structures and 70% of vital infrastructure are located less than 100 meters from the shore (Sovacool, 2012). But it is not just these coastal areas that are threatened. For example, the islands of the Maldives make up one of the flattest countries on Earth, with no land rising more than three meters above sea level (Khan, Dewan Quadir, Murty, Kabir, & Sarker, 2002). At the same time, coral mining has weakened the natural protection afforded by the surrounding reefs (Brown & Dunne, 1988). The Maldives and other island nations face the real prospect of being entirely submerged in the ocean. At the same time, economic limitations in these countries often prevent them from implementing the complex adaptations necessary to avoid this fate.

Natural Disasters

Natural disasters, which dramatically affect public health, also reflect changing climate conditions. An average of 114,992 people died each year due to natural disasters from 2003 to 2012 (Vinck, 2013), and the number of people affected by natural disasters is two orders of magnitude greater than the number killed (Centre for Research on the Epidemiology of Disasters, 2015). In addition to deaths and injuries, disruption of health care, and lasting health impacts such as mental health disorders, disasters can halt or reverse economic growth and profoundly disrupt social structures. Climate change has made such events, with their potentially catastrophic impacts on health, more likely to occur.

Floods are the most common form of natural disaster worldwide, with between 150 and 200 major floods occurring annually (Vinck, 2013). In addition to coastal flooding from sea level rise, flooding occurs as a result of heavy rainstorms, which have increased in severity and frequency. In the United States, total precipitation increased by 7% over the last century; the amount of precipitation in the heaviest 1% of rain events increased by 20%. Over the same interval, the upper Midwest experienced a 50% increase in the frequency of days with precipitation over four inches (Kunkel, Easterling, Redmond, & Hubbard, 2003). Such severe storms may cause floods that result in death, injury, and population displacement.

Ocean surface temperatures have steadily increased, and have done so sharply over the last 35 years, with 2014 the warmest year yet recorded. Although the relationship between ocean temperatures and hurricane frequency is unclear, the evidence does suggest that more extreme hurricanes may occur (IPCC, 2013; Bender et al., 2010). As previously discussed, sea level rise will also expose more coastal areas to risk and worsen the impact of storm surges.

Wildfires are another natural event that reveals the influence of climate change. Four times as many extensive wildfires (fires that burn over 400 hectares) occurred in the western United States from 1987 to 2003 as compared to 1970 to 1986 (Westerling, Hidalgo, Cayan, & Swetnam, 2006). Several consequences of climate change may have been factors in the heightened incidence of wildfires, such as droughts drying out trees or higher springtime temperatures hastening snow melt and as a result lowering soil moisture (Running, 2006; Westerling et al., 2006). For these reasons, forecasts project an increased risk of wildfires in many areas throughout the 21st century (Moritz et al., 2012). Wildfires threaten health directly and also reduce air quality. Fire smoke carries a large amount of fine particulate matter that exacerbates cardiac and respiratory problems. One study on worldwide mortality estimated that between 229,000 and 600,000 premature deaths each year could be attributed to pollution from forest fires (Johnston et al., 2012).

Food Production

One of the most urgent, widespread health concerns in the context of climate change is its impact on food security and nutrition. Climate change negatively impacts food security in three ways: reduced crop yields, increased crop losses, and decreased nutritional content. Hotter temperatures will affect food production in the tropics, as most crops are already growing at close to optimal conditions. Water shortages will also contribute to the loss of food production, especially in regions that are dependent on glacial melt. More than 800 million people currently experience chronic hunger, concentrated where productivity could likely be most affected (Food and Agriculture Organization [FAO], 2013; Wheeler & von Braun, 2013). Wheat, maize, sorghum, and millet yields are estimated to decline by approximately 8% across Africa and South Asia by 2050 (Porter et al., 2014). By 2050, around 25 million more children might be undernourished due to climate change, and rates of growth stunting could increase substantially (Nelson et al., 2009; Lloyd, Sari Kovats, & Chalabi, 2011). Climate-related food price shocks, especially for staples such as corn and rice, could more than double by mid-century, placing impoverished populations at further risk (Bailey, 2011). On average, climate change is projected to reduce global food production by up to 2% per decade, even as demand increases 14% (Porter et al., 2014).

Climate change may substantially increase the occurrence of plant disease, which is already responsible for a 16% crop loss (Chakraborty & Newton, 2011). In addition, climate change favors the growth of weeds that compete with crops (Ziska & McConnell, 2015). These conditions also diminish the nutrient value of crops that do survive. High concentrations of carbon dioxide can reduce the protein content in wheat and rice, and the iron and zinc content in crops such as rice, soybeans, wheat, and peas (Myers et al., 2014).

The production of **biofuels**, itself a response to climate change, also impacts the food supply. In order to meet increased demand for biofuel products, farmland and crops may be diverted from food to fuel. Although the impacts are controversial, it is possible that biofuel production contributes to unintended consequences such as food shortages and rising food prices (Harvey & Pilgrim 2011; Tirado, Cohen, Aberman, Meerman, & Thompson, 2010; High Level Panel of Experts, 2013).

Climate change does not threaten food security only through its impact on crops; it also affects fisheries and aquaculture. Globally, 540 million people depend on wild fisheries and aquaculture as sources of protein and income (FAO, 2013). For the poorest 80% of these people, fish represents at least half their intake of animal protein and dietary minerals. There are many ways in which climate change will affect river and marine ecosystems and impact the availability of fish, most significantly **ocean acidification**. Oceans have absorbed about 30% of human-produced carbon dioxide, and the surface pH has become 0.1 more acidic since the beginning of the industrial era. The IPCC (2013) predicts that global ocean surface pH will drop between .14 and 0.35 units over the course of the 21st century. In particular, ocean acidification threatens shell-forming organisms such as coral and the species that depend on them. Fisheries can expect to face a number of other climate-induced challenges, including altered river flows, destructive coastal storms, and the spread of diseases (Cochrane, De Young, Soto, & Bahri, 2009; Porter et al., 2014).

Air Quality

Climate change may increase exposure to air pollution, as it influences both the levels of pollutants formed in the air and the ways in which these pollutants are dispersed. In general, air quality is likely to suffer with a warmer, more variable climate (Bernard, Samet, Grambsch, Ebi, & Romieu, 2001). The concentration of some pollutants, such as ozone, increases in warmer climates. The "ozone season" for affected cities occurs during the summer, when higher temperatures promote ozone formation. Likewise, climate change may prompt increases in pollen levels. Higher levels of carbon dioxide promote growth and reproduction by some plants, including many that produce allergens. Recently, the allergy season has lengthened as some species begin to flower earlier, and levels of allergens have risen—both predictable effects of higher temperatures and carbon dioxide levels (Zhang et al., 2015). Hotter temperatures also lead to an increased demand for energy to power air conditioning, which results in more air pollution if fossil fuels supply the power. However, the relationship between climate change and air pollution is complicated. For example, some particles in the air actually reflect radiant energy and help cool the atmosphere, such as in the cooling that follows volcanic eruptions. Air pollution chemistry is complex, and many other factors—from changing vegetation to policies that reduce methane emissions—also play a role, leading to variability from place to place (Fiore, Naik, & Leibensperger, 2015).

In the case of China, there is a clear connection. China is the world's largest emitter of carbon dioxide and faces the world's worst air pollution (Kan, Chen, & Tong, 2012). In megacities such as the capital of Beijing and the economic hub of Shanghai, air pollution heightens the risk of morbidity and mortality, especially from respiratory and cardiovascular problems (Kan et al., 2012). Several studies in China have suggested that traffic exhaust—a pervasive pollutant—negatively impacts neurobehavioral function, especially in children (Liu et al., 2001; Wang, Zhang, Zeng, Zeng, & Chen, 2009). In this context, sustainable development and efforts to reduce emissions are not simply environmentally friendly measures but critical steps to averting a public health crisis.

Infectious Disease

Climate conditions influence a number of infectious diseases. The diseases most sensitive to climate influence are those contracted from water, food, or vectors such as rodents and insects. Because all of these are highly sensitive to small shifts in weather conditions, exposure to water-borne and vector-borne disease will likely change in a warmer world (Patz & Hahn, 2013; Mills, Gage, & Khan, 2010).

Water-borne diseases are likely to become a greater problem as climate change disrupts freshwater and marine ecosystems. Climate change affects both the quantity and quality of water in freshwater systems; in marine waters, changes in temperature and salinity affect coastal ecosystems in ways that may increase the risk of certain diseases, such as cholera.

As discussed earlier, climate change will contribute to more frequent and more severe flooding and rainstorms—both of which put strain on community water systems. As a result, the risk of water-borne diseases is expected to rise (Patz & Hahn, 2013). Flooding can contaminate drinking water with runoff and overwhelm sewage systems, which then discharge wastewater into rivers and lakes. Using a 6 cm (2.5 in) threshold of daily precipitation for initiating combined sewer overflows (CSOs) for metropolitan Chicago, downscaled climate models show that the frequency of these events may rise by 50–120% by the end of this century (Patz, Vavrus, Uejio, & McClellan, 2008).

Outbreaks of diseases such as cryptosporidiosis and giardiasis are associated with prior heavy rainstorms (Curriero, Patz, Rose, & Lele, 2001; Cann, Thomas, Salmon, Wyn-Jones, & Kay, 2013). In the United States and India, heavy rainfall has been linked to gastrointestinal illness in children (Uejio et al., 2014; Bush et al., 2014). One Dutch study showed a 33% increase in gastrointestinal illness associated with sewage overflow following heavy rain, as flood water contained numerous diseases (De Man et al., 2014). After heavy storms, these diseases can spread quickly. For example, in 1993 an estimated 400,000 people were exposed to cryptosporidia in Milwaukee, an outbreak that killed at least 100 (Rose, 1997). Rainfall can also increase the risk of illness through the contamination of recreational waters (Schuster et al., 2005). Heavy runoff leads to higher bacteria counts at coastal beaches, especially those near river outflows (Dwight, Semenza, Baker, & Olson, 2002).

Warm water provides a favorable environment for blooms of algae, including several varieties that release toxins. These **harmful algal blooms** can cause acute poising in humans as wells as contribute to the death of fish, mammals, and birds that rely on the marine ecosystem for food. Over recent decades, the frequency and global distribution of harmful algal blooms appear to have increased, and more human intoxication from algal sources has occurred (Anderson, Cembella, & Hallegraeff, 2012). For example, in the summer of 2012, a group of vacationers on the Washington coast were diagnosed with paralytic shellfish poisoning after harvesting and eating mussels. The mussels were contaminated with saxitoxin, an algal product more toxic than sodium cyanide (Hurley, Wolterstorff, MacDonald, & Schultz, 2014). The number of cases reported that summer was substantially higher than in previous years, which was attributed to unusually warm temperatures. Climate change is predicted to increase the frequency of these incidents; in addition, ocean acidification may increase the toxicity of some algal species (Fu, Tatters, & Hutchins, 2012; Glibert et al., 2014). Ciguatera, another kind of poisoning caused by ingesting fish that contain algal toxins, could also expand its range. This condition has been linked to sea surface temperatures; as the oceans warm, according to one projection, ciguatera fish poisoning could increase two- to fourfold over the next hundred years (Gingold, Strickland, & Hess, 2014).

Some bacteria also proliferate in warm marine waters (Pascual, Rodó, Ellner, Colwell, & Bouma, 2000). Planktons that feed on algae can serve as a reservoir for pathogens. In Bangladesh, cholera follows the seasonal warming of sea surface temperatures, which can enhance plankton blooms (Colwell, 1996). Warmer marine waters also expand the range of bacteria species. For example, in 2004 an outbreak of shellfish poisoning was reported from Prince William Sound in Alaska. The pathogenic species, *V. parahaemolyticus,* had not previously been observed in Alaskan shellfish due to the coldness of the waters. However, water temperatures during the 2004 shellfish harvest remained above 15°C and mean water temperatures were significantly higher than the previous six years (McLaughlin et al., 2005). This suggests the potential for warming sea surface temperatures to increase the geographic range of shellfish poisoning and bacterial infections.

It is difficult to distinguish precisely between water-borne and food-borne illnesses, because contaminated water often contaminates food. However, greater warmth, humidity, and other climate factors affect food-borne pathogens in many ways and can increase the risk of food-borne infectious diseases (Hellberg & Chu, 2015). Data from many parts of the world show a strong association between temperature and the incidence of food poisoning, with the effect most pronounced at the highest temperatures (Kovats et al., 2004; Naumova et al., 2007). Models of climate change suggest a sharp increase in food-borne illness: for instance, a study focused on Beirut projected a 16%–28% increase by 2050 and an increase of up to 42% by 2100 (El-Fadel, Ghanimeh, Maroun, & Alameddine, 2012).

Vector-borne diseases are infectious diseases spread by organisms such as insects or rodents. Because the life cycle of these pathogens involves a significant amount of time outside the human host, vector-borne diseases are especially subject to the influence of climate conditions. The incubation time of an infectious agent within its vector organism is typically very sensitive to changes in temperature and humidity (Patz et al., 2003). Climate change can shift the distribution of populations, affect biting rates and survival, and alter pathogen development—all factors which determine infectivity.

Temperature and other weather factors influence ticks, which carry Lyme disease (Ostfeld & Brunner, 2015). Their range is already expanding, and warming temperatures are projected to shift the range limit for this tick 200 kilometers northward by the 2020s and 1,000 km by the 2080s (Ogden et al., 2006). Rodents can transmit diseases including hantavirus, leptospirosis, and plague. Hantavirus emerged in the Southwest United States in 1993, after an El Niño brought heavy rains that led to growth in rodent populations (Glass et al., 2000). Events that increase exposure to rodents, such as extreme flooding, can greatly increase the risk of contracting leptospirosis (Lau, Smythe, Craig, & Weinstein, 2010). Plague also varies with weather and across seasons. Historical tree-ring data suggest that during the major plague epidemics of the Black Death, climate conditions were becoming both warmer and wetter (Ben-Ari et al., 2011; Stenseth et al., 2006).

Mosquitoes carry malaria as well as arboviruses such as dengue fever, chikungunya, Rift Valley fever, and West Nile virus. An increase in temperature of just half a degree Celsius can translate into a 30%–100% increase in mosquito abundance in highland East Africa (Pascual, Ahumada, Chaves, Rodo, & Bouma, 2006). Extreme rainfall or drought can also contribute to growth in mosquito populations, as pools of stagnant water created by flooding or human water storage provide breeding grounds (Stewart Ibarra et al., 2013; Trewin, Kay, Darbro, & Hurst, 2013). Most models forecast an increase in malaria risk over the next century (Caminade et al., 2014). The Zika virus also appears sensitive to the effects of climate change—a combination of drought and warmer temperatures in Brazil coincided with, and may have contributed to, the emergence of Zika (Muñoz, Thomson, Goddard, & Aldighieri, 2016). Although mosquito-borne arboviruses differ in their effect and have distinct geographic ranges, they share common traits: there is evidence that climate conditions affect their spread; their geographic range has expanded recently; and models project the potential for further spread with continued climate change (Martin et al., 2008; Dhiman, Pahwa, Dhillon, & Dash, 2010; Weaver & Reisen, 2010; Morin, Comrie, & Ernst, 2013; Campbell et al., 2015; Paz, 2015). Each disease reflects the interplay of behavior, land use, mosquito control strategies, and other factors. Disease control in the context of climate change will require an approach that recognizes the relationship between environmental and public health and makes use of those connections to tackle the complex challenges presented.

Mental Health

Climate change and its consequences have the potential to negatively impact mental health in several ways. In the aftermath of natural disasters, mental health consequences such as posttraumatic stress, depression, and anxiety are common and may represent a major part of the resulting health burden (North & Pfefferbaum, 2013; Goldmann & Galea, 2014). Mental health consequences do not stem only from these rapid, traumatic events. During a prolonged drought in Australia, researchers found increased anxiety, depression, and possibly suicidality among rural populations (Berry, Hogan, Owen, Rickwood, & Fragar, 2011). Environmental degradation may cause a sense of loss or distress; this has been observed among indigenous populations in the Arctic that put high cultural value on place (Berry et al., 2011). In addition, climate change may force populations to relocate after an acute disaster or when needed resources become increasingly scarce, creating a considerable mental health burden (United Nations High Commissioner for Refugees, 2009; Loughry, 2010).

War, Refugees, and Population Displacement

A growing body of evidence links climate change and violence, from self-inflicted and interpersonal harm to armed conflict (Levy & Sidel, 2014). One recent study found that each standard deviation of increased rainfall or warmer temperatures increases the likelihood of intergroup conflict by 14% on average (Hsiang, Burke, & Miguel, 2013). Strategic analyses by military authorities such as the Center for Naval Analysis Military Advisory Board (2014) and the US Department of Defense (2014) have warned that climate change could catalyze instability and conflict.

Climate-related disasters and conflicts may trigger broad displacement, often to places ill-prepared for the quantity and needs of refugees. Even with baseline support, displaced groups commonly experience a range of public health threats, including violence, sexual abuse, and mental illness (McMichael, McMichael, Berry, & Bowen, 2010). Rising sea levels will also force populations to shift as coastal areas and island chains become uninhabitable. The encroaching oceans may be more predictable than conflict and disaster, but the advance warning does not lessen the burden of those in soon-to-be-uprooted communities. The Pacific island nation of Kiribati has encouraged its citizens to migrate to other, safer nations, and recently purchased a parcel of less vulnerable land in Fiji for that purpose. These countries, however, might not readily accept an influx of migrants. In 2015, New Zealand deported a migrant from Kiribati who sought asylum as a "climate refugee" (Ives, 2016). The questions raised in these circumstances will only become more pressing as the number of people forced to relocate increases.

Public Health Responses to Climate Change

The wide range of threats that climate change poses to public health requires a variety of actions to be taken in response. Such efforts might include programs that curb the negative health impact of climate change, regulations to stabilize climate conditions, and initiatives that seek to reverse trends projected to cause significant future harm.

Mitigation, Adaptation, and Health Cobenefits

Two kinds of strategies are relevant to formulating a public health response to climate change: mitigation and adaptation. These strategies are best seen not as separate approaches but as residing on the same spectrum of prevention methods; it is important to consider them as complementary responses to public health threats.

Mitigation, which corresponds to primary prevention, aims to stabilize or reduce the production of greenhouse gases. Some key mitigation strategies focus on more efficient energy production and reduced energy demand. More efficient production might come from wind and solar energy, which do not produce greenhouse gases. Reduced demand could come from transportation policies that incentivize walking, biking, mass transit, or fuel-efficient automobiles. Some efforts to reduce demand might involve environmentally friendly buildings or more efficient electronic appliances. Other mitigation strategies, rather than preventing greenhouse gas production, seek to remove it from the atmosphere more quickly—for example, through land use policies that preserve and expand forests.

Adaptation, which corresponds with secondary prevention or preparedness, aims to reduce the public health impacts of climate change. For example, authorities can anticipate that certain natural disasters may occur more frequently or increase in severity, and can direct strategies accordingly to minimize the effects of these events on health. Adaptation might also involve improvements to infrastructure focused on the effects of climate change. City planners might utilize white roofs or vegetation as well as building placement and design to reduce the urban heat island effect. Some efforts at adaptation require trade-offs that make it difficult to identify optimal strategy. Air conditioning is an important adaptation to urban heat islands, but a recent study found that waste heat from AC units can warm outdoor air more than 1°C—in other words, air conditioning actually contributed to the same effect it was meant to combat (Salamanca, Georgescu, Mahalov, Moustaoui, & Wang, 2014). Rather than engineering single solutions, developing a holistic, ecological approach has the potential to obtain multiple benefits as well as cost savings. For example, seawalls are often employed to stabilize shorelines as sea levels rise. However, planting mangroves to protect against storm surges costs a fraction of what it would to build and maintain a wall, while also preserving wetlands and marine food chains that support local fisheries (Arkema et al., 2013).

An important concept in the discussion of mitigation and adaptation strategies is that of **health cobenefits**. Although some steps necessary to respond to climate change may seem expensive or complicated, sophisticated solutions often have the potential to result in multiple benefits. An appraisal of these benefits can make efforts to address the health threats posed by climate change attractive, cost-effective, and politically viable. Many health cobenefits have been carefully investigated and quantified. For example, the production of meat accounts for as much as 18% of global greenhouse gas emissions (FAO, 2006). A British study found that lowering the consumption of red and processed meat in that country could reduce its greenhouse gas emissions by 3%, while cutting the risk of coronary heart disease, diabetes, and colorectal cancer by fractions ranging up to 12% (Aston, Smith, & Powles, 2012). Similarly, a study in the midwestern United States found that replacing short car trips with bicycling could reduce air pollution and increase physical activity enough to avoid 1,295 deaths per year in a region of 31.3 million people—and save approximately $8 billion each year from reduced mortality and health care costs (Grabow et al., 2012).

Climate Change Policy

Policy solutions that address climate change, and specifically carbon emissions, have been put forward, but often face difficult paths to implementation. Many of these proposals rely on market mechanisms to incentivize positive behaviors. This is necessary because the individuals and firms that benefit from emissions do not bear the costs of those emissions. There are two major policy approaches designed to encourage reduced emissions and efficient technologies. The **cap-and-trade** approach creates a system in which the government sets a cap on total emissions and distributes permits to companies, who would then buy and sell those permits at market prices. The government could then progressively lower the emissions ceiling to reach its objectives. The United States has successfully employed a cap-and-trade system to reduce sulfur dioxide and nitrous oxide emissions, and greenhouse gas cap-and-trade systems exist in places such as Tokyo, California, and the European Union. The second major approach is a **carbon tax** in which the government places a tax on emissions. Carbon taxes are utilized in a number of places, including Sweden, Ireland, British Columbia, Quebec, and Boulder, Colorado. Although economists and policy experts debate the relative merits of these two approaches, the importance of carbon pricing as a matter of health policy is clear (Aldy & Stavins, 2012; Goulder & Schein, 2013; Howden-Chapman, Chapman, Capon, & Wilson, 2011). The NGO Citizens Climate Lobby advocates a price on carbon with proceeds that are returned to citizens rather than collected by the government—an arrangement called **carbon fee and dividend**.

Under most governments, these approaches rely on legislative action and often encounter substantial political obstacles, such as lobbying from fossil fuel companies and other interests (Jenkins, 2014). Perceptions of climate change in the general public reflect a number of political and cultural factors, and even those who believe that climate change occurs and is the result of human activity express a tendency to envision it as a remote, less urgent problem (Pew Research, 2014). In the United States, this has prevented action at the federal level; in Australia, a carbon tax was repealed in 2014 just two years after its implementation. In the United States, action instead takes the form of regulation from the Environmental Protection Agency (EPA). In 2007, the Supreme Court ruled in *Massachusetts v. EPA* that greenhouse gases met the definition of "air pollutants" under the Clean Air Act. The EPA was required to make a scientific determination known as an **endangerment finding** that greenhouse gas emissions could be expected to pose a threat to public health. The EPA made this determination in 2009, empowering the agency to regulate greenhouse gas emissions from vehicles, factories, and power plants.

International Efforts

International efforts to address climate change are carried out under the **United Nations Framework Convention on Climate Change** (UNFCCC), adopted in 1992. The UNFCCC sought to stabilize the concentration of greenhouse gases in the atmosphere in order to prevent "dangerous interference" with the earth's climate. In 1997, its third meeting resulted in the **Kyoto Protocol**, which committed developed countries and emerging market economies to reduce their overall emissions of six greenhouse gases by at least 5% below 1990 levels over the period between 2008 and 2012, with specific targets varying from country to country. However, the United States—at the time the largest emitter of greenhouse gases, though now China has surpassed it—did not sign the Kyoto Protocol. By 2007, it was apparent that many signatory nations were not on pace to achieve the relatively modest emission reductions set forth in the protocol. This reveals some of the issues facing attempts to develop robust international climate agreements. Some wealthy countries, such as the United States, have been unwilling to accept binding limits. Meanwhile, less wealthy nations are eager for economic development and believe that wealthy countries, which are responsible for the majority of greenhouse gas emissions, should take on most of the responsibility.

In November 2014, talks between the United States and China led to the **U.S.-China Joint Announcement on Climate Change and Clean Energy Cooperation**. Together, the two countries produce over a third of the world's greenhouse gas emissions. President Barack Obama announced that the United States would cut emissions 28% below 2005 levels by 2025, while President Xi Jianping of China pledged to reach a target peak of carbon dioxide by 2030 and increase the share of renewable energy by 20% over the same interval. If the two nations follow through on these commitments, it would represent a significant breakthrough in efforts to address climate change at the international level.

In December 2015, the 21st conference of parties to the UNFCCC resulted in the **Paris Agreement**. The goals of the agreement are to hold the increase in global average temperature to below 2°C above preindustrial levels, to increase the ability to adapt to the impacts of climate change, and to direct financial efforts toward low greenhouse gas emissions and climate-resilient development. Each participating country will set its own **nationally determined contribution (NDC)** toward the worldwide target. However, the agreement lacks a binding enforcement mechanism, and according to one study, the current pledged NDCs are too low to keep temperature rise under the stated limit of 2°C warming (Rogelj et al., 2016).

Who Feels the Impact? Ethical and Moral Considerations

The struggle to implement policy solutions and international agreements illustrates some of the ethical issues climate change presents. Those responsible for the majority of greenhouse gas emissions or in position to alter public policy are often not those who will bear the brunt of climate change's impact. On a global scale, the nations responsible for the majority of emissions account for a small proportion of the world's population and are relatively resilient to the effects of climate change. For example, the United States produced 25% of the world's total annual greenhouse gas emissions with just 5% of the world's population. Populations in the developing world contribute only a fraction of the greenhouse gases per capita, but their capacity to protect themselves against the adverse consequences of what are mostly others' emissions is quite limited

(Shue, 2014). Similar disparities exist within nations, as disadvantaged and marginalized groups have the least protection from climate impacts (Patz, Gibbs, Foley, Rogers, & Smith, 2007). In the United States, Hurricane Katrina drastically demonstrated this in 2004. Racial and class stratifications played a major role in human and institutional responses to the disaster (Elliott & Pais, 2006). Poorer residents of New Orleans and the Gulf Coast region were disproportionately likely to fail to evacuate, to suffer catastrophic disruption following the storm, and to be unable to recover in its aftermath (Dyson, 2007; Pastor et al., 2006). Growing awareness of these issues has given rise to the concept of **climate justice**, which focuses on local impacts and experience, inequitable vulnerabilities, and the importance of community voice in addressing the consequences of climate change (Schlosberg & Collins, 2014). A full ethical consideration also weighs our responsibility to future generations, who will have no choice but to navigate the consequences of today's actions.

Chapter Summary

It is clear that climate change poses a wide range of threats to global health. The increase in global average temperatures presents physical risks such as heat, rising seas, and natural disasters. Communities also face potential impacts as environmental conditions affect food production, disease, air quality, and mental health. The public health response to these issues must utilize elements of both mitigation and adaptation. The failure to address climate change is not only an environmental crisis but also a public health crisis that has the potential to impact millions of people worldwide. Although current domestic and international policy initiatives face a number of obstacles, some signs of progress point to a future in which responsible human behavior can limit the negative effects of climate change.

Key Terms

Adaptation
Biofuels
Cap-and-trade
Carbon tax
Climate change
Climate justice
Endangerment finding
Greenhouse gases
Harmful algal blooms
Health cobenefits

Heat island

Kyoto Protocol

Mitigation

Nationally determined contribution (NDC)

Ocean acidification

Paris Agreement

United Nations Framework Convention on Climate Change

U.S.-China Joint Announcement on Climate Change and Clean Energy Cooperation

Vector-borne diseases

Review Questions

1. How does climate change occur?
2. What are some of the public health risks of climate change?
3. Which populations are the most vulnerable to climate change health risks?
4. What is the difference between mitigation and adaptation as responses to climate change?
5. What are some possible cobenefits of public health actions taken in response to climate change?
6. What can be done on the personal, local, and global levels to address the public health impacts of climate change?

References

Aldy, J. E., & Stavins, R. N. (2012). Using the market to address climate change: Insights from theory & experience. *Daedalus, 141*(2), 45–60.

Anderson, D. M., Cembella, A. D., & Hallegraeff, G. M. (2012). Progress in understanding harmful algal blooms: Paradigm shifts and new technologies for research, monitoring, and management. *Annual Review of Marine Science, 4*(1), 143–176.

Arkema, K. K., Guannel, G., Verutes, G., Wood, S. A., Guerry, A., Ruckelshaus, M., . . . Silver, J. M. (2013). Coastal habitats shield people and property from sea-level rise and storms. *Nature Climate Change, 3*, 913–918.

Aston, L. M., Smith, J. N., & Powles, J.W. (2012). Impact of a reduced red and processed meat dietary pattern on disease risks and greenhouse gas emissions in the UK: A modelling study. *BMJ Open, 2*(5). doi:10.1136/bmjopen-2012-001072

Bailey R. (2011). Growing a better future: Food justice in a resource-constrained world. *Oxfam Policy and Practice: Agriculture, Food and Land, 11*, 93–168.

Ben-Ari, T., Neerinckx, S., Gage, K. L., Kreppel, K., Laudisoit, A., Leirs, H., & Stenseth, N. C. (2011). Plague and climate: Scales matter. *PLOS Pathogens, 7*(9), e1002160.doi:10.1371/journal.ppat.1002160

Bender, M. A., Knutson, T. R., Tuleya R. E., Sirutis, J. J., Vecchi, G. A., Garner, S. T., & Held, I. M. (2010). Modeled impact of anthropogenic warming on the frequency of intense Atlantic hurricanes. *Science, 327*, 454–458.

Bernard, S. M., Samet, J. M., Grambsch, A., Ebi, K. L., & Romieu, I. (2001). The potential impacts of climate variability and change on air pollution-related health effects in the United States. *Environmental Health Perspectives, 2001, 109*(Suppl. 2), 199–209.

Berry, H. L., Hogan, A., Owen, J., Rickwood, D., & Fragar, L. (2011). Climate change and farmers' mental health: Risks and responses. *Asia Pacific Journal of Public Health, 23*(Suppl. 2), 119s–132.

Brown, B., & Dunne, R. P. (1988). The environmental impact of coral mining on coral reefs in the Maldives. *Environmental Conservation, 15*, 159–165. doi:10.1017/S0376892900028976

Bush, K. F., O'Neill, M. S., Li, S., Mukherjee, B., Hu, H., Ghosh, S., & Balakrishnan, K. (2014). Associations between extreme precipitation and gastrointestinal-related hospital admissions in Chennai, India. *Environmental Health Perspectives, 122*, 249–254.

Caminade, C., Kovats, S., Rocklov, J., Tompkins, A. M., Morse, A. P., Colon-Gonzalez, F. J., . . . Lloyd, S. J. (2014). Impact of climate change on global malaria distribution. *Proceedings of the National Academy of Sciences, 111*, 3286–3291.

Campbell, L. P., Luther, C., Moo-Llanes, D., Ramsey, J. M., Danis-Lozano, R., & Peterson, A. T. (2015). Climate change influences on global distributions of dengue and chikungunya virus vectors. *Philosophical Transactions of the Royal Society of London B: Biological Sciences, 370*(1665). doi:10.1098/rstb.2014.0135

Cann, K., Thomas, D. R., Salmon, R., Wyn-Jones, A., & Kay, D. (2013). Extreme water-related weather events and waterborne disease. *Epidemiology & Infection, 141*, 671–686.

Centers for Disease Control and Prevention. (2013). Heat-related deaths after an extreme heat event—Four states, 2012, and United States, 1999–2009. *Morbidity and Mortality Weekly Report, 62*, 433–436.

Centre for Research on the Epidemiology of Disasters. (2015). The human cost of natural disasters: A global perspective. Brussels: Université catholique de Louvain. http://reliefweb.int/sites/reliefweb.int/files/resources/PAND_report.pdf

Chakraborty, S., & Newton, A. C. (2011). Climate change, plant diseases and food security: An overview. *Plant Pathology, 60*, 2–14.

CNA Military Advisory Board. (2014). *National security and the accelerating risks of climate change.* Alexandria, VA: CNA.

Cochrane, K., De Young, C., Soto, D., & Bahri, T. (2009). *Climate change implications for fisheries and aquaculture.* Rome: Food and Agriculture Organization. http://www.fao.org/docrep/012/i0994e/i0994e00.htm

Colwell, R. R. (1996). Global climate and infectious disease: The cholera paradigm. *Science, 274*, 2025–2031.

Curriero, F., Patz, J. A., Rose, J., & Lele, S. (2001). The association between extreme precipitation and waterborne disease outbreaks in the United States, 1948–1994. *American Journal of Public Health, 91*, 1194–1199.

De Man, H., van den Berg, H.H.J.L., Leenen, E.J.T.M., Schijven, J. F., Schets, F. M., van der Vliet, J. C., . . . de Roda Husman, A. M. (2014). Quantitative assessment of infection risk from exposure to waterborne pathogens in urban floodwater. *Water Research, 48*, 90–99.

Dhiman, R. C., Pahwa, S., Dhillon, G. P., & Dash, A. P. (2010). Climate change and threat of vector-borne diseases in India: Are we prepared? *Parasitology Research, 106*, 763–773.

Dunne, J. P., Stouffer, R. J., & John J. G. (2013). Reductions in labour capacity from heat stress under climate warming. *Nature Climate Change, 3*, 563–566.

Dwight, R. H., Semenza, J. C., Baker, D. B., & Olson, B. H. (2002). Association of urban runoff with coastal water quality in Orange County, California. *Water Environment Research, 74*(1), 82–90.

Dyson, M. E. (2007). *Come hell or high water: Hurricane Katrina and the color of disaster.* New York, NY: Basic Books.

El-Fadel, M., Ghanimeh, S., Maroun, R., & Alameddine, I. (2012). Climate change and temperature rise: Implications on food- and water-borne diseases. *Science Total Environment, 437,* 15–21.

Elliott, J. R., & Pais, J. (2006). Race, class, and Hurricane Katrina: Social differences in human response to disaster. *Social Science Research, 35,* 295–321. http://dx.doi.org/10.1016/j.ssresearch.2006.02.003

Etheridge, D. M., Steele, L. P., Francey, R. J., & Langenfelds, R. L. (1998). Atmospheric methane between 1000 A.D. and present: Evidence of anthropogenic emissions and climatic variability. *Journal of Geophysical Research, 103*(D13), 15979–15993.

Fiore, A. M., Naik, V., & Leibensperger, E. M. (2015). Air quality and climate connections. *Journal of the Air Waste Management Association, 65,* 645–685.

Food and Agriculture Organization of the United Nations. (2006). *Livestock's long shadow: Environmental issues and options.* Rome: Food and Agriculture Organization. http://www.fao.org/docrep/010/a0701e/a0701e00.HTM

Food and Agriculture Organization of the United Nations. (2013). *The state of food insecurity in the world 2013. The multiple dimensions of food security.* Rome: Food and Agriculture Organization.

Fu, F. X., Tatters, A. O., & Hutchins, D. A. (2012). Global change and the future of harmful algal blooms in the ocean. *Marine Ecology Progress Series, 470,* 207–233.

Gingold, D. B., Strickland, M. J., & Hess, J. J. (2014). Ciguatera fish poisoning and climate change: Analysis of National Poison Center Data in the United States, 2001–2011. *Environmental Health Perspectives, 122,* 580–586.

Glass, G. E., Cheek, J. E., Patz, J. A., Shields, T. M., Doyle T. J., Thoroughman, D. A., . . . Bryan, R. (2000). Using remotely sensed data to identify areas of risk for hantavirus pulmonary syndrome. *Emerging Infectious Diseases, 63,* 238–247.

Glibert, P. M., Icarus Allen, J., Artioli, Y., Beusen, A., Bouwman, L., Harle, J., . . . Holt, J. (2014). Vulnerability of coastal ecosystems to changes in harmful algal bloom distribution in response to climate change: projections based on model analysis. *Global Change Biology, 20,* 3845–3858.

Goldmann, E., & Galea, S. (2014). Mental health consequences of disasters. *Annual Review of Public Health, 35,* 169–183.

Goodess, C. M. (2013). How is the frequency, location and severity of extreme events likely to change up to 2060? *Environmental Science Policy, 27,* S4–S14.

Goulder, L. H., & Schein, A. (2013). Carbon taxes versus cap and trade: A critical review. *Climate Change Economics, 4*(3), 1–28.

Grabow, M. L., Spak, S. N., Holloway, T., Stone, B., Mednick, A. C., & Patz, J. A. (2012). Air quality and exercise-related health benefits from reduced car travel in the midwestern United States. *Environmental Health Perspectives, 120,* 68–76.

Gulluk, T., Slemr, F., & Stauffer, B. (1998). Simultaneous measurements of CO_2, CH_4, and N_2O in air extracted by sublimation from Antarctica ice cores: Confirmation of the data obtained using other extraction techniques. *Journal of Geophysical Research–Atmospheres, 103,* 15971–15978.

Habeeb, D., Vargo, J., & Stone, B. (2015). Rising heat wave trends in large US cities. *Natural Hazards, 76,* 1651–1665.

Harvey, M., & Pilgrim, S. (2011). The new competition for land: Food, energy, and climate change. *Food Policy, 36*(Suppl. 1), S40–S51.

Hellberg, R. S., & Chu, E. (2015). Effects of climate change on the persistence and dispersal of foodborne bacterial pathogens in the outdoor environment: A review. *Critical Reviews in Microbiology, 42*, 548–572.

High Level Panel of Experts. (2013). *Biofuels and food security: A report by the high level panel of experts on food security and nutrition of the Committee on World Food Security*. Rome: Committee on World Food Security.

Howden-Chapman, P. L., Chapman, R. B., Capon, A. G., & Wilson, N. (2011). Carbon pricing is a health protection policy. *Medical Journal Australia, 195*, 311–312.

Hsiang, S. M., Burke, M., & Miguel, E. (2013). Quantifying the influence of climate on human conflict. *Science, 341*(6151). doi:10.1126/science.1235367

Hurley, W., Wolterstorff, C., MacDonald, R., & Schultz, D. (2014). Paralytic shellfish poisoning: A case series. *Western Journal of Emergency Medicine, 15*, 378–381.

Intergovernmental Panel on Climate Change. (2001). *Climate change 2001: Impacts, adaptation and vulnerability. Contribution of Working Group II to the Third Assessment Report of the Intergovernmental Panel on Climate Change*. J. McCarthy, O. F. Canziani, N. A. Leary, D. J. Dokken, & K. S. White (Eds.). New York, NY: Cambridge University Press.

Intergovernmental Panel on Climate Change. (2007). *Climate change 2007: The physical science basis. Contribution of Working Group I to the Fourth Assessment Report of the Intergovernmental Panel on Climate Change*. S. Solomon, D. Qin, M. Manning, Z. Chen, M. Marquis, K. B. Averyt . . . H. L. Miller (Eds.). Cambridge, England: Cambridge University Press.

Intergovernmental Panel on Climate Change. (2013). *Climate change 2013: The physical science basis. Contribution of Working Group I to the Fifth Assessment Report of the Intergovernmental Panel on Climate Change*. T. F. Stocker, D. Qin, G.-K. Plattner, M. Tignor, S. K. Allen, J. Boschung . . . P. M. Midgley (Eds.). New York, NY: Cambridge University Press.

Intergovernmental Panel on Climate Change. (2014). *Climate change 2014: Impacts, adaptation, and vulnerability. Contribution of Working Group II to the Fifth Assessment Report of the Intergovernmental Panel on Climate Change*. C. B. Field, V. R. Barros, D. J. Dokken, K. J. Mach, M. D. Mastrandrea, T. E. Bilir . . . L. L. White (Eds.). New York, NY: Cambridge University Press.

Ives, M. (2016, July 2). A remote Pacific nation, threatened by rising seas. *New York Times*. http://www.nytimes.com/2016/07/03/world/asia/climate-change-kiribati.html

Jenkins, J. D. (2014). Political economy constraints on carbon pricing policies: What are the implications for economic efficiency, environmental efficacy, and climate policy design? *Energy Policy, 69*, 467–477.

Johnston, F. H., Henderson, S. B., Chen, Y., Randerson, J. T., Marlier, M., DeFries, R. S., . . . Brauer, M. (2012). Estimated global mortality attributable to smoke from landscape fires. *Environmental Health Perspectives, 120*, 695–701.

Kan, H., Chen, R., & Tong, S. (2012). Ambient air pollution, climate change, and population health in China. *Environment International, 42*, 10–19. doi:10.1016/j.envint.2011.03.003

Khan, T., Dewan Quadir, T. S., Murty, A., Kabir, F. A., & Sarker, M. (2002). Relative sea level changes in Maldives and vulnerability of land due to abnormal coastal inundation. *Marine Geodosy, 25*, 133–143.

Kilbourne, E. M. (2008). Temperature and health. In R. B. Wallace (Ed.), *Maxcy-Rosenau-Last public health and preventive medicine* (15th ed., pp. 725–734). New York, NY: McGraw-Hill Medical.

Kjellstrom, T., Holmer, I., & Lemke, B. (2009). Workplace heat stress, health and productivity—An increasing challenge for low and middle-income countries during climate change. *Global Health Action, 2*. doi:10.3402/gha.v2i0.2047

Kovats, R. S., Edwards, S. J., Hajat, S., Armstrong, B. G., Ebi, K. L., & Menne, B. (2004). The effect of temperature on food poisoning: A time-series analysis of salmonellosis in ten European countries. *Epidemiology and Infection, 132*, 443–453.

Kunkel, K. E., Easterling, D. R., Redmond, K., & Hubbard, K. (2003). Temporal variations of extreme precipitation events in the United States: 1895–2000. *Geophysical Research Letters, 30,* 1900.

Lau, C. L., Smythe, L. D., Craig, S. B., & Weinstein, P. (2010). Climate change, flooding, urbanisation and leptospirosis: Fuelling the fire? *Transactions of the Royal Society of Tropical Medicine and Hygiene, 104,* 631–638.

Levy, B. S., & Sidel, V. W. (2014). Collective violence caused by climate change and how it threatens health and human rights. *Health and Human Rights International Journal, 16*(1), 32–40.

Liu, P., He, C. Y., Yin, J. X., Wang, Q., Yang, H., & Li, W. M. (2001). A survey of the psychological state and neurobehavioral function of traffic policemen. *China Occupational Medicine, 28,* 7–9.

Lloyd, S. J., Sari Kovats, R., & Chalabi, Z. (2011). Climate change, crop yields, and undernutrition: Development of a model to quantify the impact of climate scenarios on child undernutrition. *Environmental Health Perspectives, 119,* 1817.

Loughry, M. (2010). Climate change, human movement and the promotion of mental health: What have we learnt from earlier global stressors? In J. McAdam (Ed.), *Climate change and displacement: Multidisciplinary perspectives* (pp. 221–238). Portland, OR: Hart.

Luber, G., & McGeehin, M. (2008). Climate change and extreme heat events. *American Journal of Preventive Medicine, 35,* 429–435.

Martin, V., Chevalier, V., Ceccato, P., Anyamba, A., De Simone, L., Lubroth, J., . . . Domenech, J. (2008). The impact of climate change on the epidemiology and control of Rift Valley fever. *Revue Scientifique et Technique, 27,* 413–426.

Matsueda, M. (2011). Predictability of Euro-Russian blocking in summer of 2010. *Geophysical Research Letters, 38*(6). doi:10.1029/2010GL046557

McLaughlin, J. B., DePaola, A., Bopp, C. A., Martinek, K. A., Napolili, N. P., Allison, C. G., . . . Middaugh, J. P. (2005). Outbreaks of *vibrio parahaemolyticus* gastroenteritis associated with Alaskan oysters. *New England Journal of Medicine, 353,* 1463–1470.

McMichael, A., McMichael, C., Berry, H., & Bowen, K. (2010). Climate-related displacement: Health risks and responses. In J. McAdam (Ed.), *Climate change and population displacement: Multidisciplinary perspectives* (pp. 191–219). Portland, OR: Hart.

Mills, J. N., Gage K. L., & Khan A. S. (2010). Potential influence of climate change on vector-borne and zoonotic diseases: A review and proposed research plan. *Environmental Health Perspectives, 118,* 1507–1514.

Morin, C. W., Comrie, A. C., & Ernst, K. (2013). Climate and dengue transmission: Evidence and implications. *Environmental Health Perspectives, 121,* 1264–1272.

Moritz, M. A., Parisien, M. A., Batllori, E., Krawchuk, M. A., Van Dorn, J., Ganz, D. J., & Hayhoe, K. (2012). Climate change and disruptions to global fire activity. *Ecosphere, 3*(6), art. *49.* doi:10.1890/ES11-00345.1

Muñoz, A. G., Thomson, M. C., Goddard, L., & Aldighieri, S. (2016). Analyzing climate variations at multiple timescales can guide Zika virus response measures. *GigaScience, 5*(41). doi:10.1101/059808

Myers, S. S., Zanobetti, A., Kloog, I., Huybers, P., Leakey, A.D.B., Bloom, A. J., . . . Usui, Y. (2014). Increasing CO2 threatens human nutrition. *Nature, 510*(7503), 139–142.

National Academies of Sciences, Engineering, and Medicine. (2016). *Attribution of extreme weather events in the context of climate change.* Washington, DC: National Academies Press. doi:10.17226/21852.

Naumova, E. N., Jagai, J. S., Matyas, B., DeMaria, A., Jr., MacNeill, I. B., & Griffiths, J. K. (2007). Seasonality in six enterically transmitted diseases and ambient temperature. *Epidemiology & Infection, 135,* 281–292.

Nelson, G. C., Rosegrant, M. W., Koo, J., Robertson, R., Sulser, T., Zhu, T., . . . Lee, D. (2009). *Climate change: Impact on agriculture and costs of adaptation.* Washington, DC: International Food Policy Research Institute. http://www.ifpri.org/publication/climate-change-impact-agriculture-and-costs-adaptation

North, C. S., & Pfefferbaum, B. (2013). Mental health response to community disasters: A systematic review. *Journal of the American Medical Association, 310,* 507–518.

Ogden, N. H., Maarouf, A., Barker, I. K., Bigras-Poulin, M., Lindsay, L. R., Morshed, M. G., . . . Charron, D. F. (2006). Climate change and the potential for range expansion of the Lyme disease vector ixodes scapularis in Canada. *International Journal for Parasitology, 36*(1), 63–70.

Ostfeld, R. S., & Brunner, J. L. (2015). Climate change and ixodes tick-borne diseases of humans. *Philosophical Transactions of the Royal Society of London B: Biological Sciences, 370*(1665). doi:10.1098/rstb.2014.0051

Pascual, M., Ahumada, J. A., Chaves, L. F., Rodo, X., & Bouma, M. (2006). Malaria resurgence in the East African highlands: Temperature trends revisited. *Proceedings of the National Academy of Sciences, 103,* 5829–5834.

Pascual, M., Rodó, X., Ellner, S. P., Colwell, R., & Bouma, M. J. (2000). Cholera dynamics and El Niño-Southern Oscillation. *Science, 289*(5485), 1766–1769.

Pastor, M., Bullard, R. D., Boyce, J. K., Fothergill, A., Morello-Frosch, R., & Wright, B. (2006). *In the wake of the storm: Environment, disaster and race after Katrina.* New York, NY: Russell Sage Foundation.

Patz, J. A., Frumkin, H., Holloway, T., Vimont, D. J., & Haines, A. (2014). Climate change: Challenges and opportunities for global health. *Journal of the American Medical Association, 312,* 1565–1580.

Patz, J. A., Gibbs, H. K., Foley, J. A., Rogers, J. V., & Smith, K. R. (2007). Climate change and global health: Quantifying a growing ethical crisis. *EcoHealth, 4,* 397–405.

Patz, J. A., Githeko, A. K., McCarty, J. P., Hussein, S., Confalonieri, U., & de Wet, N. (2003). Climate change and infectious diseases. In A. J. McMichael, D. H. Campbell-Lenddrum, C. F. Corvalán, K. L. Ebi, A. K. Githeko, J. D. Scheraga, & A. Woodward (Eds.), *Climate change and human health: Risks and responses* (pp. 103–132). Geneva, Switzerland: World Health Organization.

Patz, J. A., & Hahn, M. B. (2013). Climate change and human health: A one health approach. In J. S. Mackenzie, M. Jeggo, P. Daszak, & J. A. Richt (Eds.), *One health: The human-animal-environment interfaces in emerging infectious diseases* (pp. 141–171). New York, NY: Springer.

Patz, J. A., Vavrus, S., Uejio, C., & McClellan, S. (2008). Climate change and waterborne disease risk in the Great Lakes region of the US. *American Journal of Preventive Medicine, 35,* 451–458.

Paz, S. (2015). Climate change impacts on West Nile virus transmission in a global context. *Philosophical Transactions of the Royal Society of London. Series B: Biological Sciences, 370.* doi:10.1098/rstb.2013.0561

Petkova, E. P., Bader, D. A., Anderson, G. B., Horton, R. M., Knowlton, K., & Kinney, P. L. (2014). Heat-related mortality in a warming climate: Projections for 12 U.S. cities. *International Journal of Environmental Research and Public Health, 11,* 11371–11383.

Pew Research. (2014). Climate change: Key data points from Pew Research. http://www.pewresearch.org/key-data-points/climate-change-key-data-points-from-pew-research/

Porter, J. R., Xie, L., Challinor, A. J., Cochrane, K., Howden, M., Iqbal, M. M., . . . Travasso, M. I. (2014). Food security and food production systems. In C. B. Field, V. R. Barros, D. J. Dokken, K. J. Mach, M. D. Mastrandrea, T. E. Bilir, . . . L. L. White (Eds.), *Climate change 2014: Impacts, adaptation and vulnerability. Part A: Global and sectoral aspects. Contribution of Working Group II to the Fifth Assessment Report of the Intergovernmental Panel on Climate Change* (pp. 485–533). New York, NY: Cambridge University Press.

Robine, J. M., Cheung, S. L., Le Roy, S., Van Oyen, H., Griffiths, C., Michel, J. P., & Herrmann, F. R. (2008). Death toll exceeded 70,000 in Europe during the summer of 2003. *Comptes Rendus Biologies, 331*, 171–178.

Rogelj, J., den Elzen, M., Höhne, N., Fransen, T., Fekete, H., Winkler, H., . . . Meinshausen, M. (2016). Paris Agreement climate proposals need a boost to keep warming well below 2°C. *Nature, 534*, 631–639. doi:10.1038/nature18307

Rose, J. B. (1997). Environmental ecology of cryptosporidium and public health implications. *Annual Review of Public Health, 18*(1), 135–161.

Running, S. W. (2006). Is global warming causing more, larger wildfires? *Science, 313*, 927–928.

Russo, S., Marchese, A. F., Sillmann, J., & Immè, G. (2016). When will unusual heat waves become normal in a warming Africa? *Environmental Research Letters, 11*(5). doi:10.1088/1748-9326/11/5/054016

Salamanca, F., Georgescu, M., Mahalov, A., Moustaoui, M., & Wang, M. (2014). Anthropogenic heating of the urban environment due to air conditioning. *Journal of Geophysical Research: Atmospheres, 119*, 5949–5965.

Schlosberg, D., & Collins, L. B. (2014). From environmental to climate justice: Climate change and the discourse of environmental justice. *Wiley Interdisciplinary Reviews: Climate Change, 5*, 359–374.

Schuster, C. J., Ellis, A. G., Robertson, W. J., Charron, D. F., Aramini, J. J., Marshall, B. J., & Medeiros, D. T. (2005). Infectious disease outbreaks related to drinking water in Canada, 1974–2001. *Canadian Journal of Public Health, 96*, 254–258.

Shue, H. (2014). *Climate justice: Vulnerability and protection.* Oxford, England: Oxford University Press.

Sovacool, B. K. (2012). Expert views of climate change adaptation in the Maldives. *Climatic Change, 114*, 295. doi:10.1007/s10584-011-0392-2

Stenseth, N. C., Samia, N. I., Vilijugrein, H., Kausrud, K. L., Begon, M., Davis, S., . . . Chan, K. (2006). Plague dynamics are driven by climate variation. *Proceedings of the National Academy of Sciences, 103*, 13110–13115.

Stewart Ibarra, A. M., Ryan, S. J., Beltrán, E., Mejía, R., Silva, M., & Muñoz Á. (2013). Dengue vector dynamics (Aedes aegypti) influenced by climate and social factors in Ecuador: Implications for targeted control. *PLOS One, 8*(11). doi:10.1371/journal.pone.0078263

Tirado, M. C., Cohen, M. J., Aberman, N., Meerman, J., & Thompson, B. (2010). Addressing the challenges of climate change and biofuel production for food and nutrition security. *Food Research International, 43*, 1729–1744.

Trewin, B. J., Kay, B. H., Darbro, J. M., & Hurst, T. P. (2013). Increased container-breeding mosquito risk owing to drought-induced changes in water harvesting and storage in Brisbane, Australia. *International Health, 5*, 251–258. doi:10.1093/inthealth/iht023

Uejio, C. K., Yale, S. H., Malecki, K., Borchardt, M. A., Anderson, H. A., & Patz, J. A. (2014). Drinking water systems, hydrology, and childhood gastrointestinal illness in central and northern Wisconsin. *American Journal of Public Health, 104*, 639–646.

United Nations High Commissioner for Refugees. (2009). *Climate change, natural disasters and human displacement: A UNHCR perspective.* http://www.unhcr.org/refworld/docid/4a8e4f8b2.html

US Department of Defense. (2014). *2014 Climate Change Adaptation Roadmap.* http://www.acq.osd.mil/ie/download/CCARprint_wForeword_c.pdf

Vinck, P. (2013). *World disasters report: Focus on technology and the future of humanitarian action.* Geneva, Switzerland: International Federation of Red Cross and Red Crescent Societies. http://worlddisastersreport.org/en/

Wang, S., Zhang, J., Zeng, X., Zeng, Y., & Chen, S. (2009). Association of traffic-related air pollution with children's neurobehavioral functions in Quanzhou, China. *Environmental Health Perspectives, 117*, 1612–1618.

Weaver, S. C., & Reisen, W. K. (2010). Present and future arboviral threats. *Antiviral Research, 85*, 328–345.

Westerling, A. L., Hidalgo, H. G., Cayan, D. R., & Swetnam, T. W. (2006). Warming and earlier spring increase western U.S. forest wildfire activity. *Science, 313*, 940–943.

Wheeler, T., & von Braun, J. (2013). Climate change impacts on global food security. *Science, 341*, 508–513.

Zhang, Y., Bielory, L., Mi, Z., Cai, T., Robock, A., & Georgopoulos, P. (2015). Allergenic pollen season variations in the past two decades under changing climate in the United States. *Global Change Biology, 21*, 1581–1589.

Ziska, L. H., & McConnell, L. L. (2015). Climate change, carbon dioxide, and pest biology: Monitor, mitigate, manage. *Journal of Agricultural Food Chemistry.* doi:10.1021/jf506101h

CHAPTER 11

INFORMATION COMMUNICATION TECHNOLOGY AND HEALTH

Laura E. Jacobson, MPH

Alain B. Labrique, PhD, MHS, MS

Technology made large populations possible; large populations now make technology indispensable.

—Joseph Wood Krutch

LEARNING OBJECTIVES

- Discover the field of mobile digital health (mHealth) and learn about its history
- Understand the role mobile phones have played in health care globally
- Become familiar with the 12 essential mHealth functions and explore some case examples
- Discuss benefits and challenges to the global expansion of electronic health records
- Understand the role data play in global health understand the promise of open data, interoperable data, and "big data"
- Recognize some limitations to information communication technology and global health

The rapid developments in **information communication technology (ICT)** have transformed almost every aspect of life in recent decades. With little to no investment from the global health community, nearly every population across the globe has witnessed a vast expansion in low-cost mobile device ownership, ubiquitous wireless networks, far-reaching connectivity, and increased access to both smart and Internet-connected devices. With the spread of technological connectivity comes opportunity for better health outcomes through increased access to information, more avenues for communication, reduced distance between patients and providers, and better data to leverage resources. Most important, the speed with which information can now move through a health system is

Foundations for Global Health Practice, First Edition. Lori DiPrete Brown.

© 2018 John Wiley & Sons, Inc. Published 2018 by John Wiley & Sons, Inc.

unprecedented; test results from a laboratory or data collected in the field can be available to inform decisions in near-real time. This phenomenon, best described as "time-compression," can be instrumental in improving health outcomes in the management of clinical emergencies as well as in the diagnosis and care of chronic disease.

This chapter provides an overview of the origins of ICT in the health setting and how it has evolved with the expansion of mobile phones worldwide, the various health challenges ICT can address, and the vast opportunities for ICT to strengthen health systems globally.

The Landscape

We will cover the early examples of ICT in the health system, how they evolved with technological advancements, and applications of these advancements for global health.

Telemedicine

Telemedicine literally means "healing at a distance" (from Latin *medicus* and Greek *tele*). The origins of modern telemedicine applications date back to the early 20th century when a Dutch physiologist named Willem Einthoven developed an electrocardiograph and transmitted heart rhythm data along telephone wires. This was followed by the use of radio consultations in Norway, Italy, and France in the 1920s through 1940s to aid patients at sea (Bashshur & Shannon, 2009).

The Cover of Science and Invention In 1925

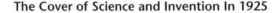

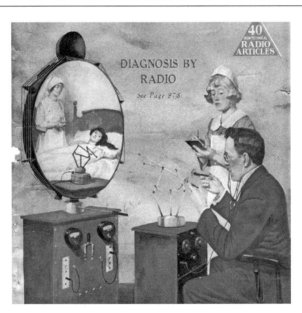

In the late 1960s, researchers conducted remote medical consultations for employees and travelers at Logan International Airport in Boston from their research center at Massachusetts General Hospital almost three miles away. Independent physician observers conducted evaluations of the diagnosis and treatment of the participating patients and the accuracy of the microwave transmission of medical information. This was one of the first conducted studies to demonstrate that diagnosis at a distance can successfully increase the availability of medical care to a remote location (Murphy & Bird, 1974).

Today, telemedicine is used all over the world to shorten the distance between patients and providers. Telemedicine is particularly useful for rural or underserved communities where distance is a significant barrier to accessing quality health care. Health care professionals use ICT for the exchange of information required for the diagnosis, treatment, and prevention of disease and injuries; for research and evaluation; and to support continuing education of health care providers (World Health Organization [WHO], 2010). Early telemedicine evolved beyond signal transmission by telephone or microwave to include a broad array of techniques and services.

Telemedicine can be broken down into several categories depending on how it is used. *Specialist referral services* involve a specialist assisting a general practitioner to advise or provide a diagnosis much like the early experiments at Massachusetts General. In this scenario, a patient might "see" a specialist by video or transmission of images. A cancer specialist reviewing images and discussing a case with a general practitioner is another example of this type of telemedicine. In other cases, a provider may offer *direct patient care* by exchanging audio, video, and/or medical information to diagnose, develop a treatment plan, prescribe medication, or provide clinical advice. If a patient resides in a region where no psychiatrists practice, for example, they could use video conferencing to have a virtual consultation without leaving their home or a nearby clinic. Providers may also use medical devices to *monitor remote patients*, collecting data and sending it to a central location for evaluation and interpretation. Remote monitoring of blood pressure, blood glucose, or other vital signs at home can help providers detect changes in a patient's health without requiring an expensive clinic or hospital visit. Experts can also use similar remote technology to *exchange their expertise and knowledge* with other practitioners without incurring expensive travel costs. In the same way, *consumer engagement* provides opportunities for individuals to discover specialized health information online or to participate in peer-group discussions for support (American Telemedicine Association, 2006).

Although telemedicine is useful in regions where geographic barriers to accessing care persist and critical clinician shortages (in particular, specialists) compromise care, earlier generations of technology require a certain level of connectivity. In many low- and middle-income countries (LMICs), lack of reliable Internet coverage, power outages, and limitations to audio and video equipment limit the effectiveness of these telemedicine strategies. However, the rapid proliferation of the mobile phone has allowed some LMICs to leapfrog beyond basic infrastructure limitations and extend the reach of telemedicine worldwide.

Digital Health or Connected Health

The vision of telemedicine has changed along with the underlying technologies that support it. The advent of mobile technology has forced a rethinking of what telemedicine can do—no longer requiring fixed sites. **Digital health** or **connected health** describes the current paradigm of ICT in health, where in addition to developing new innovations that take advantage of mobile and cloud-based solutions, we now recognize the importance of bridging earlier generations of fixed-site technologies, such as hospital computer systems and servers, with compatible and complementary mobile platforms. The goal of this new era of digital and connected health is to create functional bridges across the three main layers of the health system (patient, provider, and system). This is enabled by information technologies that reduce inefficiency and facilitate a patient-centered approach to care (Labrique, Vasudevan, Kochi, Fabricant, & Mehl, 2013). In the next section, we'll take a look at how digital health can impact these layers of the health system and walk through specific examples of digital health functions.

mHealth

Mobile digital health, or **mHealth**, encompasses a broad range of medical and public health practices supported by mobile devices, such as mobile phones, patient monitoring devices, personal digital assistants (PDAs), and other wireless devices (WHO, 2010). Underserved populations in LMICs see much higher rates of important development indicators such as infant and maternal mortality related to disparities in health system quality and access to care. The evolution of telemedicine to mHealth was motivated by these disparities to address persistent factors in many LMICs, such as a high burden of disease, shortages in the health workforce, and a large rural population. A dramatic increase in access and reduction of cost of mobile phones made this shift possible (Mehl & Labrique, 2014).

Despite the opportunities that mHealth presents, governments in LMICs are challenged by budget limitations, competing priorities, and gaps in technical infrastructure that impede widespread adoption of innovations. For this reason, credible evidence, guidance, and a systematic framework with which to adopt emerging technology are critical to incentivize and support decision makers as they consider integrating new tools to address specific health system constraints (Labrique et al., 2013). Recognizing that mHealth should be integrated into existing health system functions and not treated as stand-alone solutions, mHealth researchers and implementers at WHO, the Johns Hopkins University Global mHealth Initiative, the United Nations Children's Fund (UNICEF), and frog Design created an mHealth and ICT Framework that systematically describes the components of an mHealth strategy and defines the relationships between common applications of mHealth and ICT and the health system constraints that they address. (See http://www.ghspjournal.org/content/1/2/160.full.pdf±html for the full framework.)

We will walk through the 12 common mHealth and ICT applications described in this framework and discuss some selected examples from the field (Table 11.1).

Table 11.1   Twelve Common mHealth and ICT Applications

Application	Examples of Mobile Phone Functions
1. Client education and behavior change communication	• Short message service • Multimedia messaging service • Interactive voice response • Video clips • Images
2. Sensors and point-of-care diagnostics	• Mobile phone camera • Tethered accessory sensor, devices • Built-in accelerometer
3. Registries and vital events tracking	• Short message service • Voice communication • Digital forms
4. Data collection and reporting	• Short message service • Voice communication • Digital forms
5. Electronic health records	• Digital forms • Mobile web
6. Electronic decision support (information, protocols, algorithms, checklists)	• Voice communication • Mobile web • Stored information "apps" • Interactive voice response
7. Provider-to-provider communication (user groups, consultation)	• Short message service • Multimedia messaging • Mobile phone camera
8. Provider work planning and scheduling	• Interactive electronic client lists • Short message service • Mobile phone calendar
9. Provider training and education	• Short message service • Multimedia messaging service • Interactive voice response • Voice communication • Audio or video clips
10. Human resource management	• Web-based performance dashboards • Global positioning service • Voice communication • Short message service
11. Supply chain management	• Web-based supply dashboards • Global positioning service • Digital forms • Short message service
12. Financial transactions and incentives	• Mobile money transfers and banking services • Transfer of airtime minutes

Source: Adapted from "mHealth Innovations as Health System Strengthening Tools: 12 Common Applications and a Visual Framework," by Labrique et al., 2013, *Global Health, Science and Practice, 1,* p. 164.

Client Education and Behavior Change The first set of mHealth and ICT applications focuses primarily on the client (often the patient) and are intended to provide a channel to deliver timely educational content or actionable health information, with the goal of improving knowledge, modifying attitudes, and influencing health behavior. These messages are often delivered by short message service (SMS), audio, or video. The Mobile Alliance for Maternal Action (MAMA) is an example of an organization that uses mHealth for client education and behavior change.

Sensors and Point-of-Care Diagnostics Medical sensor technologies are developed to supplement or complement diagnostic tests through the use of mobile phones. Just as in earlier-stage telemedicine, these technologies allow providers to monitor the condition of their patients remotely in situations where there is great distance between patients and their providers. The newer generation of sensors, now operating on a mobile device, expands reach further while performing relatively simple tests, such as blood glucose measurements for diabetes management as well as sophisticated assays, such as electrocardiograms (Labrique et al., 2013).

BOX 11.1

MOBILE ALLIANCE FOR MATERNAL ACTION

Mobile Alliance for Maternal Action (MAMA) began in 2011 as a three-year, public-private partnership between USAID, Johnson & Johnson, the United Nations Foundation, mHealth Alliance and babycenter with the goal of delivering critical health messages to new and expectant mothers in developing countries via their mobile phones. MAMA ran programs in Bangladesh, India, South Africa, and Nigeria and created free, adaptable, evidence-based mobile messages informed by experts in maternal, newborn, and child health.

The MAMA model is based on the expectation that when women and families have greater access to relevant health information, this improved knowledge will lead to changes in behaviors and practices and ultimately translate to better health outcomes.

Evaluations of the MAMA programs showed that they reached millions of mothers, developed partnerships in over 50 countries, and contributed to a growing body of evidence supporting the effectiveness of mHealth initiatives. In 2015, MAMA ended its global coordinating and turned over operations to their in-country partners. MAMA tools and resources are free and available here: http://www.mobilemamaalliance.org/tools-and-resources.

Mobile Messages Put the Power of Health in Every MAMA's Hand

GLOBAL MOBILE PHONE ACCESS

 3 out of 4 people have access to mobile phones.

WOMEN'S MOBILE PHONE ACCESS

 Approximately 1 billion women in low and middle income countries own mobile phones.

1 billion

MATERNAL & INFANT MORTALITY

 800 each day — Every day, there are 800 women that do not survive child birth or pregnancy.

 2 out of 5 child deaths occur within the first month of life.

 About 29,000 children under the age of five — 21 each minute — die every day mainly from preventable causes.

How MAMA Messages Work

Mom receives personalized, stage-based messages 2–3 times a week.

• Encouragement   • Warning Signs   • Reminders

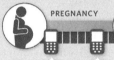 PREGNANCY
 BIRTH
 1 YEAR
 3 YEARS

"Dizziness, headaches and tiredness are all symptoms of low iron. Take a daily iron and folic acid supplement. This should help."

"Baby kicking? Try tickling him when he kicks. He can feel your touch now. If his movements slow down, talk to your midwife."

"Look out for signs of illness. If your baby vomits more than five times during a day, go to the clinic. Give her plenty of extra breastfeeds."

"Give your baby a big smile or scrunch up your nose: watch and your baby will copy you. You are the center of his world!"

"Your child will take her first steps soon, if she hasn't already. All children are different. She will develop at her own pace."

 Moms are empowered to make health decisions for themselves and their babies.

MAMA Mobile Alliance for Maternal Action

Bangladesh
South Africa
India

www.mobilemamaalliance.org

partners

 USAID FROM THE AMERICAN PEOPLE   Johnson&Johnson   UNITED NATIONS FOUNDATION   mHealth Alliance   babycenter

Source: Mobile Alliance for Maternal Action, http://www.mobilemamaalliance.org/
Material courtesy of the United Nations Foundation © 2015 United Nations Foundation or its licensor.

Registries and Vital Events Tracking Enumeration of a country's population, a government responsibility, is important for constructing an accurate denominator for which a health system is accountable. Many LMICs rely on paper-based registration systems that are often inaccurate and slow to update (Mehl et al., 2014). The tracking of vital events such as births and deaths by a mobile phone–based registration system can bolster population enumeration and demographic information needed to support program development; identify patients in need of specific services; and provide insight into health disparities. Mobile population registries can provide data on key development indicators; and, in settings where high proportions of births and deaths may occur in remote villages or at home, mobile registries can extend the infrastructure and engage front-line health workers to register these vital events in communities once on the periphery of the health system (Frøen et al., 2016).

Data Collection and Reporting *The Roadmap for Health Measurement and Accountability,* a joint effort of the World Bank Group, USAID, and WHO (2015), provides an outline for LMIC countries to harness the data they need to plan and manage their health priorities and deliver safe, high-quality health care in a cost-effective manner.

Policymakers need accurate and timely health information to ensure that planning priorities align with the needs of the population. As mentioned, mobile registries can supply better data needed to enumerate populations, characterize the burden of disease within a population, and monitor and track epidemics and outbreaks. With access to more reliable data, countries can design better policies, monitor and evaluate initiatives, and leverage resources to achieve broader development goals (United Nations, 2013).

Open data, or open source data, are data that are available for all to access, analyze, and publish without restriction. With the initiation of the Sustainable Development Goals in 2015, open data have been recognized as necessary components to better meet these goals. UN member states can use data, freely available online from governments. For more information, go to http://blogs.worldbank.org/ic4d/sustainable-development-goals-and-open-data.

As health systems make progress collecting electronic data and making such data available for analysis, it is imperative that these data are structured such that disparate data sets can be aggregated and integrated for larger, more meaningful analysis. These types of data are known as **interoperable data**.

"Big data" are data sets that are large enough that sophisticated analytics can produce new insight. There is much excitement about the prospects of the role of big data in both the private sector and in the global health community. However, many questions remain about the practicality and predictability of such endeavors. Currently most data sets large enough to reveal insight are held by private corporations such as Facebook, Google, and China's largest search engine, Baidu, so private-public partnerships are an important component to unlocking the promise of large data sets.

Google used big data to attempt to reveal influenza trends in the United States (see Box 11.2). This early exploration of the use of big data in public health revealed some important lessons to inform future studies.

BOX 11.2

GOOGLE FLU TRENDS

In 2007, a small team of software engineers at Google began searching for ways to use the company's vast stores of data to predict real-world phenomena. The team analyzed aggregated search queries, compared their data to official data provided by the Centers for Disease Control and Prevention (CDC), and discovered a strong correlation between the frequency of certain searches and the actual number of people who reported flu-like symptoms each week. They used this correlation to launch Google Flu Trends in 2008, a "nowcasting" dashboard listing daily influenza-related activity estimates for each US state.

This early warning system was able to provide estimated results weeks before the official CDC data became available, making it possible for public health officials to respond more quickly to outbreaks. The team also anonymized and aggregated the input search data to protect the privacy of searchers on Google. By 2014, Google had extended the system to nearly 30 countries and added coverage for other diseases like dengue fever. But the early promise of the system soon turned into a more complicated reality. In 2012 and 2013, the tool significantly overpredicted actual flu trends. An updated model improved performance in 2014 by incorporating CDC data throughout the season. A year later, though, Google shut down its public reporting dashboard and began providing model results directly to the CDC and other institutions.

The story of Google's foray into the prediction of outbreaks shows both the promise of advanced technology and its peculiarities. Flu Trends offered a faster way to detect and respond to influenza outbreaks. But even Google, with its immense (and proprietary) stores of data and legions of the best and brightest engineers, had to invest in continuous improvement of its modeling. Search queries that had strong predictive power one year led to overpredictions the next, especially as media coverage of influenza changed the way individuals turned to Google to search for health information. Privacy advocates remained skeptical of Google's aggregation and anonymization techniques, concerned that the system might still reveal highly personal data. And until it began providing data directly to the CDC and other groups in 2015, only Google could maintain and improve its model. So seven years after its small team started their exploration, Google and its partners are still looking for the right way to collaborate across the private and public sectors to actually improve health outcomes related to influenza (Butler, 2013; Ginsberg et al., 2009; Flu Trends Team, 2015; Lazer, Kennedy, King, & Vespignani, 2014; Stefansen, 2014).

Electronic Health Records An **electronic health record (EHR)** (or electronic medical record) is a digital version of a patient's health record or chart. EHRs typically contain a patient's medical history, diagnoses, medications, treatment plans, immunization records, allergies, and other test results. EHRs have become the standard in developed countries over the past decade, but in LMICs, a number of barriers prevent wide-scale adoption of these tools. Many EHR products are expensive and require a network of computers with consistent power and Internet access. Some countries have adopted EHRs but have not been able to scale these electronic health products beyond a few hospitals or clinics.

Mobile phone–based EHRs are making it possible for health systems to centralize the collection and maintenance of a patient's health data such that providers in other clinics, villages, or cities can more easily provide consistent and continuous care. Digital reporting in EHRs of medical events can offer clinicians real-time information to reduce response lag for urgent and time-sensitive matters (Mehl et al., 2014).

Electronic Decision Support: Information, Protocols, Algorithms, Checklists Ensuring all health workers' adherence to clinical protocols is critical for implementing complex care guidelines. Shifting tasks from clinicians to frontline health workers has been a strategy of many resource-limited health settings to ameliorate health worker shortages. When clinical procedures are adapted for health workers with limited formal training, mHealth initiatives that incorporate point-of-care decision support tools with algorithms and checklists that are easily accessible on a mobile device can ensure quality of care and reduce the potential for error or delay (Labrique et al., 2013). One example is Electronic-Integrated Management of Childhood Illness (e-IMCI), a product that provides an electronic step-by-step algorithm to aid in triage and treatment decisions for children according to WHO protocols for the diagnosis and treatment of common childhood diseases (DeRenzi et al., 2008). In South Africa, Essential Medical Guidance disseminates clinical guidelines and health system information to health care workers in a specific geographic location (see Box 11.3).

BOX 11.3
ESSENTIAL MEDICAL GUIDANCE

"We believe that through Innovation, Collaboration and Technology, we will overcome significant healthcare challenges in the developing world." These few words outline the underlying premise of the South Africa–based nonprofit organization the Open Medicine Project. The company's founders, Dr. Mohammed Dalwai and Dr. Yaseen Khan, define their goals as "dissemination of relevant clinical guideline and health system information to frontline healthcare workers, helping facilitate free and open access to critical health information and support—aiming to use mobile technology to disseminate life-saving information, in the best format to where it is needed the most." Dalwai and Khan have spent the last five years developing and implementing innovative clinical applications, such as the Mobile Triage application, the Primary Health Care Clinical Guide and the HIV Clinical Guide application for the South African National Department of Health and such organizations as Médecins Sans Frontiers/Doctors Without Borders.

In 2014, the pair partnered with Dr. Janis Tupesis of the University of Wisconsin–Global Health Institute to further develop this idea, forming the Essential Medicine Guidance (EMGuidance) platform. The group aimed to further develop an application that would provide users instant, mobile access to local clinical information. By partnering with hospitals in South Africa's Western Cape province, the group was able to collate accurate and relevant clinical content into an elegant mobile application. By using self-identified user data and geolocating capabilities, the group hopes to revolutionize how clinical care will be provided in developing health care systems. The group envisions a scenario where the clinical application will be able to give accurate, updated clinical information to a provider in a specific geographic locale, whether they are practicing at a large, academic hospital or a rural health outpost. The group envisions a time where their EMGuidance application on a user's mobile telephone will be able to provide the clinician optimal clinical guidelines, even if they change hospitals, provinces, or regions. By tracking usage profiles, the group also hopes to provide feedback to individuals, hospitals, and governments about what data are being accessed, helping formulate optimal clinical protocols and educational programs.

The group's applications have been accessed more than 3.4 million times by 150,000 health care workers in 200 countries worldwide. The group has just released their free, open-access application in South Africa's Android and Apple app stores. Further information can be obtained at www.emguidance.com and www.openmedicineproject.org.

Provider-to-Provider Communication: User Groups, Consultation Although it is easy to take for granted in developed nations, simple voice communication by mobile phone is perhaps one of the most transformative mHealth applications. Direct provider-to-provider communication, which was once unavailable, can now coordinate care, provide expert assistance, allow for discussion, and provide a diagnosis and treatment plan when and where it is needed. Furthermore, mobile phones can also allow for the exchange of images or sounds to allow for real-time remote consultation (Labrique et al., 2013).

Provider Work Planning and Scheduling Work planning and scheduling tools on mobile platforms can assist busy health workers by sending reminders of upcoming or overdue services and creating a structure to organize their calendar or other work tools.

Because health care worker shortages in limited-resource settings persist, mHealth systems have the potential to ease some of the burden of traditional paper-based workflow practices and provide extra support tools (Labrique et al., 2013).

Provider Training and Education Mobile devices provide continued training and support to frontline and remote providers through educational videos and messaging as well as interactive exercises such as quizzes and case study examples that reinforce skills much like those that would be provided in a typical in-person medical continuing education training (Labrique et al., 2013).

Human Resource Management Many health centers in resource-limited settings lack robust human resource departments dedicated to staff operations and oversight. When community health workers are embedded in or deployed to remote villages, they may have limited contact with supervisory staff. mHealth tools have the potential to bridge some of these gaps through tracking of remote work with web-based dashboards or real-time GPS. These tools can not only provide oversight and accountability of staff but also allow for avenues of recognition for exemplary work (Labrique et al., 2013).

Supply Chain Management Keeping remote health clinics stocked with essential medicines and supplies can be challenging for many LMICs. Delays in stockout reporting and inefficient allocation of supplies can increase costs for already burdened health systems. mHealth tools that track and manage these stocks are based on relatively simple technologies that allow remote clinics or pharmacies to report daily levels of drugs and supplies and send requests for additional materials electronically (Labrique et al, 2013).

Financial Transactions and Incentives Often, health systems in developing countries rely on cash transactions, which contributes to inefficiencies and potential security risks. mHealth and mobile money are converging rapidly and may increase patients' access to health care by lowering financial barriers via platforms that facilitate quick access to funds at crucial times. Further, mobile money has the potential to expand access to financial services such as insurance as account-based enrollment become more available (www.hfgproject.org).

Considerations

Innovators are developing strategies to harness the power of mobile technologies for the benefit of public health. Due to the complex and context specific nature of health system constraints in LMICs, it can be difficult to develop "one-size-fits-all" solutions. However, these 12 common mHealth and ICT applications are informed by system-level thinking that favors addressing multifunctional layers over narrow-scope or "Band-Aid" solutions. Sustainable adoption of new technology that leads to improved health outcomes depends on strategic and systematic design, development, and integration. When technology is constructed without context-specific evaluations, cost-effectiveness analysis, or input from end users, or is based on assumptions, the opportunity for sustainable system-wide benefit is lost.

BOX 11.4

A GRADUATE STUDENT'S EXPERIENCE

LAURA JACOBSON

As a graduate student in public health, I embarked on a field experience in western Uganda to conduct a qualitative evaluation of the role of mobile phones in the health system. This was at a time when mHealth pilot projects were rapidly expanding. I interviewed health workers and policymakers and asked participants to describe their current workflow and documentation practices, their perceptions of technology in the health system, and their thoughts on barriers to improving ICT and health in their community. Qualitative research is an important aspect of developing a deep and rich understanding of a particular topic or problem. This experience showed that although respondents perceived a role for mobile phones in their health system, they also noted some important considerations. Some were concerned about the cost, sustainability, and operability of mobile phones, and many felt that they were not included in the discussion around the product design or development of the tools.

In addition, respondents highlighted a tension around the idea that existing wide-scale mobile phone ownership was the key to mHealth success. Some indicated that workers and community members participating in mHealth interventions often see device ownership as an entitlement or an incentive to adopt this technology and that they would expect new phones to be supplied and maintained. However, if implementers of mHealth projects anticipate that the phones are already in place and users expect that new phones will be supplied, this disconnect in expectations could potentially have significant budgetary implications or cause conflict.

From this research, I learned that clarifying and establishing expectations around who is purchasing and maintaining the devices are critical to the success of mHealth work in the future. Having the end users, such as the health workers and policymakers, involved in the development of the mHealth tools will ensure that the tools are designed to meet the needs of those who may eventually use them (Jacobson et al., 2015).

Conclusion

Global health agendas strive to expand the reach of health services to achieve universal health coverage. mHealth tools that aid in enumeration, registration, communication, and record keeping have the potential to facilitate better health system performance (Mehl & Labrique, 2014). The arc of development from early telemedicine to mobile digital strategies to vast stores of data and beyond shows that ICT has embedded itself into the health system in many ways. Mobile technologies are becoming more sophisticated and less costly, continuing to provide fuel to the ever-evolving technical landscape that supports and promotes global public health. With the spread of technological connectivity comes opportunity for better health outcomes through increased access to information, more avenues for communication, reduced distance between patients and providers, and better data to leverage resources. However, this goal is achieved only when partnership, capacity building, and the intentional creation of tools that serve end users and enhance and support current systems are prioritized over developing the newest high-tech, innovative products. With a structure and framework to guide investment and adoption of mobile technology into existing health systems, we move closer to expanding health care access, reducing inefficiency, and improving health outcomes.

Mobile phones have been a transformative addition to the landscape of global health. We can imagine them making their way into the core set of tools carried by all health workers or supplied to expectant mothers, connecting them to key services and health information. In the not-so-distant future, these tools that connect us may be fully integrated, making the whole system stronger and shortening the distance between us.

Chapter Summary

In this chapter, we have described the role of information communication technology (ICT) in the health system. We have focused on the evolution and development of telemedicine and mobile digital health (mHealth) and described how they are enhancing and improving the health system. We've explored the expansion of data in the health system globally and discussed the importance of electronic, standardized, and accessible data. Further, we have emphasized the need to develop technology intentionally and systematically, to engage leaders and build capacity, and to create ICT tools that are compatible with current systems and that leverage the needs of the end users.

Key Terms

"Big data"
Digital health or connected health
Electronic health records
Information communication technology (ICT)
Interoperable data
mHealth
Open data
Telemedicine

Review Questions

1. Why is information communication technology important in the health system globally?
2. Come up with an example of a public health problem that could be supported by the use of a mobile phone. Explain the problem and how mobile technology could help.
3. Describe the benefits of electronic health records (EHRs) in LMICs. What are some drawbacks?
4. Why are data important in public health? What types of public health problems could be improved with better data and why?

References

American Telemedicine Association. (2006). *Telemedicine, telehealth, and health information technology: An ATA issue paper.* Retrieved from www.who.int/entity/goe/policies/countries/usa_support_tele.pdf

Bashshur R. L., & Shannon G. W. (2009). *History of telemedicine: Evolution, context, and transformation.* New Rochelle, NY: Mary Ann Liebert.

Butler, D. (2013). When Google got flu wrong. *Nature, 494,* 155–156. doi:10.1038/494155a

DeRenzi, B., Parikh, T., Mitchell, M., Chemba, M., Schellenberg, D., Lesh, N., . . . Borriello, G. (2008). e-IMCI: Improving pediatric health care in low-income countries. In *Conference on human factors in computing systems—Proceedings* (pp. 753–762). doi:10.1145/1357054.1357174

Flu Trends Team. (2015, August 20). The next chapter for flu trends. [Web blog post]. *Google Research Blog.* Google. Retrieved from https://research.googleblog.com/2015/08/the-next-chapter-for-flu-trends.html

Frøen, J. F., Myhre, S. L., Frost, M. J., Chou, D., Mehl, G., Say, L., Cheng, S., . . . Flenady, V. J. (2016). eRegistries: Electronic registries for maternal and child health. *BMC Pregnancy and Childbirth, 16,* 11. doi:10.1186/s12884-016-0801-7

Ginsberg, J., Mohebbi, M. H., Patel R. S., Brammer, L., Smolinski, M. S., & Brilliant, L. (2009). Detecting influenza epidemics using search engine query data. *Nature, 457*, 1012–1014. doi:10.1038/nature07634

Jacobson, L. E., Bajunirwe, F., Vonasek, B. J, Twesigye, L., Conway, J. H., Grant, M. J., & Sethi, A. K. (2015). Characterizing the flow of health information in rural Uganda: Is there a role for mobile phones? *Journal of Public Health in Developing Countries, 1*(1), 4–13.

Labrique, A. B., Vasudevan, L., Kochi, E., Fabricant, R., & Mehl, G. (2013). mHealth innovations as health system strengthening tools: 12 common applications and a visual framework. *Global Health, Science and Practice, 1*, 160–171. doi:10.9745/GHSP-D-13-00031

Lazer, D., Kennedy, R., King, G., & Vespignani, A. (2014). The parable of Google Flu: Traps in big data analysis. *Science, 343*, 1203–1205.

Mehl, G., & Labrique, A. B. (2014). Prioritizing integrated mHealth strategies for universal health coverage. *Science, 345*, 1284–1287.

Mehl, G., Vasudevan, I., Gonsalves, L., Berg, M., Seimon, T., Temmerman, M., & Labrique, A. (2014). Harnessing mHealth in low-resource settings to overcome health system constraints and achieve universal access to health. In L. A. Marsch, S. E. Lord, & J. Dallery (Eds.), *Behavioral healthcare and technology: Using science-based innovations to transform practice* (pp. 239–264). Oxford, United Kingdom: Oxford University Press.

Murphy, R.L.H., & Bird, K. T. (1974). Telediagnosis: A new community health resource. *American Journal of Public Health, 64*, 113–119.

Stefansen, C. (2014, October 31). Google Flu Trends gets a brand new engine. [Web blog post]. *Google Research Blog.* Google Inc. Retrieved from https://research.googleblog.com/2014/10/google-flu-trends-gets-a-brand-new-engine.html

United Nations. (2013). *A new global partnership: Eradicate poverty and transform economies through sustainable development.* The report of the High-Level Panel of Eminent Persons on the post-2015 development agenda. New York, NY: United Nations Publications. Retrieved from https://sustainabledevelopment.un.org/content/documents/8932013-05%20-%20HLP%20Report%20-%20A%20New%20Global%20Partnership.pdf

World Bank, USAID, & World Health Organization. (2015, June). *The roadmap for health measurement and accountability.* Retrieved from http://www.who.int/entity/hrh/documents/roadmap4health-measurement_accountability.pdf

World Health Organization. (2010). *Telemedicine: Opportunities and developments in Member States: Report on the second global survey on eHealth* (Global Observatory for eHealth Series, 2). Retrieved from http://whqlibdoc.who.int/publications/2010/9789241564144_eng.pdf

CHAPTER 12

SCALING UP IN GLOBAL HEALTH
LESSONS FROM PRACTICE

Richard Cash, MD, MPH
Sophie Broach

Small is beautiful, but large is necessary.
—**Sir Fazle Hasan Abed, founder of BRAC**

LEARNING OBJECTIVES

- Define scale-up and the different forms it can take
- Become familiar with the story of programs successfully scaled up by BRAC
- Become familiar with a range of successful scale-up examples
- Become aware of common challenges and key considerations for program scale-up
- Consider scale-up implications for your own work

Although some excellent ideas spread on their own, others do not, including many public health solutions. Interventions to tackle many of the biggest problems in global health already exist, but bringing these to the people who need them, particularly the poor and underserved, presents serious challenges. The global health community is becoming increasingly aware that many promising, effective innovations fail to spread on a large scale. According to USAID (2015), hastening the adoption of existing key high-impact health interventions between 2015 and 2020 could prevent the deaths of 600,000 mothers and 15 million children.

Foundations for Global Health Practice, First Edition. Lori DiPrete Brown.
© 2018 John Wiley & Sons, Inc. Published 2018 by John Wiley & Sons, Inc.

How can a promising intervention that has performed well in a bounded area be made ubiquitous? How long should it take for such interventions to spread from one to many? Examples of successfully scaled-up public health programs offer key insights into how to navigate the challenges inherent in bringing an intervention from one community to many.

What Is Scale-Up?

This section defines scale-up, including the different forms it can take and phases of the scale-up process.

Definition and Overview of Types of Scale-Up

Scaling up refers to the process of effectively implementing a standardized, low-cost health intervention nationwide to reach the majority of the population. An intervention can be extended to a greater number of people by either (1) expanding availability to increase **coverage** or (2) increasing uptake by raising demand for and use of services among the target population. In general, scale-up involves identifying an effective intervention, honing it to improve its impact and cost-benefit ratio, and then rolling out the program at a larger scale. BRAC founder Sir Fazle Hasan Abed summarized his organization's model for scale-up as "effective, efficient, expand" (Haddad, 2011). For scale-up to be successful, the intervention should continue to produce results similar to what was achieved during the pilot phase, and the key features of the intervention should be preserved as it grows.

Deliberate, guided scale-up proceeds in two major ways: horizontally and vertically (Simmons, Fajans, Ghiron, & Johnson, 2011). In **horizontal scale-up**, an intervention expands to new geographic areas and new populations. Horizontal scale-up is usually what people's thoughts turn to when they think of scale-up, but it alone cannot ensure strong results or sustainability. **Vertical scale-up**, which refers to the building of legal, political, policy, or institutional changes necessary for the large-scale implementation of an intervention, is also crucial. Through vertical scale-up, an intervention can be integrated into the institutions that will be involved in its implementation.

Scale-up can unfold through several different methods. The organization that led the pilot can itself lead the scale-up, or a new organization with the capacity to deliver at scale can take over the project after the pilot phase. The piloting organization can also join forces with other organizations to deliver the intervention at scale. The pace and timing of scale-up can also vary. Programs can go to scale from the start of implementation or later, and can increase coverage rapidly or through incremental steps

(Abed, 2011). **Diversification** is a form of scale-up in which interventions are tested and added into an existing package of services already being delivered by an organization or institution (Simmons et al., 2011).

Spontaneous scaling up, a rare phenomenon in public health, occurs when innovations spread on their own, without any guidance from implementers, due to an organic demand from the population. Although this can be a positive phenomenon, it can also result in people taking up certain aspects of the innovation and not others, hurting impact and reflecting negatively on the innovation itself (Simmons et al., 2011).

Phases of Scale-Up

Scaling up is a multidimensional activity. Ideally the concept should be taken into account from the beginning—it should be a "before thought," not an "after thought." Scaling up a public health program is a dynamic and iterative process that includes the following steps: piloting for feasibility; experimentation, planning, capacity building, rollout, advocacy, and institutionalization (Kohl, 2011). The aim of the pilot is to demonstrate on a small scale that an intervention is effective, evidence based, and able to work in a range of settings. During the pilot, the intervention is also refined to simplify the process of implementation and reduce costs.

In the planning phase, clear goals should be set that are specific, achievable, measurable, and time-bound, yet ambitious, and strategies to reach them should be determined. Identifying sources of funding is also critical during this phase, as is delineating the roles and responsibilities of the actors that will be involved in implementation.

Once the intervention has been identified and the scale-up has been planned, the program can be rolled out to new populations and areas, while being adapted to local conditions. Successful rollout demands strong management capacity and coordination, as well as effective monitoring, evaluation, and research to provide timely feedback to inform ongoing program design and implementation. Management should be as simple as possible to achieve the desired results. **Monitoring and evaluation** are crucial to discovering whether scale-up is working as anticipated and uncovering obstacles that need to be overcome. **Capacity building** is also a critical component of scale-up. Through capacity building, the necessary infrastructure, human resources, skills, equipment, and supervision for implementing the model are developed. Program staff must be able to carry out **knowledge transfer**, teaching the technical and operational elements of the intervention to other implementers.

Budgetary resources are always limited, and there are always numerous policies and programs competing for priority. Thus, effective advocacy, which fosters the perception that a program is legitimate and addresses an important need, is critical to ensuring a program's success as it scales up.

The Story of BRAC: Experiences in Successfully Scaling Up Public Health Programs

BRAC, the world's largest and top-rated NGO, has become known as a global leader in scaling up public health programs. BRAC's experiences in scaling up programs to combat child diarrhea; improve maternal, neonatal, and child health; and reduce tuberculosis offer valuable insights into how to scale up successfully.

What Is BRAC?

Perhaps no other organization in the world has had greater success in scaling up public health programs than **BRAC**. In the way that it implements its programs, BRAC has expertly embodied the belief that "small is beautiful but large is necessary," as articulated by its founder Sir Fazle Hasan Abed. Small organizations and programs can adapt quickly to meet new challenges and develop deep, nuanced understandings of local needs. As organizations and programs grow, they risk becoming rigid and bureaucratic and losing touch with realities on the ground in the communities they serve. BRAC has recognized the benefits of being small, but has heeded the call to bring its services to greater numbers of people in need. As the organization has expanded, it has worked to stay innovative and has continued to emphasize the value of local expertise.

BRAC has grown dramatically since it was founded in 1972, becoming the world's largest development NGO. In 2016, its programs covered 138 million people around the world; employed 111,000 staff; and supported 117,000 community health workers ("BRAC at a Glance," 2015). BRAC, which began as a relief organization distributing emergency aid in Bangladesh, now works at all levels of development including microfinance, education, legal aid, agriculture, community development, and health.

BRAC has achieved remarkable results by designing programs to ensure their replicability, adjusting them during the pilot phase to improve efficiency and effectiveness, and then implementing the refined programs across broad swathes of the country using a network of highly decentralized staff and a "learning by doing" approach. For example, BRAC implemented a microfinance program early in its existence through village organizations. It treated each village organization as a business experiment, creating approaches intended to produce specific results and then measuring their actual effects on the ground and making adjustments as necessary. BRAC has subsequently leveraged these village organizations to deliver programs in health and other areas.

BRAC delivers health interventions through a cadre of community health workers, known as **Shasthya Shebikas** and *Shasthy Kormis*. The *Shasthya Shebikas*, female community health volunteers who receive training in the provision of essential health care services, are the frontline workers who are embedded in the communities where they deliver health services. The typical *Shasthya Shebika* is a married woman between ages 25 and 35 who does not have children under two years old. Often *Shasthya Shebikas* are members of BRAC village organizations and have received some schooling. BRAC offers *Shasthya Shebikas* performance-based incentives and supportive supervision through interactions with BRAC health staff. *Shasthya Kormis* carry out supervision and management activities. They receive more extensive health training, enabling them to deal with more complicated conditions. BRAC also works with governments, forming partnerships with public health facilities and government health workers.

Oral Therapy Extension Program

The Lancet once hailed the discovery of **oral rehydration solution** (ORS) as "potentially the most important medical advance" of the 20th century. The knowledge that sugar enables the gut to absorb more fluid had enormous implications for efforts to combat child diarrhea. However, 10 years after this groundbreaking discovery in the 1960s, diarrheal disease remained the leading killer of children. Although ORS appeared to be a simple and easy solution to a deadly problem, its use remained limited. Coaxing a child who has diarrhea to drink more liquid seemed intuitively to many parents to exacerbate the problem (Gawande, 2013).

In 1980, BRAC began implementing the Oral Therapy Extension Program (OTEP) to teach parents how to use ingredients in their own homes to combat child morbidity and mortality from diarrhea. The OTEP would become the first BRAC program taken to scale. It started as a small pilot aiming to reach only 60,000 women. Within three years, the program had been scaled up to reach 2.5 million households, and in 10 years, it had reached nearly 12 million households, with 90 percent retaining correct knowledge (Chowdhury & Cash, 1996).

Through door-to-door outreach, *Shasthya Shebikas* taught caregivers how to make lifesaving ORS by simply mixing a handful of brown sugar, a pinch of salt, and a half-liter of water together. These women traveled on foot, methodically covering all homes in a village until they had talked to every mother. Lacking high levels of education themselves, the *Shasthya Shebikas* adopted simple messages to convey to parents. BRAC limited *Shasthya Shebikas* to visiting 10 mothers per day after finding that fewer visits each day appeared to improve the quality of their teaching.

Ongoing research led to modifications to the program to achieve optimal results. Researchers examined questions including who the target groups for health education should be, how trainers' skills should be developed, what the key educational messages should be and how they should be disseminated, and how support for ORS could be mobilized among the community, and particularly among men.

BRAC searched for ways to ensure that presentations by the health workers actually resulted in caregivers' learning how to use ORS correctly. They arrived at using **performance-based incentives** to improve the quality of teaching by *Shasthya Shebikas*. To test how effective *Shasthya Shebikas* were at communicating messages about ORS, an evaluator later tested the knowledge of a subset of the mothers who had been counseled. *Shasthya Shebikas* were then paid according to caregivers' knowledge during the follow-up visits. This pressure led the workers to make sure the lessons stuck, and they adopted innovative strategies to do so. For example, they taught mothers in a hands-on manner, having them make the ORS themselves rather than simply hearing how to make it.

Eventually, the knowledge of how to use ORS became integrated into Bangladeshi culture, being passed along by word of mouth. Between 1980 and 2005, deaths from diarrhea among children in Bangladesh dropped by 80 percent. Even decades after the program, national surveys found that nearly 90 percent of children experiencing severe diarrhea received ORS (Gawande, 2013). Today Bangladesh has the highest ORS use rate of any country in the world.

Maternal, Neonatal, and Child Health Interventions

At the time BRAC began implementing maternal, neonatal, and child health (MNCH) interventions in Bangladesh, maternal and child health indicators were dismal. In 2007, under-five child mortality stood at 65 per 1,000 live births (Bangladesh Demographic and Health Survey, 2009, cited by Afsana, 2011). Only about half of pregnant women attended three or more antenatal checkups, and about 80 percent of births occurred at home. Maternal and child health indicators were often even worse in urban slums than in rural areas. In 2006, one third of Bangladesh's urban population, and 3.4 million people in Dhaka alone, resided in slums (Centers for Urban Studies, 2006, cited by Afsana, 2011).

BRAC developed an MNCH intervention by drawing from knowledge produced in other countries, testing the intervention in a rural district in 2005 and then in a slum in Dhaka in 2007, and then expanding it throughout the country (Afsana, 2011). BRAC's extensive human resources, which spanned villages all over Bangladesh, and its strong existing platform on which to add more interventions helped set up the program for success.

Through the program, *Shasthya Shebikas* conducted house-to-house visits to identify pregnancies and births in their target areas, provide antenatal and postnatal checkups and education, attend deliveries, and facilitate women's visits to immunization centers. The program also strengthened the capacity of birth attendants and established a referral system for women with pregnancy complications. By 2008, maternal deaths in the district had dropped to 220 per 100,000 as compared to 320 nationwide (Afsana, 2011).

After refining the program in the rural district, BRAC adapted the program to Bangladesh's urban slums. With support from the Bill and Melinda Gates Foundation, the program, called Manoshi, began with a phased scaling up in Dhaka and then moved to other cities. The program encouraged women to give birth at "birthing huts," delivery centers staffed by urban birth attendants and midwives. Manoshi set up 241 birthing huts in

Dhaka catering to between 10,000 and 15,000 people each. These were designed to provide a hygienic environment, privacy, and gender-sensitive care and to enable rapid referrals to hospitals in the event of birth complications. Manoshi also developed a community support network comprising local stakeholders and community leaders who were educated about MNCH issues and encouraged to promote Manoshi's services to potential beneficiaries.

The referral system developed through Manoshi was an important innovation to reduce maternal mortality in the event of complications. It relied on partnerships with both public and private health facilities. When an emergency occurred, a BRAC staff member would be contacted and would then issue a referral slip and arrange for care at a hospital, while a community health worker would simultaneously assist in arranging emergency transport.

BRAC developed innovative responses to several challenges confronting the program. Women were often reluctant to make decisions about whether to go to a hospital for complications without their husbands' input, leading to dangerous delays in receiving care. Manoshi addressed this issue by informing men about possible complications and the hospital referral system ahead of time. Delays also occurred at the facilities. At the start of the program, some NGO clinics were not accepting patients referred by BRAC. In response, BRAC conducted outreach to these NGOs and included them in workshops to secure their support. There was also a dearth of skilled personnel at hospitals able to respond to complications. To reduce delays, BRAC stationed its own staff at the referral facilities to assist with patients referred through its program. Low retention rate of *Shasthya Shebikas* presented another obstacle. The dropout rate for *Shasthya Shebikas* was 31 percent in slums, more than three times the rate in rural areas. BRAC lost *Shasthya Shebikas* to migration and other job opportunities, which were more plentiful in urban areas. To combat this problem, BRAC began giving out performance-based incentives and increasing supervision.

Research, monitoring, and evaluation played a key role in the program's success. At the start of the Manoshi program, formative research guided strategy development, and a baseline provided a snapshot of the situation at the beginning of the project. Ongoing monitoring and evaluation captured the program's progress and highlighted its shortcomings. Findings about successes and challenges were shared quickly within BRAC, and data were fed into a management information system on a monthly basis.

In the end, the Manoshi program has achieved remarkable results, reaching 2.9 million people in Dhaka and the surrounding area within two years. After the first year, 95 percent of pregnant women were identified, up from 39 percent at the baseline. The percentage of women receiving three or more antenatal care visits rose from 45 to 73, far above the national average of only one antenatal visit for 73 percent of women. More women also gave birth at delivery centers. Whereas at the baseline, 84 percent of births took place at home, that number dropped to 32 percent after the program. Hospital births also rose from 16 to 23 percent (Afsana, 2011).

Moving forward in phases had allowed implementers to test what would work in a new area and adjust implementation accordingly. The approach also increased uptake of services by catering to women's needs—for example, by providing antenatal and post-natal care at women's homes and holding special meetings for expectant mothers to prepare them for their deliveries.

Tuberculosis Directly Observed Treatment Short Course Program

In the 1980s, the prevalence of tuberculosis in Bangladesh was 870 per 100,000 (Islam & May, 2011). Most of the population was rural and poor, making accessing facilities to seek treatment very difficult. When people did reach facilities, they often found them understaffed and with limited services.

In 1984, the National Tuberculosis Control Program (NTP) had begun operating in urban areas, but no outreach to rural populations was occurring. BRAC stepped up to address this gap, launching a community-based **Directly Observed Treatment Short Course (DOTS)** pilot program in the rural subdistrict Manikganj Sadar, which had a population of 220,000 (BRAC Health Program, 2011, Islam & May, 2011). It partnered with the NTP, which provided free medications and employed door-to-door outreach through *Shasthya Shebikas* who at this point were known in these communities. They were trained to do active case findings, visiting homes to determine if residents had symptoms associated with TB, particularly a persistent cough lasting more than three weeks, and recording suspected TB cases in a logbook. They also collected sputum samples and accompanied people to smearing centers to provide their final samples. The *Shasthya Shebikas* received notification of results and relayed them to people in their communities. Patients testing positive would go to the house of a *Shasthya Shebika* each day to take medications under her supervision, ensuring that drugs were taken in the correct manner for the required duration of treatment.

BRAC stayed in the pilot phase and refined the model until strategies for success were realized before implementing DOTS at scale. Decentralized management allowed adjustments to be made rapidly to the program as it expanded into new areas, and strong monitoring and evaluation allowed BRAC to uncover what was and was not working. BRAC leveraged its existing strengths and infrastructure, utilizing the village organization and *Shasthya Shebika* model that had been successful in delivering other interventions.

BRAC devised innovative methods to address challenges during scale-up. For example, *Shasthya Shebikas* dropped out 10–15 percent of the time, draining resources when new women were required to be trained. In response, BRAC made its requirements for becoming a *Shasthya Shebika* stricter. It also gave *Shasthya Shebikas* the chance to earn additional money by selling other medications, and increased supervision and training for them. Ensuring adherence to the treatment regime presented a major challenge. Patients often dropped out after the first few weeks once their symptoms abated. To combat high patient dropout rates, the program began requiring a bond from patients of US$3, the equivalent of about a week's worth of wages, during the pilot phase of the project. This was collected by the *Shasthya Shebikas*, who would return half of this amount after the patient successfully completed the treatment course. The other half of the bond covered the costs of the *Shasthya Shebikas*.

BRAC's nationwide expansion of the pilot began in 1995 through a public-private partnership with the NTP, which provided supplies, technical advice, and monitoring and conducted clinic-based activities. Due to government capacity constraints and the inability to test the influx of incoming sputum samples, BRAC established some of its own lab facilities. After 10 years of implementing its TB DOTS program, BRAC had expanded the program to an area with a population of roughly two million people. Over this time, it had brought down costs and produced high cure rates. In 2008, BRAC expanded the program once again after receiving a grant from the Global Fund for AIDS, TB, and Malaria. At this point, BRAC was able to begin paying its roughly 10,000 *Shasthya Shebikas* for successful treatments. TB cases treated by BRAC rose from 1,496 in 1995 to 90,000 in 2008, nearly two thirds of all TB cases treated in the country. Using *Shasthya Shebikas* to treat TB patients was also less costly than using government facilities, at US$64 compared to US$96 per case (Islam & May, 2011). With support from the Global Fund, the DOTS model eventually expanded to all districts in the country, with BRAC supplying services in 42 districts and a network of 27 NGOs covering the remaining 22 districts (Abed, 2011).

At scale, the DOTS program covered over 100 million people and contributed to slashing TB prevalence. Cure rates and treatment compliance rates both increased after the pilot phase, reaching the global targets of a 70 percent case detection rate and an 85 percent successful treatment rate for positive cases (Abed, 2011). The key features and impact of the pilot intervention had remained intact as the program was expanded from one subdistrict to the entire nation.

Engaging in Global Health Practice with Scale in Mind

Scaling up presents many challenges, particularly in developing countries with poor transportation infrastructure, limited Internet access, and underresourced public health facilities (McCannon, Schall, Perla, & Barker, 2011). However, challenges to scale-up can be overcome if they are anticipated and the plans and resources to attack them are assembled. The following key insights about scaling up are drawn from the book *From One to Many: Scaling Up Health Programs in Low Income Countries* (Cash, Chowdury, Smith, & Ahmed, 2011).

First, it is critical that programs be piloted for feasibility prior to scale-up. Interventions may work very well during the pilot phase and then collapse when expanded. Thus an intervention must be tested in different contexts to ensure that it can be replicated successfully across new areas with differing sociocultural and geographic features. The intervention may also turn out to be too expensive to be implemented at a large scale, so the pilot must unearth ways to bring down costs without limiting impact. Inadequate evaluation of the pilot, such as evaluation overly focused on technical components of the program, can fail to capture intangible elements key to the program's success.

Scaling up is a complex, multifaceted process that requires negotiating with political, social, and economic institutions. The skills required to create an innovation and execute a pilot project differ greatly from those needed for scaling up a health program, and an organization that successfully pilots an approach may not be well suited to rolling it out. In particular, scale-up demands efficient and effective management structures, as managing scale-up can be far more complex than managing routine programs. Bureaucratic and logistical issues and heavy reporting requirements can slow implementation when programs expand, which points to the need to continuously search for efficiencies and ways to streamline the program as much as possible.

It is vital that scale-up be led by an entity with strong capacity to deliver programs at scale efficiently. Working through the public health system, though often bringing political legitimacy and reach, may require programs to grapple with overworked staff with poor capacity for implementation. The alternative of building new institutions through which to deliver a program also takes time and funds and can result in a lack of critical political support for the intervention and even in clashes with existing institutions (Kohl, 2011).

During scale-up, it may become apparent that service providers lack the capacity to implement the program adequately. Incentives and adequate supervision can help improve performance, as can celebration of program victories and recognition of good work (McCannon et al., 2011). Staff turnover can lead to the deterioration of skills and the quality of services provided, so systems must be set up to transfer skills and knowledge to new personnel and monitor their performance.

BOX 12.1
CASE STUDY OF PROBLEMATIC SCALE-UP

Not all programs are well suited for scale-up. For example, the Bangladeshi government and UNICEF partnered to construct tube wells across the country in an effort to reduce water-borne diseases. By the end of the 1980s, there were over one million such wells in Bangladesh. However, since the early 1980s, scientists had connected arsenic poisoning to tube well water in nearby areas of India. Although program implementers were aware of these findings, the program continued, perhaps because changing or stopping it would have jeopardized its financial resources and political support. To this day, many communities in Bangladesh must contend with arsenic-contaminated wells.

Although funders often demand quick results, program managers should be aware that scaling up takes time, often longer than originally planned, and should attempt to set realistic time frames. Preparing for scale-up should begin in the pilot period by establishing systems that can serve as springboards for scaling-up activities (Cash et al., 2011). In general, slower scale-up over the course of multiple phases tends to be more effective than rapid scale-up, which can result in only some components of an intervention being spread while other important components suffer, such as quality of care. A slower pace allows for adjustments to be made along the way to improve program effectiveness.

Simultaneous horizontal and vertical scale-up are key to achieving sustainability (Simmons et al., 2011). Advocacy work is needed to cultivate the political will to support the program and mobilize necessary resources to ensure its longevity. If support for scale-up is secured from only one individual or group, the program will be in jeopardy in the event of a change in power. In addition, potential sources of opposition to the intervention should be identified early on and won over. Linking an intervention to issues already widely regarded to be high priority and leveraging international pressure can help in this regard. Including potential allies in setting program goals and developing strategies can foster motivation and help them encourage support for the program. Creating a shared story placing the program scale-up in the context of a larger narrative of improvement also helps bring participants onboard (McCannon et al., 2011).

Internal advocacy work to inspire implementers should also not be overlooked in scale-up. Securing support for the program from low-level implementers will improve the program's prospects, as these implementers deal directly with beneficiaries on the ground and will likely be ineffective in promoting the intervention if they do not believe in it themselves.

Research, monitoring, and evaluation are essential to guiding program implementation and expansion. In particular, the experiences of "frontline" participants are crucial to understand. Data collected must be useful to program participants and point to areas for improvement. Both quantitative and qualitative measures, which can capture participants' reflections and lessons learned, are necessary. At the same time, data submission must be as easy and not feel unduly burdensome. Program managers should determine how best to disseminate knowledge of better practices among those involved in implementing the program—for example, through structured annual meetings, extension agents who deliver information to different participating sites, or cascading sequences of trainings (McCannon et al., 2011).

Overall, scaling up requires self-criticism and the honesty to assess what is not working and to learn how to address these problems. Trial and error is a normal part of scaling up. Because context matters deeply, programs must be flexible and able to be modified in response to evidence of what works effectively in different linguistic, cultural, and institutional contexts.

Chapter Summary

The magnitude of global health problems today is large, so the scale of the interventions addressing them must be large as well. Although discovering new lifesaving techniques is crucial in the field of public health, spreading interventions already known to be evidence based and cost-effective is equally, if not more, important. Interventions already exist that could save the lives of millions of people worldwide. The challenge now is to spread those interventions. Scaling up successful health programs is a process that demands different types of work than routine program management, but successful scale-up is certainly possible, as BRAC's experiences in Bangladesh clearly demonstrate. There are at least six principles that are part of any scaling-up activity: it is multidisciplinary; it should be considered from the very beginning of any pilot program; workers should be trained in anticipation of increasing activity; management should be appropriate and simple, and address the key issues; and it should involve evaluation, adaptation, and advocacy.

Key Terms

BRAC
Capacity building
Coverage
Directly Observed Treatment Short Course (DOTS)
Diversification
Horizontal scale-up
Knowledge transfer
Monitoring and evaluation
Oral rehydration solution
Performance-based incentives
Scaling up
Shasthya Shebikas
Spontaneous scaling up
Vertical scale-up

Review Questions

1. What are the different forms of scale-up? *or* What is the difference between horizontal and vertical scale-up?
2. Describe common challenges that arise when working to scale up public health programs.

3. What factors contributed to BRAC's success in scaling up public health programs?

4. What key considerations must be taken into account when scaling up public health programs?

References

Abed, F. H. (2011). Foreword. In R. A. Cash, M. R. Chowdury, G. B. Smith, & F. Ahmed (Eds.), *From one to many: Scaling up health programs in low income countries* (pp. xxi–xxv). Dhaka, Bangladesh: University Press Limited.

Afsana, K. (2011). Scaling up BRAC's maternal, neonatal, and child health interventions in Bangladesh. In R. A. Cash, M. R. Chowdury, G. B. Smith, & F. Ahmed (Eds.), *From one to many: Scaling up health programs in low income countries*. Dhaka, Bangladesh: University Press Limited.

BRAC at a glance. (2015). BRAC. Retrieved from http://www.brac.net/partnership

BRAC Health Program. (2011). *Making tuberculosis history: Community-based solutions for millions*. Dhaka, Bangladesh: University Press Limited.

Cash, R. A., Chowdhury, M. R., Smith, G. B., & Ahmed, F. (Eds.). (2011). *From one to many: Scaling up health programs in low income countries*. Dhaka, Bangladesh: University Press Limited.

Chowdhury, M., & Cash, R. (1996). *A simple solution*. Dhaka, Bangladesh: University Press Limited.

Gawande, A. (2013, July 29). Slow ideas. *New Yorker*. Retrieved from http://www.newyorker.com/magazine/2013/07/29/slow-ideas

Haddad, L. (2011). Scaling up "scaling up" for health. In R. A. Cash, M. R. Chowdury, G. B. Smith, & F. Ahmed (Eds.), *From one to many: Scaling up health programs in low income countries* (pp. 255–260). Dhaka, Bangladesh: University Press Limited.

Islam, A., & May, M.(2011). Decentralized management in the expansion of BRAC's rural tuberculosis program (DOTS). In R. A. Cash, M. R. Chowdury, G. B. Smith, & F. Ahmed (Eds.), *From one to many: Scaling up health programs in low income countries* (pp. 207–214). Dhaka, Bangladesh: University Press Limited.

Kohl, R. (2011). An analytical framework for scaling up pilots in public health. In R. A. Cash, M. R. Chowdury, G. B. Smith, & F. Ahmed (Eds.), *From one to many: Scaling up health programs in low income countries* (pp. 241–254). Dhaka, Bangladesh: University Press Limited.

McCannon, J. C., Schall, M. W., Perla, R. J., & Barker, P. (2011). Planning for scaling up. In R. A. Cash, M. R. Chowdury, G. B. Smith, & F. Ahmed (Eds.), *From one to many: Scaling up health programs in low income countries* (pp. 15–31). Dhaka, Bangladesh: University Press Limited.

Simmons, R., Fajans, P., Ghiron, L., & Johnson, B. R. (2011). Managing scaling up. In R. A. Cash, M. R. Chowdury, G. B. Smith, & F. Ahmed (Eds.), *From one to many: Scaling up health programs in low income countries* (pp. 3–13). Dhaka, Bangladesh: University Press Limited.

USAID. (2015). *Acting on the call: Ending preventable maternal and child deaths*. Retrieved from https://www.usaid.gov/sites/default/files/documents/1864/USAID-2015-Acting-on-the-Call.pdf

GLOBAL HEALTH PRACTICE

CHAPTER 13

GLOBAL HEALTH EXPERIENCES
PREPARING FOR GLOBAL HEALTH PRACTICE

Katarina M. Grande, MPH
Lori DiPrete Brown, MS, MTS

If you have come here to help me, you are wasting your time. But if you have come because your liberation is bound up with mine, then let us work together.

—Lila Watson at the 1995 UN Decade for Women, reflecting the collective wisdom of the Aboriginal activist groups in Queensland in the 1970s

---

LEARNING OBJECTIVES

- Understand the intentions and purposes of student global health experiences
- Describe various types of global health experiences and the kinds of students who can benefit from them
- Prepare a comprehensive country profile about the country you will visit

---

Global health students are often asked by friends, mentors, and teachers, "Where do you want to go?" and "What type of work do you want to do?" Initially, driven by curiosity, a spirit of adventure, and a desire to be part of change, these students may answer, "I'll go anywhere!" "I'll do anything!" However, as global health study progresses, students begin to discern which type of global health work aligns best with their values

Foundations for Global Health Practice, First Edition. Lori DiPrete Brown.
© 2018 John Wiley & Sons, Inc. Published 2018 by John Wiley & Sons, Inc.

and strengths. They develop specific geographic and topical interests. They realize the complexity and ethical considerations surrounding global health. It is at this point that they are ready to begin planning their first global health learning experience.

This chapter and the seven chapters that follow provide guidance about global health learning and practice from your undergraduate training through graduate school and the early years of your career. Chapter 14 presents global health competencies that can help you plan your engagement for maximum learning. Chapter 15 gives an overview of community-based research and action principles that can be applied in both global health educational experiences and subsequent global health practice. Chapter 16 provides insights and useful exercises to practice transformational leadership skills. Chapter 17 provides guidance for instructor-led field experiences, which can help faculty and students select, design, and evaluate their fieldwork. Chapter 18 focuses on the unique learning and leadership opportunities offered by global health student organizations, with a strong focus on respectful and ethical practice. An overview of standard health and safety precautions is provided in Chapter 19. Finally, Chapter 20 outlines a global health career path, with information about skills needed, the job search, and networking within the global health community.

Global Health Experiences: A Focus on Learning

Global health education experiences center on learning, rather than on helping. Global health work in a country other than your own can often encompass the well-intentioned idea, "I want to go to [insert destination] to help people." This thinking is full of assumptions. It assumes that the population that you aim to serve needs help; it assumes that you are equipped with the skills and knowledge needed to provide this help; and it assumes that you are the best person to do the "helping." It is important to remember that the central goal of your early global health experiences is to *learn*. These global health field experiences can prepare you to advocate for equitable public policies and can provide you with an experiential understanding of the social determinants of health. The benefits—during, immediately after, and in the distant future—of a global health field experience can be immense. But understand that "relationships with institutions, organizations, communities, and people in international service-learning contexts can both disrupt and reproduce inequitable power dynamics and historical global relations" (Crabtree, 2013, p. 61). Approach your planning process with a conscious focus on humility, respect, and an openness to listening and learning.

A community of practice can help you develop perspectives that will help you make the most of your global health experience. Building a community of globally minded friends, colleagues, and mentors ensures that you will have a much-needed support system when you see difficult situations firsthand (you will), need to process ethical dilemmas, or want to discuss a new project. Start with your classmates in this course:

Who is asking the deep questions? Who seems to have an extensive network from which you could learn? This cultivation of strategic friendships can be viewed as an alternative to more traditional "networking"—cold-calling or introducing oneself to leaders in the field. If an opportunity for global health fieldwork arises, chances are your network of colleagues will share the opportunity within the group before sending it on to others.

By cultivating a diverse and broad network of mentors, you can get a sense of the types of skill sets you'll want to gain as you explore the global health field. Finding mentors and role models with experience in or connections to the global health field can be immensely useful. Think strategically about cultivating these relationships; it is unlikely that just one person will serve all your needs. Seek out global health professionals across the career spectrum—early career, midlevel, and senior. Connect with people who *aren't* global health professionals but have qualities you admire: a dynamic leader, a deeply reflective listener, a logistics guru, or an amazing project manager. To broaden your mentor network, look for people who you "want to be," but also seek out those whose backgrounds are different than yours—for example, if you identify as a member of a historically underrepresented group, it can be advantageous to have mentors and role models from both within and outside your group.

Types of Global Health Experiences

There are many forms of experiential learning in global health. What is best for you will depend on your goals, the extent of your prior experience and knowledge in the setting that you are choosing, and the time and resources you are able to devote to the experience. This chapter will describe different types of global health experiences and provide guidance to help you discern the type of experience that matches your interests and skill sets. We will profile the following categories of experiences:

1. Short-term group immersion experience with an instructor ("field" course)
2. Mentored independent experience for individuals or small teams (internship)
3. Study abroad with a focus on community engagement
4. Making the global connection locally
5. Global engagement and experiential learning from a distance
6. Social impact venture/competition courses
7. Conferences
8. Postgraduate fellowship or service
9. Volunteer experiences

Short-Term Group Immersion Experience with an Instructor (Field Course)

A **field course** takes the classroom to the community. It may be led by a university instructor or a place-based expert and may include traditional lectures alongside visits to organizations, institutions, households, or projects. For example, in a course titled Public

Health 550: Health Systems and Tuberculosis [TB] in Uzbekistan, you may read about TB diagnostic systems in the morning, visit a TB clinic and ask a lab technician questions in the afternoon, and discuss local innovations and challenges in TB diagnostics with your course mates in the evening. See chapter 17 for a discussion of global health field courses and an example of a curriculum for a global health field course in Nepal.

Some field courses will have prerequisites, such as a political science, language, or history course related to the region you will visit. Although the trip is usually planned out for you, you should expect to do some place-based orientation and study before departure. Good questions to ask about a field course before enrolling are, "How long has this course been running?" "Does the instructor have extensive expertise working with this community?" and "What has been the experience of others who have taken this course?"

A field course is an ideal first global health experience. Even if you have prior global experience, a field course can be a good way to be introduced to a new region of the world. In a field course, you will have the mentorship and guidance of someone who knows the country well, as well as administrative support from the university that makes logistic and health and safety matters easy. A field course may also be a stepping-stone to doing independent work in the same country in the future.

Mentored Independent Experience for Individuals or Small Teams (Internship)

Internships are typically more aligned with a framework of job training. Whereas volunteer experiences are often (though not always) designed primarily with the needs of the host organization in mind, internships may be mutually beneficial to the student and the host; thus internships require more focus on finding a match in values and skills. Examples of internship titles include fundraising management intern, community health worker outreach intern, administrative support to deputy country director intern, refugee services coordination intern, or social media and communications intern.

Like volunteering, internships can span a range of tasks and skill sets. Some interns may do more administrative or clerical work to help fill organizational gaps; others may be assigned a specific project with concrete deliverables and time frames. For the internships requiring a specific skill set, such as website development, the applicant is expected to already have the specified expertise. The Akili Initiative (http://www.mappinghealth.com/akili/) is a comprehensive database that sorts internship and job opportunities by topic, countries in which the organization operates, whether or not the site accepts undergraduate students, and whether the site is open to internships.

Independent global health experiences may require more active planning and vetting than a university-led field course. Students are therefore encouraged to think deliberately about a regional focus and type of global health experience that best fits with their skill set and interests. As part of the deliberation process, the following activities can be useful: conducting a literature review to understand prominent health issues facing the region, researching potential placement sites to understand examples of available internships or volunteer experiences, practicing writing a query letter to an organization to elaborate on why a particular position is a good match, completing a country profile to become familiar with the culture and history of a specific placement site, and planning strategies for supporting oneself financially during an unpaid internship or volunteer experience.

Study Abroad with a Focus on Community Engagement

Study abroad programs can offer a rich opportunity to learn in an international setting. Most universities provide access to a broad range of experiences to dozens of countries and include courses from many disciplines. Generally, these are semester or yearlong programs in which students take classes and earn credit at an international university. The degree to which these programs provide global health learning opportunities varies greatly. Some programs are taught in English by faculty from the home institution and enroll students in separate courses with other international students. Others are taught in the local language, and students are integrated with students from the home country. Some programs provide independent dorm or apartment housing; others arrange for a home stay with a family. Many programs do not have immersion learning components.

Each of these types of programs has value, and you need not make global health content the primary factor in choosing a program. Given the duration of these programs, you will find that, whichever type of study abroad program you choose, it is possible to seek out learning opportunities that will engage you with the local community and expose you to the social determinants of health. This might mean shadowing or volunteering with a local organization, participating in cultural activities, or engaging in a local sport or pastime that has a link to health. Conduct research prior to committing to a study abroad program. Speak with program representatives or your study abroad office about the level of engagement the program has with the community in which it resides. Inquire about possibilities for volunteering for a local organization during your study abroad time.

Making the Local to Global Connection

Globally contextualized study can take place anywhere, which means that your immersion learning experience can be done in your community, your state, or elsewhere in the United States. You might work in areas of health disparity in the cities or rural areas of your state. Or you might engage with communities that have an international heritage, either as an end in itself or as a step toward working in that country of origin. You might engage with Native American/American Indian populations that are within our borders but sovereign nations. In each case, you can adopt a global perspective. Frame these experiences with such questions as "What are the global root causes of health and disease?" "What are the impacts?" "What are the strengths, assets, and sources of resilience in the community?"

Global Engagement and Experiential Learning from a Distance

Again, traveling to another place is not the only way to build your global experience. There are plenty of opportunities to engage globally from home, particularly with the help of technology. For example, a university course may partner with a grassroots organization abroad to conduct work directly with the organization in the form of fundraising, advocacy, or research on an identified need of the community. Often these types of courses require frequent email or Skype communication with the organization with which you will work, which can provide important lessons in cross-cultural communication and work styles for both you and your partner. With these types of international deliverable-based projects, students may also gain skills applicable to "consulting"—short-term contract work assignments. Another example of university-based global engagement is a "competition course," which is further described in the next section.

Social Impact Venture/Competition Courses

Many universities are realizing the need to build **systems thinking** skills—the practice of studying linkages and interactions among disciplines and issues—among students who are seeking to solve complex challenges by working in interdisciplinary, international teams. In contrast to traditional lecture-style courses, "competition courses," which incorporate business-minded approaches to tackle social issues (including global health issues), are becoming more prevalent. In these courses—under the names of social entrepreneurship, social innovation, social enterprise, or social ventures, among others—student teams compete with each other in tackling real-world problems with real clients. The prize may include start-up funding to pilot the venture. An example is the University of Minnesota Institute on the Environment's Acara Challenge (http://environment.umn.edu/leadership/acara/competitions/acara-challenge/), in which students from any academic major team up with students at a partner university across the world to address a specific global challenge, such as how to provide clean water to a slum in Dharavi, Mumbai, India. Also see Harvard's Social Enterprise project list (http://www.hbs.edu/newventurecompetition/social-enterprise-track/Pages/teams.aspx) for more examples. As these courses grow in popularity, the number of social enterprises that are sustained "in the real world" as businesses or nonprofits will increase. Although not all social ventures competition courses take participants physically outside the walls of the university, deep collaboration with potential clients or students from universities located where the challenge is taking place can be a type of global health field experience.

Conferences

Conferences are great places to learn about the latest developments in global health. The Consortium of Universities for Global Health (www.cugh.org) hosts an annual conference that brings together students and academia alongside global health practitioners and leaders to present and discuss what programs, innovations, and ideas are working in global health and what is needed. The American Public Health Association, the largest association of public health practitioners in the United States, also hosts a yearly conference and has an International Health Section (https://www.apha.org/topics-and-issues/global-health). In these subsets of presentations, a broad range of global public health topics are addressed, ranging from program implementation strategies to large-scale analyses of government policies. Numerous topic-based conferences (such as the International AIDS Conference) are also held regularly.

In addition to offering excellent insight into current global health trends, conferences can provide a platform for connecting with like-minded individuals to add to your network and for discussing potential opportunities. Most conferences have discount registration pricing for students, and some offer free live streaming of events and enable people to participate in discussions via social media. Many conferences also offer discounted or waived registration fees in exchange for volunteering at the conference.

BOX 13.1
ILLUSTRATIVE LIST OF GLOBAL HEALTH CONFERENCES

- Consortium of Universities for Global Health (http://www.cugh.org/)

- American Public Health Association Annual Meeting (http://www.apha.org/annualmeeting)

- Clinton Foundation Health Matters Summit (U.S.-focused) (https://www.clintonfoundation.org/our-work/clinton-health-matters-initiative)

- Clinton Global Initiative (https://www.clintonfoundation.org/clinton-global-initiative/)

- Unite for Sight's Global Health and Innovation Conference (http://www.uniteforsight.org/conference/)

- International AIDS Conference (http://www.iasociety.org/)

- Social Good Summit (http://mashable.com/sgs/)

- Connected Health Conference (http://www.pchaconference.org/)

- Harvard's International Development Conference (http://harvardidc.com/)

- Women Deliver Conference (held every three years) (http://womendeliver.org/)

Postgraduate Fellowship or Service

The principles set forth in part 2 of this textbook can also be used to prepare for longer-term postgraduate global fellowships or service work, such as with the Peace Corps, Global Health Corps, AgriCorps, Atlas Corps, Doctors Without Borders, or Mercy Corps. Frequently, such organizations will strongly recommend experience with global work prior to applying. Global Health Corps has an excellent list of links to fellowship opportunities: http://ghcorps.org/connect/join-the-movement/other-opportunities/. For more examples, see chapter 20, Global Health Professional Skills and Careers.

Volunteering for Experiential Learning and Service

Volunteer experiences are unpaid (or pay-to-volunteer) arrangements in which a person provides time to an organization or entity. Individuals can connect directly with a volunteer site, or they can seek opportunities with volunteer-sending organizations that set up experiences for them with specific organizations. These volunteer-sending organizations may be nonprofit (such as VSO, WorldTeach, and Global Volunteers) or for-profit (such as Global Crossroad, ProWorld, and i-to-i). Sometimes an organization will provide free housing or meals to volunteers, and sometimes the volunteer must pay for these expenses. Some organizations utilize volunteers for a very specific project or task; others host volunteers as generalists. Volunteer tourism, or **voluntourism**, combines a volunteer experience with traditional tourism. These experiences can vary greatly in quality and in terms of ethical considerations.

One example of problematic voluntourism is orphanages that prey on individuals living in poverty to send their children to a facility at which tourists pay to volunteer (Pattisson, 2014). By contrast, other voluntourism experiences work to support local organizations to the point that they can operate sustainably without foreign volunteers (Blackledge, 2013). Regardless of the type of volunteer experience, you should conduct careful research prior to selecting an arrangement.

BOX 13.2

TEN QUESTIONS TO ASK A VOLUNTEER ORGANIZATION

- What is the organization's mission?

- How long have you worked with international volunteers?

- Does your organization have any specific political or religious affiliation?

- Why are international volunteers needed for this work? (Listen for an answer that names the benefit for both the community and you)

- What do you think are the greatest challenges for international volunteers at this organization? Is there anything I can do in advance to prepare for them?

- Do you engage local volunteers?

- How are local citizens involved in determining what projects to do?

- Who will volunteer projects benefit? What are the goals of the project?

- Do you need the skills and experience I can bring to the project?

- How do you match volunteers to projects, both in terms of skills and interest?

Source: Adapted from "Ways to Volunteer Abroad," by Action Without Borders, 2017. Retrieved from http://www.idealistvolunteering.org/ways-to-volunteer-abroad/

Applying for and Funding Global Health Experiences

As you research types of experiences, create space and time for personal reflection to discern whether a particular opportunity embodies ethical principles of global health practice, is a good match for both you and the organization, and is a sound personal financial investment. A helpful exercise, described in the following section, can be to write a query letter. The action of writing a letter that carefully connects your intentions with the organization and opportunity can help you think through these considerations. Finally, a necessary exercise is to plan wisely around the cost implications of a global health experience. Such opportunities can be life changing, but there can also be significant financial implications.

Writing a Query or Letter of Introduction

Most global health internships and volunteer experiences will require that you write a query letter or letter of introduction. The letter should establish a positive rapport and make it clear why you want to work with this organization. It should tell the reader who you are, what your strengths are, and what you hope to do, learn, and contribute. It also should clarify your availability and provide contact information. When possible, have a classmate or advisor review the letter and provide you with feedback. The letter should not exceed one page.

BOX 13.3

TIPS FOR QUERIES AND LETTERS OF INTRODUCTION

- Address the communication to a specific person, rather than a generic "Dear Sir or Madam." Be sure you are directing the communication to the correct person.

- Use a formal, accurate title when addressing the recipient (i.e., Dr., Mr., Ms.).

- Do not send a letter in English unless you have verified that the recipient can read English. If a second language is required and you are not fluent, first consider whether you are a good fit for the organization; if you are, have a native speaker help you review the letter.

- In the first paragraph, make a specific personal connection to (1) the organization and its mission and (2) the individual and their role.

- Summarize your skills and interests, what you hope to learn, and what activities you are interested in. What can you contribute? What are you most interested in? Indicate that although you have specific interests and preferences, you are flexible and eager to learn.

- Clarify the dates and duration of your availability, and your expectations regarding payment and logistical arrangements. For example, state that you will pay for room and board or that you might need assistance with arrangements for lodging or with arranging transport to and from the site.

- Make it clear how and when you can be reached. Be flexible and respectful of the person's time, offering email, phone, and Skype contact information.

- Do not exceed one page.

Funding Your Global Health Experience

Depending where you decide to go or where an opportunity arises, a global health field experience can be an expensive endeavor. Most volunteer and internship experiences are unpaid; and many have additional costs beyond a plane ticket, such as housing, transportation, and administrative support related to the work you do for them. In planning for your field experience, start thinking about cost implications early so that you can identify options for funding. Many universities have scholarships that can be used specifically for global health experiences; ask your program administrators for details and deadlines for applying. Private foundations are another funding option, although the funding tends to be research focused. Personal fundraising efforts are another option—through community groups with which you may be involved, a church, or online fundraising platforms like GoFundMe. You can also consider paying your own way, if possible. Given the impact a global health experience can have on your career trajectory, such expenses could be considered a professional investment. Check with your student loan officer to determine whether student loans can be used for global health experience travel expenses.

Chapter Summary

Global health learning experiences are the first steps toward becoming a global health practitioner. These experiences can take many forms, such as volunteerism, field courses, and internships. It is also helpful to cultivate a network of global health classmates and professionals, continuously learn about global health issues, and seek mentors and role models who can provide you with guidance and opportunities. The country profile activity that follows can be another preparatory tool for global health engagement.

Activity: Develop a Country Profile

Developing a country profile provides structure and guidance for preparatory learning that enables you to take full advantage of the opportunities to learn and share during your global health experience. The country profile is useful for first-time travelers or seasoned international advisors who want to inform their fieldwork with broad contextual information.

The profile can be prepared individually or in a group. The goal is both to learn about the country and to learn *how* to gather this kind of information so that you have the mastered the skill of place-based preparation.

This exercise can be done in preparation for a global health learning trip, or, alternatively, it can be used in a global health course as a group assignment in preparation for a virtual trip (distance-based engagement with international communities) or for engagement with local populations who have an international heritage.

BOX 13.4

COUNTRY PROFILE WORKSHEET

COUNTRY _____

Please describe briefly why you chose this country. Do you have relevant prior experience, language skills? Is this country part of your heritage?

TOPIC _____

Conduct a literature review to identify key resources that summarize the most current scholarship related to your global health focus topic in the country or region where you wish to work. Strive to find 2–3 social science articles as well as 2–3 health science articles that address your topic in a regional context. These articles can be a mixture of gray literature (i.e., they may be organizational reports or policy briefs) and peer-reviewed literature.

Health Science Articles

1.

2.

3.

Social Science Articles

1.

2.

3.

Organizations That You Will Work With or Visit

Provide a summary description of each organization that you will visit or work with. In your summary, answer the following six questions: (1) What type of organization is it (NGO, government, private sector, civil society, faith-based organization, or community)? (2) What are the organization's goals, history, and mission? (3) Whom does the organization primarily aim to serve? (4) What are its sources of funding? (5) What are the core values that drew you to want to work with this organization? (6) What challenges might you face in working in this organization? Also identify the key contact person with whom you would be working and list the organization's website.

Comparative Population Characteristics

Fill out the following chart completely for the **nine indicators named** and **three additional indicators** that are particularly relevant for your work. The comparative data from the region, the United States, and the world will give you a comparative perspective.

	Focus Country	Geographic Region of Focus Country	United States	World
Population				
Birth rate				
Death rate				
Fertility rate				
Infant mortality rate				
Child mortality rate				
Literacy rate				
Per capita income				
Social development index				

Basics

Capital city: _____

Locate on a map (list adjacent countries and bodies of water):

Name of president/leader: _____

Currency and exchange rate: _____

Language(s) spoken: _____

Word for "Hello": _____

Word for "Please": _____

Word for "Thank you": _____

Current Events

Identify two online sources that you can use to monitor news in the country of study. Monitor these sources for 2–4 weeks and list five articles (titles and links) that you found to be interesting and relevant for you.

News Sources

1. _____

2. _____

Articles

1. _____

2. _____

3. _____

4. _____

5. _____

Historical Time Line

Review historical information or existing time lines (for example, BBC News includes historical time lines for many countries in the world. List **10 key events/moments** in the history of this country. Consider reading in more detail about one or two of these events that are of particular interest to you.

Year	Event

Year	Event

Leading Causes of Morbidity and Overall Disease Burden (GBD 2015 Country Profiles, WHO Country Profiles)

Morbidity (Type of Condition)	Overall Disease Burden (Number of People Impacted in the Country)

Food and Nutrition

1. What are the staple foods in the country?

2. What kinds of foods are grown locally?

3. What are the rates of malnutrition and/or food insecurity?

4. Describe the local cuisine and/or a national dish that you hope to try.

Economy

1. What are the most important resources and sources of income in this country?

_____

2. What percentage of the population lives in poverty?

_____

The Health System

1. Countrywide, who has access to health care?

_____

_____

2. What is covered?

_____

_____

3. How are services financed?

_____

_____

4. How does the country address disparities and ensure service quality?

_____

_____

5. What are the current governmental priorities related to health?

_____

_____

6. What is one government policy in relation to your topic?

_____

_____

Environment

List the environmental challenges that this country faces (water access and quality, air quality, vulnerability to the impacts of climate change, deforestation, biodiversity, soil erosion, depletion of other natural resources).

1.

_____

_____

2.

_____

_____

3.

_____

_____

4.

_____

_____

Infrastructure

Answer the following infrastructure questions for the country and communities that you will visit.

Transportation: How do local people travel? What are the risks associated with travel? How do you plan to travel?

_____

_____

Energy: What systems are in place? Will you have regular access to electricity?

_____

_____

Parks and public spaces: What are the parks and public spaces that you will have access to? Are they well maintained and safe? Will you visit them?

_____

_____

Education: What is the average level of educational attainment in the country and community in which you will work? What is the structure of the education system (i.e., length of primary school, secondary school, etc.)?

_____

_____

Works of Literature

Identify and read works of literature from the country. Include the **author, title, and a brief description.**

1.

_____

_____

_____

_____

2.

_____

_____

_____

_____

Films

Identify and view two films from or about this country. Include the **title, director, and a brief description.**

1.

_____

_____

_____

_____

2.

_____

_____

_____

_____

Famous People from the Country

List and describe three famous people from the country. These can be people who are well known within the country and/or internationally.

1.

_____

2.

_____

3.

_____

Sports

What sports are popular in the country? What are the names of the teams? Are there any important competitions that will occur during your visit?

_____

_____

_____

_____

Music

Describe traditional and contemporary music traditions in this country. Is the country known for a particular musical style or type of instrument? (Add a link to a traditional or contemporary song.)

_____

_____

_____

_____

Link 1:

_____

Link 2:

_____

Travel Information

Review the State Department travel information (https://travel.state.gov) for the country you will visit. List any concerns you may have and actions you will take to address them to be as safe as possible.

1.

_____

_____

_____

2.

_____

_____

_____

3.

_____

_____

_____

Your Network

List people you know who might have contacts for you in country. (Ask these individuals to provide you with emails or phone numbers of people you might like to visit with in country.)

1. _____

2. _____

Possible Funding Sources

See the section "Funding your Global Health Experience" in this chapter. List possible funding sources to help you pay for your specific global health experience.

1. _____

2. _____

3. _____

Key Terms

Field course
Systems thinking
Voluntourism

Suggested Reading and Resources

The Akili Initiative: http://www.mappinghealth.com/akili/

Birrell I. 13 November 2010. Before you pay to volunteer abroad, think of the harm you may do. *Guardian*. Accessed from https://www.theguardian.com/commentisfree/2010/nov/14/orphans-cambodia-aids-holidays-madonna

Blackledge S. 25 February 2013. In defence of "voluntourists." *Guardian*. Accessed from https://www.theguardian.com/world/2013/feb/25/in-defence-of-voluntourism1

Crabtree RD. 2013. The intended and unintended consequences of international service-learning. *Journal of Higher Education Outreach and Engagement, 17*(2), 43–66.

The Ethical Volunteer. 2016. The 7 deadly sins that make for bad volunteering. Accessed from http://www.theethicalvolunteer.com/7-deadly-sins.html

Hammersley LA. 2016. A reply to the response by Mark Griffiths to the *JOST* special issue on volunteer tourism. *Journal of Sustainable Tourism, 24*(2), 179–181. doi:10.1080/09669582.2015.1109838

Idealist.org. 2017. Guidelines for international volunteering. Accessed from http://www.idealist volunteering.org/guidelines-international-volunteering/

Kushner J. 22 March 2016. The voluntourist's dilemma. *New York Times Magazine.* Accessed from http://www.nytimes.com/2016/03/22/magazine/the-voluntourists-dilemma.html?_r=0

Pattisson P. 26 May 2014. Nepal's bogus orphan trade fuelled by rise in "voluntourism." *Guardian.* Accessed from https://www.theguardian.com/global-development/2014/may/27/nepal -bogus-orphan-trade-voluntourism

Ruiz A, Khoshnood K, Ackerman J, et al. 2013. *Global health field experience guide.* Yale College Center for International and Professional Experience. Accessed from http://globalhealth. yale.edu/sites/default/files/files/GlobalHealth_YaleCIPE_Dec2013_V6.pdf

References

Blackledge S. 25 February 2013. In defence of "voluntourists." *Guardian.* Accessed from https:// www.theguardian.com/world/2013/feb/25/in-defence-of-voluntourism1

Crabtree RD. 2013. The intended and unintended consequences of international service-learning . *Journal of Higher Education Outreach and Engagement, 17*(2), 43–66.

Pattisson P. 26 May 2014. Nepal's bogus orphan trade fuelled by rise in "voluntourism." *Guardian.* Accessed from https://www.theguardian.com/global-development/2014/may/27/nepal -bogus-orphan-trade-voluntourism

CHAPTER 14

GLOBAL HEALTH COMPETENCIES FOR THE HEALTH SCIENCES

Gabrielle A. Jacquet, MD, MPH
Jessica Evert, MD
Kevin Wyne, PA-C, MPAS, MSc

Cultural competency is not an abdominal exam.
—**Arno Kumagai and Monica Lypson**

LEARNING OBJECTIVES

- Describe the development of global health competencies and their importance for global health work
- Describe how competencies can be used by students and faculty to evaluate global health experiences and student skill development
- Discuss elements that should be included in global health competencies, including work as a part of interprofessional teams, justice, equity, ethics, and sociopolitical awareness
- Discuss the importance of input from local health partners in developing competencies for global health experiences

---

Competency-based education is common within higher education. Educational competencies are used to set assessable standards for knowledge and performance, and are critical to curriculum development, evaluation, and integrity (Gebbie, 2004). Put another way, identification of competencies makes explicit the knowledge and skills that students gain through an educational experience and allows for assessment of

Foundations for Global Health Practice, First Edition. Lori DiPrete Brown.
© 2018 John Wiley & Sons, Inc. Published 2018 by John Wiley & Sons, Inc.

their achievements and shortfalls (Frenk et al., 2010). For global health, traditional notions of competency must be expanded to include not only "knowledge, skills, and attitudes" but also "a critical consciousness of oneself, others, and the world" (Kumagai & Lypson, 2009). Hence the epigraph that opens this chapter. Cultural competency is not an abdominal exam because, in Kumagai and Lypson's words, "It is not a static requirement to be checked off some list." Rather, it is a continued process of learning and reflection that enables a person to function effectively within a specific cultural context. In this context, an abdominal exam is never just an abdominal exam. It exists within a specific context; not only a biological context, but a cultural one that is full of meanings, history, power dynamics, and social nuances.

Global health practice does not occur in isolation, but always in relationship with others (Koplan et al., 2009). Thus global health competencies must include a reflective awareness of the power and privilege embedded in social relationships and foster a reorientation of perspective to focus on issues of social justice (Kumagai & Lypson, 2009). This chapter will discuss the ongoing development of global health competencies and their importance for learners and host communities.

Background

Despite the rapid expansion of global health programs for undergraduate and graduate students, until recently there were no standard competencies for global health training. Many health care disciplines had created individualized competencies for learners in international settings, though often these discipline-specific competencies failed to address interprofessional teams or account for the complex interplay of variables that affect the health of individuals and communities (Jogerst et al., 2015). This problem was addressed at the 2013 annual conference of the Consortium of Universities for Global Health (CUGH), where members of the CUGH Education Committee developed a set of interprofessional global health competencies, a framework that could be used to help prepare students to become global citizens and global health practitioners (Jogerst et al., 2015).

The rise of agreed-on global health competencies allows schools to create appropriate learning objectives and professional development tracks in global health. Ideally, these competencies also benefit global communities by prioritizing those needs that the communities themselves identify as important, rather than those recognized by volunteers. Unfortunately, global health work has not always prioritized or even included input from local communities, and work undertaken ostensibly to benefit local communities has at times resulted in disastrous consequences, such as a recent cholera outbreak in Haiti that was traced to a United Nations peacekeeping camp (Domonoski, 2016).

Levels of Experience and Training

Because effective global health work is context specific, creating competencies that apply to students and faculty with varying levels of experience and training can be challenging. The CUGH interprofessional global health competencies attempted to address this problem by including four levels of training: Global Citizen (Level I), Exploratory (Level II), Basic Operational (Level III), and Advanced Lead (Level IV). The Global Citizen level (I) identifies competencies required of all postsecondary students pursuing any field with a bearing on global health; Exploratory level (II) identifies competencies for students who are considering future professional pursuits in global health or preparing for a global health field experience. Levels III and IV are designed for those who have acquired specific skills that apply to global health work (e.g., medical training, engineering, anthropology).

In the CUGH model, the Global Citizen level is most applicable for undergraduate students who are interested in global health. This level includes competencies that highlight the complex determinants of health and the deep community engagement required for sustainable global health endeavors (see Box 14.1).

BOX 14.1

COMPETENCIES FOR GLOBAL CITIZEN LEVEL

- Describe the major causes of morbidity and mortality around the world, and how the risk for disease varies with regions.

- Describe major public health efforts to reduce disparities in global health.

- Describe how travel and trade contribute to the spread of communicable and chronic diseases.

- Describe how cultural context influences perceptions of health and disease.

- List major social and economic determinants of health and their effects on the access to and quality of health services and on differences in morbidity and mortality between and within countries.

- Describe the effects of access to and quality of water, sanitation, food, and air on individual and population health.

- Exhibit interprofessional values and communication skills that demonstrate respect for, and awareness of, the unique cultures, values, roles and responsibilities, and expertise represented by other professionals and groups that work in global health.

- Acknowledge one's limitations in skills, knowledge, and abilities.

- Demonstrate an understanding of and an ability to resolve common ethical issues and challenges that arise when working within diverse economic, political, and cultural contexts as well as when working with vulnerable populations and in low-resource settings to address global health issues.

- Articulate barriers to health and health care in low-resource settings locally and internationally.

- Demonstrate a basic understanding of the relationships among health, human rights, and global inequities.

- Demonstrate a commitment to social responsibility.

- Describe the roles and relationships of the major entities influencing global health and development.

Source: Adapted from "Identifying Interprofessional Global Health Competencies for 21st-Century Health Professionals, by Jogerst et al., 2015, *Annals of Global Health, 81,* 239–247. Retrieved from http://www.annalsofglobalhealth.org/article/S2214-9996(15)01156-X/fulltext

It is important to understand that the competencies listed in Box 14.1 do not constitute a curriculum, but rather are a framework onto which specific global activities may be mapped to ensure that the experience is meeting the students' needs (Jogerst et al., 2015). When considering global health educational opportunities, students will do well to map the activities involved to the proposed competencies to ensure that the experiences meet their needs.

Timing of Experience

The CUGH competencies outlined here are helpful for students who are considering global health work. They adhere to the philosophy that individuals can frequently contribute more readily when they possess specific skills that can directly benefit local communities. Thus, when evaluating a possible global health experience, students should consider many factors, including their level of training, prior experience, cultural background, goals, and expectations. The level of training and preparation of a trainee will directly affect the type and timing of a global health experience. For example, if the purpose of a global health learning experience is to provide direct medical care, then the experience should be undertaken when the participant has undergone specific training and is able to contribute to a health care team. Students who have had less training will not be as capable of providing a meaningful contribution to care, and their role will likely be more observational. If participants with less training are included in an observational or other capacity, it is important that their presence does not negatively affect the ability of the team to achieve its goals.

Scope of Practice

It is also essential that students and faculty do not work in a capacity that exceeds their training or scope of practice. A 2005 report by the Federation of State Medical Board defined *scope of practice* as "the activities that an individual health care practitioner is permitted to perform within a specific profession. Those activities should be based on appropriate education, training, and experience. Scope of practice is established by the practice act of the specific practitioner's board, and the rules adopted pursuant to that act."

Standards of medical care in the United States are among the highest in the world. As a general rule, it is not appropriate for students (or providers) to treat patients in international settings if they do not have current credentials that would allow them to perform similar care in the United States. The risk to patients and potentially to the student is simply too high. The following is a good general rule for those working in global health: if you are not qualified to do something in your own community or training program, then you should not do it during your global health learning experience.

It is also important to note that, even if one is fully licensed to practice medicine in the United States, one must still acquire knowledge of local diseases and health systems in order to care for patients effectively in these settings. Moreover, what constitutes proficiency in one global health setting does not necessarily do so in another context. In all global health work, local licensure and expertise requirements must be met. In some settings where licensure systems are less formal or developed, health care workers may need to self-impose such limits. Ideally, identification of the skills and proficiencies needed to effectively practice medicine in global health settings will be done in close collaboration with local health care providers so as to prioritize the needs that the community identifies as important (Eichbaum, 2015).

Additional Competencies

Although global health work that involves direct patient care requires training and experience that most undergraduate students do not possess, participating in other global health opportunities nonetheless offers enormous benefits for these students.

Experiences with a focus on education or research (with strong supervision in an academic setting), language immersion experiences, or those that utilize a trainee's other skills can be invaluable for both students and local communities. The CUGH competencies for Global Citizens are certainly applicable for these experiences, but they may be incomplete for more participatory global health endeavors. Further, it is important to recognize that competencies will need to be adapted to evolving local conditions (Frenk et al., 2010) and should include feedback from local communities (Eichbaum, 2015). Increased focus on interprofessional teamwork, the importance of establishing a dynamic where high-income countries can also learn from low-income countries, and applying lessons learned in global settings to local ones are all important considerations for global health work and are incompletely addressed by the CUGH Global Citizen competencies.

A working group at the University of Wisconsin (UW)–Madison recently revised its own competencies that had been initially established in 2005, after students and faculty identified a need for increased focus on interprofessional teams as well as such topics as justice, equity, ethics, and sociopolitical awareness (Brown, 2014). This working group included representatives from medicine, nursing, pharmacy, physical therapy, physician assistant studies, veterinary medicine, and public health. The process of revision included feedback from students and faculty, incorporation of recent literature on the topic of global health competencies, and shared experiences with other faculty within the United States.

These competencies (listed in Box 14.2) were intended to be applicable to all international graduate learning experiences through UW's Global Health Institute, and they are highly relevant for undergraduate experiences as well. As with the CUGH competencies discussed earlier, these competencies are not necessarily easily measurable, though activities can be designed to ensure that students can gain experience in the competency area. Additional competencies based on a student's discipline, intended profession, or chosen international experience may also be required. Although these competencies are focused on the development of specific skills in individual students, a guiding principle is mutual respect and the development of understanding between the hosting community and those who are visiting. *Health* is defined broadly here to include the well-being of people, animals, and the environment. The concept of *team* is also defined broadly to include student learners, faculty members, and international partners.

These competencies will be used by instructors at UW to guide curricular development, course content, and assignments in global health. Students and faculty alike can use these competencies to establish professional development goals for experiential learning opportunities. Unlike skills or procedures that can be practiced and mastered, all of these competencies are domains of ongoing growth and development.

BOX 14.2
UW REVISED GLOBAL HEALTH COMPETENCIES

1. To demonstrate self-guided learning habits, recognizing that experiential learning opportunities exist in many forms and that learning is a lifelong endeavor
2. To interpret quantitative and qualitative information from the sciences, social sciences, and the humanities to inform global health work
3. To integrate contextually grounded information about a location's health, history, politics, culture, and environment into one's learning experiences
4. To practice directed self-assessment and reflection about one's experiences and chosen profession, including consideration of one's role as a member of an interdisciplinary team
5. To compare and contrast the practice of health-related activities in different settings, including the social production of health and well-being
6. To draw connections between global experiences and health care challenges in your home setting
7. To work effectively as a member of a diverse team to achieve shared goals
8. To effectively communicate ideas about health to other professions as well as to community leaders and members of the general public
9. To recognize valuable opportunities for high-income and low- and middle-income partners to learn from one another, and creatively evaluate assets in addressing problems
10. To employ ethical models of community-based engagement recognizing the mutual benefit to learners and to the host community

---

Students can use these competencies over the course of their training and career to continue to grow professionally. They can also be used to evaluate global health learning opportunities. It is important to highlight that these competencies are a work in progress and that the authors are planning to elicit feedback from students, faculty, and, most important, from global health partners. Nor is this list exhaustive. Additional competencies based on the specific context of the global experience should be added when indicated.

Chapter Summary

Students bring diverse cultural knowledge and assets based on their heritage and life experiences, which can both enhance and hinder their work as global health science professionals-in-training. The competencies discussed in this chapter, both those established by the CUGH and those from UW, attempt to illustrate the complex process involved in forming the critical consciousness with which global health work should be approached. Central to this process is self-reflection, cultural humility, and a willingness to learn from others. Although the desire to alleviate suffering and improve health care disparities is admirable, students should recognize that it is important to undertake global health work that is appropriate for their stage of training, and that to work outside of an established scope of practice can be harmful for both the learner and the host community.

The development of global health expertise is a lifelong process that will require frequent reevaluation of oneself in relation to others and to the world. The competencies outlined here can serve as a guide in the evolution of a critical awareness that is requisite for effective global health work.

Case Study for Group Discussion

Imagine that you are invited to join a team of health care providers who are planning to provide medical care in rural Guatemala for one week. Using the two sets of competencies listed in this chapter as a framework, create a detailed plan for how you will approach this experience. This should include activities both before and after the experience as well as those that you will do while in Guatemala. As much as possible, be specific in terms of the readings, activities, interactions, and reflection activities that you will complete. For example, to address the competency related to self-guided learning habits, create a plan for how you will maximize your learning opportunities. Box 14.3 lists a few examples of how you might approach UW competencies 1 and 2 for the Guatemala case.

BOX 14.3
EXAMPLES OF STRATEGIES TO DEVELOP COMPETENCIES: GUATEMALA

Competency 1: To demonstrate self-guided learning habits, recognizing that experiential learning opportunities exist in many forms and that learning is a lifelong endeavor

1. I will identify a person involved with the experience who is willing to serve as a point person to review these competencies and my plan for addressing them. I will meet with this person before the experience, at least once during the experience, and again after returning home.
2. During my week in Guatemala, I will shadow three different health care professionals and speak to them about their role on the health care team.
3. I will speak with at least one Guatemalan health care provider to learn about his or her day-to-day work.

> **Competency 2: To interpret quantitative and qualitative information from the sciences, social sciences, and the humanities to inform global health work**
> Before leaving for Guatemala, I will familiarize myself with Guatemala's health care infrastructure and existing needs by reading the following report, articles, and biography:
>
> *Guatemala Health System Assessment 2015 Report,* by USAID's Health Finance and Governance project. https://www.usaid.gov/sites/default/files/documents/1862/Guatemala-HSA%20_ENG-FULL-REPORT-FINAL-APRIL-2016.pdf
>
> "Health Care Issues Facing the Maya People of the Guatemalan Highlands: The Current State of Care and Recommendations for Improvement," by Sunil Bhatt (2012, August 1), *Journal of Global Health.* http://jglobalhealth.org/article/health-care-issues-facing-the-maya-people-of-the-guatemalan-highlands-the-current-state-of-care-and-recommendations-for-improvement-2/
>
> *I, Rigoberta Menchú: An Indian Woman in Guatemala,* by Rigoberta Menchú (1984). London, United Kingdom: Verso.
>
> "Duffle Bag Medicine," by Maya Roberts (2006), *Journal of the American Medical Association, 295,*1491–1492. doi:10.1001/jama.295.13.1491)

Consider how you might use these competencies in your own global health field experience. The specific ways in which you address these competencies are up to you, but you should strive to be as specific as possible in putting your plan together.

Key Terms

Competency
Global health
Interprofessional collaboration

Suggested Resources

These resources are recommended to help you develop global health competencies:

Consortium of Universities for Global Health. Global Health Modules. Available at https://www.cugh.org/resources/educational-modules

Melby, M. K., Loh, L. C., Evert, J., Prater, C., Lin, H., & Khan, O. A. (2016). Beyond medical "missions" to impact-driven short-term experiences in global health (STEGHs): Ethical principles to optimize community benefit and learner experience. *Academic Medicine, 91,* 633–638. doi:10.1097/ACM.0000000000001009

The Practitioner's Guide to Global Health. [EdX course]. https://www.edx.org/course/practitioners-guide-global-health-bux-globalhealthx
    Part 1: The Big Picture
    Part 2: Preparation and on the Ground
    Part 3: Reflection
Unite for Sight. (n.d.). Ethics and photography in developing countries. Retrieved from http://www.uniteforsight.org/global-health-university/photography-ethics
University of Minnesota-Twin Cities School. (n.d.). Global ambassadors for patient safety. Retrieved from https://www.healthcareers.umn.edu/courses-and-events/online-workshops/global-ambassadors-patient-safety

References

Brown, L. D. (2014). Towards defining interprofessional competencies for global health education: Drawing on educational frameworks and the experience of the UW–Madison Global Health Institute. *Journal of Law and Medical Ethics, 42*(Suppl. 2), 32–37. doi:10.1111/jlme.12185

Domonoski, C. (2016, August 18). U.N. admits role in Haiti cholera outbreak that has killed thousands. *NPR.* Retrieved from http://www.npr.org/sections/thetwo-way/2016/08/18/490468640/u-n-admits-role-in-haiti-cholera-outbreak-that-has-killed-thousands

Eichbaum, O. (2015). The problem with competencies in global health education. *Academic Medicine, 90,* 414–417. doi:10.1097/ACM.0000000000000665

Federation of State Medical Boards. (2005). *Changes in healthcare professions' scope of practice: Legislative considerations.* Retrieved from https://www.fsmb.org/Media/Default/PDF/FSMB/Advocacy/2005_grpol_scope_of_practice.pdf

Frenk, J., Chen, L., Bhutta, Z. A., Cohen, J., Crisp, N., Evans, T., Fineberg, H., Garcia, P., . . . Zurayk, H. (2010). Health professionals for a new century: Transforming education to strengthen health systems in an interdependent world. *The Lancet, 376,* 1923–1958. doi:10.1016/S0140-6736(10)61854-5

Gebbie, K. M. (2004). *Competency-to-curriculum toolkit: Developing curricula for public health workers.* New York, NY: Columbia University School of Nursing and Association of Schools of Preventive Medicine.

Jogerst, K., Callender, B., Adams, V., Evert, J., Fields, E., Hall, T., Olsen, J., . . . Wilson, L. L. (2015). Identifying interprofessional global health competencies for 21st-century health professionals. *Annals of Global Health, 81,* 239–247. doi:10.1016/j.aogh.2015.03.006

Koplan, J. P., Bond, T. C., Merson, M. H., Reddy, K. S., Rodriguez, M.H., Sewankambo, N. K., Wasserbeit J. N., for the Consortium of Universities for Global Health Executive Board. (2009). Towards a common definition of global health. *The Lancet, 373,* 1993–1995. doi:10.1016/S0140-6736(09)60332-9

Kumagai, A., & Lypson, M. (2009). Beyond cultural competence: Critical consciousness, social justice, and multicultural education. *Academic Medicine, 84,* 782–787. doi:10.1097/ACM.0b013e3181a42398

CHAPTER 15

WORKING WITH COMMUNITIES

Lori DiPrete Brown, MS, MTS
Sophia Friedson-Ridenour, PhD

For apart from inquiry, apart from praxis, individuals cannot be truly human. Knowledge emerges through invention and re-invention, through the restless, impatient, contriving, hopeful inquiry human beings pursue in the world, with the world, and with each other.

—**Paulo Freire,** *Pedagogy of the Oppressed*

LEARNING OBJECTIVES

- Define community-based participatory research (CBPR) and clarify its relationship to service-learning and community engagement
- Identify key CBPR principles that can be useful for global health field experiences
- Explore some of the nuances and challenges of CBPR implementation through a brief case study
- Become familiar with a mixed-methods research approach that can be used with and for communities
- Develop a walk-along approach to learning about your global health field site and developing relationships with the community

Many aspects of global health rely on community-level collaboration for change. Community-based participatory research (CBPR) methods offer practical guidance that will help you make your field experience and work with communities respectful, collaborative, community led, and productive. This chapter defines CBPR and its key principles, presents a case study for consideration and discussion, and outlines how a range of

Foundations for Global Health Practice, First Edition. Lori DiPrete Brown.
© 2018 John Wiley & Sons, Inc. Published 2018 by John Wiley & Sons, Inc.

research methods can be used with and for communities. Finally, we outline a "walk-along" approach to engaging with communities that can be used by students as they embark on global health field experiences.

Community-Based Participatory Research: Core Concepts

Community-based participatory research (CBPR) employs a mixed-methods approach to sharing information that benefits from complementary quantitative and qualitative information. It is especially useful for integrating local knowledge that relies on context, shared history, and insider perspectives with knowledge that arises from academic inquiry and scientific research. CBPR is more than just a set of methods to describe social realities in a holistic way (Cornwall & Jewkes, 1995); it also has an action orientation that focuses on the equitable relationship between researchers and community members. CBPR, well executed, involves researchers and community members working together at every step of the research process, with the goal of fostering and supporting community-led social change (Minkler & Wallerstein, 2003).

Defining CBPR

There are many definitions of CBPR, and many derive from the work of Barbara Israel, which characterizes the practice as follows: "Community-based research in public health is a collaborative approach to research that equitably involves, for example, community members, organizational representatives, and researchers in all aspects of the research process" (Israel. Schulz, Parker, & Becker, 1998, p. 176).

CBPR presents a powerful alternative to more traditional research approaches in which anonymity and objectivity are emphasized and in which researchers are largely responsible for defining research questions, methods, and interventions, and control the process of data analysis and reporting. By contrast, CBPR steps away from the power hierarchies and inequities encoded in such research processes, which value expert knowledge over community experience.

CBPR reframes the engagement from one where researchers study communities to one where researchers and community members study, learn, and act together. Community partners are equal collaborators at every step of the research process, from formulating a research question, to developing tools, to using data, to taking action. Because these efforts take place in the context of persistent inequities, this approach requires intentional recognition of, and ongoing reflection about, the unique strengths that each party brings to the process and emphasizes doing research *with* people, not *on* them (Cornwall & Jewkes, 1995; Minkler & Wallerstein, 2008). CBPR can increase the ability of individuals and communities to carry out community-led social change. In an effective CBPR process, both community members and researchers grow in their capacity to enact social change effectively in the future.

Service-Learning and CBPR

Global health field experience may take the form of study tours, internships, or immersion learning experiences. In addition to lectures, discussion, and observational and experiential learning, many of these programs include service-learning components. **Service-learning** is an educational approach in which students learn through active participation in thoughtfully organized community service. Service is combined with self-reflection so that students derive maximum learning and personal growth from the experience. Service-learning activities emphasize reciprocity or mutual benefit, meaning that service and learning occur in a two-way relationship, and that wishes and needs in the community are addressed at the same time that students are engaged in a meaningful learning opportunity. Service-learning, done well, enriches the community and develops civic responsibility and skills in students (Jacoby, 1996).

Just as not all field experiences include service-learning, not all service-learning efforts use CBPR principles. For example, field experiences may carry out effective and appropriate outreach or service projects such as tutoring, building a well, community beautification, small-scale construction projects, or cultural sharing through the arts. All of these kinds of experiences have value, but should not be classified as CBPR if they are not planned and implemented in partnership with the community.

Although not all global health field experiences need be fully realized examples of CBPR, all global health experiences can be enriched by CBPR principles and practices. Employing the key principles of CBPR in your global health work will help you develop a more participatory experience and a greater ability to appreciate and learn from local knowledge.

Key Principles of CBPR for Global Health Experiences

A range of CBPR sources have informed global health fieldwork over the years (Israel et al, 1998; Minkler & Wallerstein, 2003; Mathie & Cunningham, 2002). Here we highlight key principles for community-based participatory work that have been particularly useful in global health education and practice.

Practice Multidirectional Learning Community-based participatory approaches can help deconstruct the directionality of learning in global health work. Students, teachers, and community members learn alongside, with, and from each other. When multidirectional learning and cultural exchange are emphasized, the negative impacts of power differentials and social marginalization, which cannot be totally erased, are decreased. Community members understand themselves as teachers as well as learners, and they understand that their culture and knowledge are valued. Engaging in this kind of inclusive and collaborative exchange can be challenging for everyone, because it often requires taking risks and crossing personal and social boundaries. However, the mutual vulnerability and open-ended nature of these interactions, combined with continuous collaboration, good communication, and critical self-reflection, are precisely what make these experiences rich for personal growth, and potent ways to collaborate for change.

Value Local Knowledge CBPR is a colearning process that is meant to bring academic and community knowledge and expertise together to create social change. Engaging in community-based research means placing significant value on the knowledge generated from the life experience and self-concept of the people with whom you are partnering. This is always a rich, new, wonderful experience that, if you let it, can broaden your horizons and understanding of the many different ways there are of being in the world.

Focus on Action CBPR approaches are action oriented; and research components, even when primarily descriptive, are articulated in the context of the goals of the community. Collective assessment and description of the situation are always important, because often there is missing knowledge and perspective that can be revealed with mixed-methods participatory approaches, but research should be linked to action from the outset.

Follow the Lead of the Community Mutually respectful partnership forms the foundation of a CBPR approach. CBPR is rooted in the principle of self-determination—the idea that community members not only are best positioned to effectively evaluate their strengths and needs but also have the right to lead change in their communities (Minkler, 2004). This means that community members must be full participants at every step in the process. It is common for teachers, students, researchers, and others who want to engage in change from the position of an outsider to wonder if this is really possible. The answer is yes, but it takes time.

As representatives of universities from higher-income countries, we carry with us the power, privilege, and prestige of those institutions to our global health field learning. Even when we are well intentioned and truly listening, communities may be deferential to our ideas and plans and reticent to share their own goals. This deference can be rooted in economic need that makes communities willing to take whatever is offered, an attitude that may have developed during community members' prior experiences with health and development efforts. It may also be rooted in colonialist mind-sets, and histories of oppression, which lead people to assign less value to their own knowledge and ideas. It might just as likely be borne of a sense of hospitality and kindness or of cultural communication practices that are more nuanced than the direct approach we may be using. Finally, communities may be very aware of the trade-offs involved in what you are proposing, and have decided that the engagement on your terms is worthwhile.

Although authentic community leadership may be possible at the outset in many situations, it will often be the case that the trust and transparency needed to have truly equal partnership will develop gradually over several years. Once established, the foundation is in place for a long-term partnership with strong community leadership. For this reason, it is important to take extra care in selecting first projects and in eliciting feedback. As long-term partnerships develop, university-affiliated course leaders provide context and continuity for students.

Respect the Experience of Historically Marginalized Populations Although CBPR is effective for addressing health inequities in a range of settings, it is commonly used to work with historically marginalized and underserved communities and populations. Because CBPR is grounded in a partnership approach that emphasizes power sharing and a commitment to building the capacity, strengths, and resources of communities, it can be effective for addressing long-standing insider-outsider tensions that are grounded in complex legacies of historical trauma, racism, and oppression (Minkler, 2004). For global health learning, this principle can be best put into practice by ensuring that you include activities that allow you the time and setting for conversations that enable you to learn about community perspectives. Often these learning experiences that are arranged with students in mind end up creating opportunities for people from within the community to engage in dialogue with each other in new ways.

Value Accompaniment and Witness CBPR will bring you into dialogue with a diversity of people and situations, each with their own strengths and challenges. Your partners may experience direct suffering that is not easily addressed or ameliorated. In such instances, the fact that you have come to be and learn with people can be humanizing and provide an important kind of dignifying comfort, which is valuable in and of itself. This kind of presence is sometimes called *witness* or *accompaniment*. Although your presence may not produce a solution to suffering, a respectful approach, perspective taking, and empathy, along with sustained presence, can say, "You are seen," "Your voice is heard," "You are valued," or "You are not alone."

Structure Your Efforts to Realize Mutual Benefits When engaging in CBPR, it is important to recognize that teachers, students, and community partners should experience some kind of benefit. It is important to be mindful, transparent, and intentional about these mutual benefits. They change over time, even in the context of the same partnership, so it is recommended that you frequently reflect on and revisit these benefits to ensure that they are aligned with the community's current needs and wants. It is easy to put the label of "partnership" on something, but a true partnership requires an iterative process of ongoing review and renewal, which is strengthened by engaging in critical reflection. An essential part of CBPR, structured and frequent reflection will help lead to longer-term partnerships that are increasingly community led, and over time can allow for more complex research and educational components to be integrated into the work you do with communities.

Insights for CBPR Practice: A Case Study from Ecuador

Here we illustrate how CBPR principles provide a lens for planning, implementing, and evaluating your global engagement. Box 15.1 describes the evolution of a partnership with Sumak Muyo, a women's group in La Calera, Ecuador. As you read about the program, think about how you might tell the story of your own work with communities. Following the case is a discussion of the strengths of the program and areas for improvement. The authors prepared the first draft of this analysis, then reviewed it with Flora Yepez, who represented the perspectives of Sumak Muyo, and revised accordingly. This iterative review process is vital to the integrity of CBPR. Consider how this kind of reflective analysis can be applied to your own past, present, and future engagement.

BOX 15.1

THE WOMEN OF SUMAK MUYO: MICROENTERPRISE AND WELL-BEING IN LA CALERA, ECUADOR

LORI DIPRETE BROWN
JANET NIEWOLD

Background

The first UW–Madison visit to La Calera, a rural indigenous community in the Ecuadoran highlands, took place in 2006, during a UW–Madison global health field course led by Professor Frank Hutchins, an anthropologist who has worked in the area for many years. Lori was involved in planning and facilitating community public health activities for his program, and he thought she might want to explore working with women from the community on health and well-being matters. He introduced her to Flora Yepez, a community member who was a farmer, had training and expertise as a community health worker, and was part of a group of women leaders in her community. These leaders faced the challenges of poverty and social marginalization on a daily basis. They had worked together on projects related to child care, health, and violence against women. They worked to preserve indigenous culture—from their language and dress to their herbal medicines and birth practices—and they had challenged social norms to become leaders in local government and their regional farmers association.

Frank and Lori recognized these assets and felt that it would be a great community in which students could engage and learn. They explained what they hoped to do, and Flora agreed to coordinate activities related to health and culture for the following year. They decided to bring students to La Calera each year, and that each year they would decide together on what would be learned and shared. The community would teach the students about traditional health practices and indigenous life, and the students would work together on a project chosen by the community.

Over the next few years, they carried out a number of projects ranging from nutrition education, dental hygiene, and working with the local day-care center, to developing a community pharmacy kit. Most of these projects were the products of lists made together, with the pros and cons weighed and a conscious selection. Then, in 2009, when pharmacist Trisha Seys Ranola (see Seys Ranola and Kraus, chapter 34) was with Lori in La Calera, completing some education and clarifications that accompanied the pharmacy effort, their next project emerged in a different way.

A New Project Idea

At the end of the field course, Flora asked Lori and Trisha to wait just a few more minutes before leaving, and she disappeared into the other room. She returned with a plastic bag tied securely around a cluster of beaded necklaces made out of palm seeds and other natural materials—a product that was readily available, and perhaps even in oversupply, in the artisan marketplace in nearby Otavalo. Flora and the other women called themselves Sumak Muyo, which meant the "good seed" in their native language, and they wanted Lori to help them sell some necklaces.

Lori was not sure she would be able to sell these necklaces. And if she did, she might be expected to sell more. Wasn't this creating an economic dependency of the very kind she cautioned against? Yet this was the first time the group had been truly directive about the shared work, and Flora had become a friend. Lori decided she could not say no. She paid Flora full price in advance, then said her good-byes until next year.

The dilemma Lori faced, and her response to it, reflected differences in access to resources, opportunities, and mobility between Lori and the women of La Calera. When Flora asked her to sell jewelry, Lori's status and relative privilege in the global marketplace made it easy enough to say yes, and saying no seemed unfair. The women of Sumak Muyo needed income, and Lori had the ability to take their jewelry back to the United States and try to sell it for them out of her home to friends, neighbors, and acquaintances, on an ad hoc basis. Although the instinct to say yes came from a place of good intention, it is rooted in an imbalance of power, and, as an overall basis for the relationship, is antithetical to the principles of equality that are central to CBPR work.

When Lori returned to Madison, she did sell some of the necklaces to friends, family, and her local book group. It was slow going, but she kept her promise. Her colleague and friend Janet Niewold, who had experience buying and selling artisan work from women in Latin America, looked over the jewelry, made some observations about the quality, and had a lot of questions about the products that Lori could not answer. She suggested that a better way to engage, rather than through direct sales, would be to work with the group to define a product line, develop multiple clients, and work on quality and design. Janet offered to go to Ecuador with Lori to launch the project.

The Birth of the Microenterprise Project

Janet wanted to bring students and faculty with design and business skills into the work, and she herself wanted to relate to the women as a buyer who appreciated their skills and was willing to pay a fair price for a consistent and quality product. The relationship that Janet was proposing was a much better approach than one of being a helpful friend. What she was proposing allowed us to envision a project where students would learn a great deal and the Sumak Muyo group could earn money and develop their business.

At this writing, much of what Janet envisioned has come to pass. Janet has built a relationship as a trusted business associate, teacher, and friend with the women, and she has mentored many students through fieldwork at the site and a student organization called the Wisconsin without Borders Marketplace. Faculty members and artists from UW's School of Human Ecology—Carolyn Kallenborn, Jennifer Angus, and Dee Warmuth—have contributed their expertise. Through site visits and classroom-based exchange, and through the work of their students, they have helped the women develop needed skills in design and sales. The UW–Madison partnership has enabled the women of Sumak Muyo to grow their beadwork into a viable complementary business that can supplement their farming activities by generating additional revenue. The women have learned a great deal about art and design, and they now have a product line that is beautiful and distinct from others. They value their work for its beauty and quality and for the revenue it produces.

Jewelry making for artisans in La Calera, though, is about more than just generating additional revenue. It is also about the solidarity and community they experience when they work together. Generally they gather together in homes to work. They can talk about challenges related to the economy and the sale of their jewelry, but also the discrimination they sometimes face because of their gender and indigenous identity. The space they have created for shared artistry and income generation has become a place where they can grow as leaders as well. Although they each had leadership experience when they came to the project, and the group had worked together successfully before on community service projects, they had not successfully done an income-generating project together. They enjoyed the relationships they had with UW students and faculty. They were proud of the teaching they did about health and culture, and they were equally proud of what they were learning—about design and color, filling orders with precision, designing a product line, and striving for quality. The process of setting goals, putting plans into action, and achieving their goals increased their self-confidence and left them feeling hopeful despite ongoing challenges at the community level. Magdalena Fuentes, one of the artisans in the group who is also

traditional midwife and has served as an elected official in her local community, elo-
quently expressed her hopes for the kind of social change their work can generate:

> My hope is that women's conditions that are not equitable will improve. That
> someday women will be free to make their own decisions, and not depend on
> men. That there is an understanding between men and women. I hope that
> students grow up without forgetting about our community and the solidarity
> of our culture. That all women have employment and love for their children.
> That we care for our culture and the environment. That we have the capacity to
> improve the conditions of our lives. That our children don't follow paths towards
> vices and that they are leaders of their community and country, without losing
> the vision of our ancestors and population. That we use only what is necessary
> and don't destroy our environment for personal needs. Because without the
> earth, we have no life.

> What started as a small project is now an ongoing effort that has not only connected
> the Sumak Muyo women's group to viable local as well as international markets but also
> provided a meaningful platform for social change for women within their home commu-
> nity and a rich learning environment for students. This is an example of service-learning
> in action, informed by a community-based approach.

Strengths and Positive Outcomes

Assessing the strengths and positive outcomes of a program helps clarify what goals it
achieved and may also reveal unexpected areas of success. Here are some reflections on
what went well in the partnership with the women of La Calera.

Successful Small Business Development First and foremost, the central goal of establishing a successful small business was accomplished. Although there are still challenges,
such as markets flooded with similar goods and a troubled local economy, the women
are able to run the business on their own and change course as needed.

Some other strengths relate to the small business approach used. Whereas many
microenterprise projects focus on business skills, this team recognized that the women
of La Calera faced a very competitive market. To be successful, they needed artisan and
design skills. They developed new designs together, and the Sumak Muyo members felt
ownership of the designs, even naming them after themselves. They chose to design
higher-quality products with a higher price point, rather than cheaper products that
would result in a high demand, because they did not want to make jewelry as a full-time
job or to open a factory. They saw themselves as farmers, deeply connected to the land,
and they wanted to earn supplemental income without destroying the balance of their

lives. They valued working together in their homes, sharing meals from time to time, and integrating the work with other responsibilities.

One important insight occurred when they needed to procure funds for the first larger order that the women would fill. Because microfinance is a popular development strategy, the UW team suggested that the women might want to take out a microloan together to buy the materials needed for this first order. The women felt strongly that they did not want to take out a loan, and at first it could have seemed that they were not committed to the project. In fact, this reticence to accept indebtedness was deeply rooted in their experience as indigenous people who had a history of labor exploitation. Once this context was made clear, Janet arranged another way to fund their efforts. Initially, she provided materials up front and then deducted the price from the payment when the products were delivered. Eventually they developed a system based on a partial deposit, with payment completed upon delivery of the product. The down payment system is much preferred to requesting loans, and the women have successfully used this process with other clients.

Psychosocial Benefits   There are also clear psychosocial benefits of this collective work for the members of Sumak Muyo. They have expressed how enjoyable it is to work together, that the social time together lifts their spirits and keeps away negative feelings that they call *mal aire*. They have shared a great deal about their lives and daily struggles because of the hours spent working together. Although the group faces challenges related to keeping members engaged, getting work done on the promised schedule, and controlling quality, they seem able to problem-solve and move forward.

Good Relationships with Partners   Another strength of the program relates to the relationships that have been engendered. Rather than participating in a helping relationship that is unidirectional, members on both sides have multiple roles that are reinforcing. The women of Sumak Muyo are both teachers and learners, as are the faculty and students. While Lori remains engaged with the community as a public health professional, the microenterprise effort is led by Janet and others who have related skills and expertise.

International Exchange   In the spring of 2015, the team was able to bring three members of the group to Madison for a learning and cultural exchange. This was a full-circle experience because the UW team was finally able to reciprocate, welcoming the women of Sumak Muyo into their homes as they had welcomed us for years. The women of Sumak Muyo gave presentations on campus and in local organizations, were able to spend time with faculty and students on shared work, and participated in a cultural exchange with an indigenous community in northern Wisconsin. These shared experiences deepened and added new dimensions to the relationships.

Challenges, Missteps, and Missed Opportunities

No program is without challenges, mistakes, and missed opportunities. Here are just a few critical reflections about the work in La Calera, each with implications for the future of the partnership.

The Challenge of Authentic Representation There are many narratives about this work, one for every faculty member, student, and community member involved. And each one is different. One tempting narrative is to suggest that the UW group somehow "empowered" these women or helped them become leaders in the community through the various public health projects and then later the microenterprise effort. In fact, the women with whom we worked were already established leaders in their own right, as can be noted by the earlier descriptions of Flora and Magdalena. Another Sumak Muyo member and leader is Ines Bonilla. She has been a leader in efforts to address domestic violence in her community and, working with others, successfully changed indigenous laws to address violence against women. Her presence and skills in the group likely had a huge impact on the degree to which psychosocial support was achieved in the group, and, when family violence was raised as an issue, she had the skills to address the problem. Further, there are artisans in the community with small business experience; they weave and embroider, for example. Thus many of the women had some skills from other work that they have done with their families or other community members.

The Challenge of Cultural Preservation When working in La Calera, one is immediately aware that life there is rooted in local history, customs, and landscapes. There is a deep desire to preserve culture, especially language, dress, and annual rituals. When the artisan team agreed to work with products based on palm seeds, they did not know that it was an introduced rather than indigenous craft and that the materials were not produced locally. Although it is not necessarily wrong to work with a new product, they did not research the local assets carefully at the outset. Instead they moved forward based on the request from Flora and the others. Shortly into the effort, they came to realize that there may have been other products that would have been a better fit with the local artistic heritage. For example, there is extensive artisan expertise in relation to the embroidery that is used on traditional clothing. Sewing skills and design are a matter of pride and identity, and community members are concerned that the tradition is dying out because of the lack of financial viability. Had the team explored these issues in more detail, they might have focused on artisan products that used this skill and thus bolstered a local product that is very important culturally. We have begun to explore this as possible new product for the group.

Integrating a Gender Approach with the Complexity of the Community Setting As is obvious from the narrative, the project focused on working with a women's group in La Calera. This choice was made because livelihoods are organized by gender to a great degree in this geographic area. (Women do embroidery and work in the fields; men weave and care for animals.) However, the effort could have employed a broader gender lens that included men and women in dialogue, and other women in the community who were not part of the group. It might have been possible to buy and sell weavings that the men were making, enhancing the family economies for all and taking advantage of the men's design expertise. Many of the women's worries relate to the lack of opportunity for the youth in their community. This effort might have engaged young people as a priority. Further, there are women who leave town to work as day laborers, and some of them could be involved if demand for products grows. It is possible to explore these possibilities in the future and reframe how the work is understood in the larger community.

Economic Dependency? As the economy has weakened in Ecuador over the past few years, local jewelry sales have become more competitive. Because UW orders have provided a consistent and lucrative market, Sumak Muyo is now relying on that for the majority of its sales. It is important to continue to work toward a broader customer base. Sumak Muyo had sold goods in local shops and has obtained some orders from other international buyers. However, in order for the business to continue to be successful and eventually independent of our involvement, the women of Sumak Muyo have to make some additional efforts, such as reaching out to potential buyers regularly and making occasional trips to Quito.

True Cost of This Program? At first glance, this project looks expensive. How can the expenses be justified: faculty salary and airfare for faculty and students, in addition to the costs associated with materials and training? Why didn't the group just send money, instead of visiting this community and working together on a microenterprise project? If the benefits to the community alone are taken into account, this is not a viable development model. However, it is important to look at all the learning and growth that are happening. Faculty members are having an experience as artisans that will nourish their careers and their arts. Each year, between 10 and 20 students benefit from engagement with the program. They are learning artisan skills, small business skills, and life skills. Because of the long-term commitment to the site, undergraduate and graduate students have a very special opportunity to learn and to do challenging work. To determine the true costs and benefits, the educational value of the experience must be included, with all its ripple effects.

Failure in Success and Success in Failure

This analysis of the program in Ecuador, though partial, is intended to show that there are many layers and nuances to community experiences. There are always successes and failures, but there are also failures and shortcomings layered into successful efforts, and successes—such as lessons learned, relationships deepened, and other silver linings—embedded in the failures. In the end, negotiating tensions and constraints is an intrinsic part of doing community-based work, and ongoing critical reflection is needed. The goal is not to foresee and avoid all potential challenges and conflicts but rather to deal with them well when they arise. How do you stay in relationships that are imperfect, and work to make them more authentic and generative? CBPR requires that you be reflexive and adaptable, able to engage in an iterative process of learning with your partners as your work evolves and changes. Be ready and willing to be uncomfortable and unsure. Making change, individually and socially, is jagged and messy, challenging and rewarding.

CBPR Methods and Global Health: A Mixed-Methods Approach

In this section, we will outline a community-based participatory approach for global health field experiences. Based on methodological resources developed at UCLA (Carroll, Perez, & Toy, 2004) and through the World Conservation Union (Barton et al., 1997), as well as experience with UW–Madison global health field courses, the tools we discuss here—including informant interviews, community surveys, group interviews, transect walks (walk-alongs), and community mapping—are useful for global health fieldwork. These methods can be used in combination to provide complementary descriptive information, measures, perspectives, and possibilities. This information can be put to use in the context of a collaborative partnership to foster sustainable positive change in health and quality of life for people and communities.

Informant Interviews

Informant interviews are conducted with an identified leader whom you can talk to about a specific subject matter, yielding descriptive information, historical information, and social or cultural information. Rather than using a survey in which you ask a lot of people the same question, conducting an informant interview with one or two key people will enable you to get a greater depth of information on a particular topic. For example, a grandmother might talk about food traditions, and another elder might talk about how the community first got running water or electricity—both big moments in the history of a rural community. Key informants can provide rich information about health, education, food, water, sanitation, the local economy, culture, history, and more.

Be aware that, in the beginning, you are most likely to be introduced to or meet those who have a certain level of status, whether that be a function of age hierarchy, wealth, education, gender, or lineage. Over time, as you become more familiar with the community and as people become more comfortable with you, you will build relationships and gain access to a wider variety of people. Remember that there are multiple points of view and many histories, even in a small village. Informant interviews can help you capture a wide range of perspectives and understandings.

Surveys

Another tool that you might use is a **survey** of community members. If you want to describe population characteristics or know what percentage of people have access to health care, education, or food, a survey can answer these questions. Using a survey that has mostly closed-ended questions can be helpful because the data collected is more easily summarized and analyzed. Closed-ended questions you might use include yes-or-no questions, multiple-choice questions, or opinion questions that employ a 5-point scale. When open-ended questions are used in a community survey, they should be small in number (one or two) so that you have a manageable amount of information to summarize.

Where possible, use a **random sample**. Often health centers will have maps of all households that you can use as your sampling frame. An **intercept survey** is another efficient option. This means that, rather than going to households to find people, you go to one place where people come, such as a clinic, school, marketplace, or town square. If systematic sampling is not feasible, you can use a **convenience sample**—that is, simply interviewing people who are available. Although you must be very cautious about generalizing or inferring too much from such data, they can often provide helpful information in the formative stages of your work.

Group Interviews

A **group interview** is a dialogue with community members to explore topics of interest, with key questions to guide discussion. Group interviews emphasize dialogue with and among the community members, in which you get a depth of perspective and hear community voices building on each other. During group interviews, it can be helpful to depersonalize questions to elicit freer disclosure. For example, instead of asking "Do you need birth control?" you might say, "Do you think women in this community need birth control?" Group interviews are a rich complement to informant interviews or surveys because they allow you to hear a variety of opinions and hear how different points of view build on each other.

Community Mapping

Another method to explore is **community mapping**. With this approach, you work with a selected group of people from the community and have them draw their community, label its features, and then talk about community assets and risks. The following are some of the questions that might guide a community mapping exercise: What places are special in your community? What does your community have that you couldn't find anywhere else? What would you like to change about your community? Where do you feel safe? Where do you feel unsafe?

Community mapping can be an ongoing process; over time, you can enhance the initial map with photos, stories, and data. You can use this enriched map as a starting point to generate ideas for community action.

The Walk-Along

The **walk-along**, more formally referred to as a **transect walk**, is an observational walk and interview that is grounded in CBPR principles. This method was adapted for use in global health field courses from methods related to transect walks (Barton et al., 1997) and novel approaches to the study of health and place (Caprian, 2009). The walk-along is a respectful, natural, and enjoyable way to get to know a community. Simply defined, it is a tool that is designed to enable knowledge exchange and foster relationships in a respectful, mutual, and open way. These walks can be unstructured: you walk with people from the community, observing carefully and asking questions as you go. Or they can be structured around a particular topic, aided by the use of a checklist. You might, for example, structure a walk-along around food sources or the market, water sources and sanitation, learning about flora and fauna, health and social services, education and employment, or recreation. Or you might simply follow a linear path, taking samples of soil, water, and the natural environment to understand a place.

If you are with a large group, it can be very helpful to divide into pairs or small groups. Three or four different walk-along assessments on different topics can take place at the same time, and you can come together at the end of the day and share what you have learned. If you divide up in this way, you will have lots of stories to share, and you will have done a well-rounded rapid assessment of the community.

During a walk-along, listen, look around, observe, taste things, and touch and smell things as much as you can. Pay attention to feelings you have, your gut reactions, and what you observe in others. These will be important for reflection and follow-up later. Be ready to learn and follow cues about social behaviors. In some places, you kiss everyone; in some places, you do not touch anyone; in some places you pat people on the head; in other places, you never pat people on the head. Pay attention and let your community guide lead, follow their social cues, ask questions, and do your best to engage. People will respond to your efforts.

Be discreet about recording your experience. Although taking notes can be an important part of this activity, be careful not to let that be a distraction. Holding up or hiding behind a clipboard, or writing constantly, for example, might create distance between you and the people you are with. Only take photos or videos with permission, and try not to let this get in the way of being present.

Use appreciative questions. Appreciative or asset-based questions invite people to tell you about their strengths and stories of success, pride, and history. Too often we ask about deficits, problems, and challenges, leaving people no chance to tell us about who they really are or what they are proud of. Positive questions are a solid basis for beginning a relationship, and should precede conversations about challenges.

Use your peripheral vision. Using peripheral vision is another really important skill. While working with a community, you will experience lots of moments when you see something spectacular and completely new and out of the ordinary: a waterfall, a baby-naming ceremony, a festival, or some other wonder that you have been told about. Of course it is perfectly appropriate to focus your attention on the main event. But there is always something else happening too, and if you look around, beyond the center of attention, you will be rewarded with subtle and nuanced understandings about the place you are visiting. For example, maybe you are observing a birth. You might focus on the mother, the birth attendant, and the baby being born. But what else is happening? Who is there? Who is not there? Who is bringing water? Who is singing? Who is the first to touch the baby? All these observations that are happening on the sidelines can teach you a great deal about what it means to begin life in that community.

BOX 15.2
WALK-ALONG GUIDE

The questions here help you plan an observational walk and interview related to your global health field interests.

- Where will you do your global health fieldwork?
- What health issue do you hope to learn about from the community?
- Whom will you want to talk with?
- What three to five open questions will you ask?

- What one or two appreciative or asset-oriented questions will you begin with?

- Whom will you want to walk with?

- Whom will you ask to see?

- How will you use your other senses and peripheral vision to gain insights?

- What strategies will you use to build relationships?

- What do you hope to share about yourself?

   Answering these simple questions will help you be more intentional and present during your walk-along.

In summary, a walk-along assessment is a respectful way to get to know a community. It emphasizes local knowledge, and because it is led by community members in their own setting, it reduces power differentials and de-emphasizes social hierarchies.

Chapter Summary

CBPR principles, such as equitable partnership, mutual benefit, critical self-reflection, and an empowerment and action orientation, are vital tools for every kind of global health work. CBPR is a field that employs a mixed methodology of qualitative and quantitative data. It is, however, more than a set of methods. It is a way of approaching collaborative research which requires that community members act as equitable partners at every step of the process, with the aim of combining knowledge and action between experts and community members for social change that will improve community health and well-being.

Review Questions

1. Describe some key principles of CBPR.
2. How are service-learning projects and CBPR projects alike? How do they differ? Can you think of a situation where one might have advantages over the other?
3. Why is reflection an important part of community-based work?
4. Write one example open-ended question and one appreciative question that you might use when interviewing a community member.

Key Terms

Community-based participatory research (CBPR)

Community mapping

Community survey

Convenience sample

Group interviews

Informant interviews

Intercept survey

Random sample

Service-learning

Walk-along or transect walk

References

Barton, T., Borrini-Feyerabend, G., de Sherbinin, A., & Warr, P., with contributions from IUCN staff, members, and partners. (1997). *Our people, our resources: Supporting rural communities in participatory action research on population dynamics and the local environment.* Gland, Switzerland: IUCN—the World Conservation Union.

Caprian, R. M. (2009). Come take a walk with me: The "go along" interview as a novel method for studying the implications of place for health and well-being. *Health Place, 15*(1), 263–272.

Carroll, A. M., Perez, M., & Toy, P. (2004). *Performing a community assessment curriculum.* Los Angeles: UCLA Center for Health Policy Research, Health DATA Program Train-the-Trainer Project.

Cornwall, A., & Jewkes, R. (1995). What is participatory research? *Social Science & Medicine, 41,* 1667–1676.

Freire, P. (1972). *Pedagogy of the oppressed.* New York, NY: Herder and Herder. (Original work published 1968)

Israel, B. A., Schulz, A. J., Parker, E., & Becker, A. B. (1998). Review of community-based research: Assessing partnership approaches to improve public health. *Annual Review of Public Health, 19,* 173–202.

Jacoby, B. (1996). *Service-learning in higher education: Concepts and practices.* San Francisco, CA: Jossey-Bass.

Mathie, A., & Cunningham, G. (2002, January). *From clients to citizens: Asset-based community development as a strategy for community driven development.* Occasional Paper Series No. 4. Antigonish, Nova Scotia: Coady Institute, St. Francis Xavier University.

Minkler, M. (2004). Ethical challenges for the "outside" researcher in community-based participatory research. *Health Education & Behavior, 31,* 684–697.

Minkler, M., & Wallerstein, N. (Eds.). (2003). *Community based participatory research for health.* San Francisco, CA: Jossey-Bass.

Minkler, M., & Wallerstein, N. (2008). Introduction to community-based participatory research: New issues and emphases. In M. Minkler & N. Wallerstein (Eds.), *Community based participatory research for health: From process to outcomes* (2nd ed., pp. 5–24). San Francisco, CA: Jossey-Bass.

CHAPTER 16

TRANSFORMATIVE ENGAGEMENT AND LEADERSHIP FOR GLOBAL HEALTH

C. Perry Dougherty

The quality of light by which we scrutinize our lives has direct bearing upon the product which we live, and upon the changes which we hope to bring about through those lives.

—Audre Lorde

LEARNING OBJECTIVES

- Define transformative engagement and leadership
- Describe reasons why this approach to leadership is particularly important in global health work
- Understand key elements of a framework for practicing transformative engagement and leadership for global health by defining the practices of reflection and discernment
- Identify and apply multiple lenses of reflection and discernment: self, other, and life
- Introduce the specific importance of both historical and cultural contextual awareness and of the centrality of relationships
- Define and explore two key skills of transformative engagement and leadership: leading with vision and values and pursuing deep listening and meaningful connection

Transformative engagement and leadership is an approach to activities that identifies a need for a moral or values-based transformation within individuals, communities, and/or societal structures; envisions a path toward said transformation; and engages

Foundations for Global Health Practice, First Edition. Lori DiPrete Brown.

in relationships and activities in pursuit of such a vision. The ideal associated with the approach is to create positive, directed, step-by-step changes in pursuit of larger transformation within any given field or area of influence.

Central to this definition of transformative engagement and leadership is the concept of iterative change, because to be in pursuit of a world that better cares for and serves its people means to be in pursuit of the steps needed for dramatic transformation. To engage in transformative activities and practices is to operate with the baseline assumption that the world needs transformation, which is implemented based on positive, directed, incremental change. Such positive, directed, and incremental change is not inevitable; the job of the leader is to drive the momentum of changes toward a desired outcome or vision for transformation. Therefore, it becomes critical that we each embrace and understand the nature of change in order to harness and direct its potential for transformation.

The challenge of doing so is often overlooked, likely because on the surface, the idea of embracing change is fairly straightforward; but, in the reality of our lives, change is often difficult and uncertain even if we are seeking it. The framework and skills of transformative engagement and leadership in global health practice that are presented here aim to help us as individuals and/or groups develop purpose, connection, and resilience in the face of change, thereby enabling us to pursue the transformation we seek rather than simply allowing events to unfold around us without our awareness or intention.

The application of this framework and these skills in the field of global health practice is particularly relevant not only because the field confronts the fundamental transformation of human existence in the form of birth, illness, healing, and death but also because any notion of success in global health hinges on transformation at multiple levels of engagement. Within the field, regardless of role, people seek transformation at every level of society—from the individual patient to the population—and this requires that every level of society, from the individual to social structures to the nation to the global community, have the ability and need to find purpose, connection, and resilience in the face of change and in the pursuit of transformation.

To draw on Audre Lorde's metaphor of illumination that began this chapter, transformative engagement and leadership require, primarily, creating the space to reflect on and scrutinize our life's experiences and, secondarily, cultivating the ability to form ideas through the distillation of such experiences in order to pursue the changes we wish to bring about in the world around us.

To expand on this notion, the light we need to learn and practice transformative engagement and leadership lies within each and every one of us, regardless of our role or authority. Anyone can strive for transformative engagement and leadership in their realm of influence, no matter how small, because everyone—with the right supports, motivations, and freedoms—has the potential to reflect on life's experiences and allow new ideas to come to life.

In order to keep this idea present in our work, it can be valuable to challenge traditional models of hierarchical or authoritative leadership and begin to reframe engagement and leadership as the many movements between, and endless set of choices around, when and how leaders and followers relate and collaborate in any given moment or context (Berg, 1998). This approach moves to define leadership and followership not as rigid or fixed attributes but rather as roles that one steps into and out of continuously throughout one's pursuit of a vision or set of activities associated with that vision.

The practice of transformative engagement and leadership unlocks a cyclical inner and outer process where experiences and ideas continuously converge and diverge as we act and then reflect on that action. Therefore, it is important to note that the framework and skills presented here are dynamic and interconnected—not one of the concepts stands alone. They all intersect with one another and with the other concepts, principles, and methods presented in this textbook—in particular with the perspectives outlined in chapters that address human rights and ethics, partnership, participatory engagement, identity, and developing your career.

A Framework for Transformative Leadership

The foundational framework for transformative leadership is based on the practices and principles of reflection and discernment. To be of service to the brokenness and suffering of the systems and communities in the world demands that we offer our whole selves to leadership, which requires us to develop a deep inner and outer awareness. Such awareness is best cultivated by engaging in intentional practices and routines of reflection and discernment.

Reflection is a mental process through which individuals or groups seek clarity about truth through the integration of experience. Reflection demands consideration of our interior state and our external realities. The ultimate intent of engaging in reflection is to help us get into the habit of constructing meaning from our experiences through processes of reflective observation, connection, and integration.

Taking reflection one step further involves processes of analyzing, reconsidering, and questioning experiences within a context beyond the self or immediate experience. This process of moving beyond reflection is called critical reflection or discernment. **Discernment** involves testing the meaning made from one's reflection on an experience through assumption analysis, contextual exploration, imaginative speculation, and reflective skepticism.

Reflection and discernment together form the foundation of transformative engagement and leadership development. The processes of reflection and discernment also rest on some additional core concepts.

Three Lenses of Reflection and Discernment

There are three overlapping lenses—the lenses of self, other, and life—through which transformative leaders must cultivate awareness and understanding throughout their lives in order to effectively navigate the landscape and impact of their efforts. The ability to reflect and discern using multiple lenses is essential to building the practices of transformative leadership explored later in this chapter.

1. Self: the view that examines and tests the stories or narratives of one's self—both the inner (feelings, thoughts, sensations) and the outer (identity, behaviors, actions) realities
2. Other: the view that explores and challenges the stories or narratives of the other, which is most often defined in relationship to one's self
3. Life: the view that contemplates and confronts the stories or narratives of life, which is defined in this context as that which includes but is also greater than one's self and the other(s)

At any given moment, leaders are likely to be operating with various unconscious but influential biases in one or more of these areas, which means that being able to conceptualize these perspectives and bring them into the forefront of our awareness and understanding becomes essential to seeing any given experience clearly and to choosing right action.

Historical and Cultural Context of Your Leadership

As a field, global public health today has emerged from an undeniably complex history. Whether we are working in global health or other fields dedicated to social transformation, it is essential to both understand and work to transform the narratives of self, other, and life that are passed on through history and create implicit biases that become embedded in our cultures. This idea is perhaps best articulated by Bryan Stevenson in his exploration of how the narratives of white supremacy that were used to justify slavery in the United States have not gone away but rather have simply been used to justify new racist practices and institutions (Rushing, 2016). When leaders use reflection and discernment processes in their best modes, they can begin to open up dialogue and therefore to chart a path of action through the minefields of historical narratives and their influences on the way things unfold today.

A brief dive into history reveals that global public health today is rooted in the sordid legacy of colonial-era tropical medicine studies and practices that were often steeped in oppressive narratives of white supremacy. Those historical origins of the field of study are complemented by more recent historical legacies such as the grassroots activist and community-led movements—consider ACT UP in the United States or TASO in Uganda—that raised voices and engaged communities in fighting for the basic rights of all those suffering from HIV/AIDS.

A transformative leader is tasked with holding these multiple historical narratives and their impacts on the various cultural contexts in which the leader is operating. Such a responsibility demands both a knowledge of the robust historical context and an awareness of the various cultural dynamics at play within nations, communities, systems, organizations, teams, families, and relationships—those that the leader belongs to and those that the leader does not. The three lenses of reflection and discernment, therefore, must be paired with a robust contextual awareness of history and its influence on culture, and vice versa. These processes inevitably bring up deep existential questions of identity, privilege, and marginalization, which must be confronted both personally and relationally in pursuit of our development as transformative leaders.

Centrality of Relationship

The demand for leadership theories, development programs, and skills is high around the world. Everyone wants to be a leader, and there are a certain set of culturally nuanced but fairly universal stereotypes that get associated with the idea of the "leader" and likewise with the "follower" (Berg, 1998). As discussed before, transformative leadership is defined by its acceptance of and desire for change, so stereotypical, rigid images of the leader do not apply to the pursuit of transformative leadership. Rather, transformative leadership encompasses the acts of both leading and following, thereby enabling transformative engagement to exist in roles that do not have ultimate authority and are traditionally seen as followership roles.

With this idea in mind, it is undeniable that the practice of transformative leadership unfolds in a hierarchical world of complex relationships between individuals and collectives. Since the colonial period, global health has been developed based on the transfer of resources as well as the exertion and exchange of power in relationships among people, groups, communities, and nations across racial, social, political, economic, and religious divides. Whether we are focused on individuals' healing or population-level change, we execute ideas, programs, and interventions in collaboration with people across roles, disciplines, and systems. These relationships—as well as the lenses we use to analyze them and the historical and cultural contexts that influence them—are the central infrastructure for engaging transformative leadership's mandate to identify, envision, and enable a path to constructive change. In any approach to transformative engagement and leadership, relationships—namely, navigating the powers, postures, and privileges embedded within them—must take priority over the transactional nature of merely redistributing wealth and resources.

The acceptance of the importance of prioritizing a relational approach to engagement and leadership holds us accountable to individual and collective reflection and discernment and also serves as a reminder that positive, directed, and iterative change interpersonally and systemically is the core purpose of a transformative approach. Paying attention to relationships attunes our awareness to the ways in which we engage, experience, and integrate change as well as to the ways in which we distill and define our experiences and those of others. Although this work will not ensure that all relationships thrive, communicating and mutually engaging the elements of the transformative framework will create the possibility of relationships—at both micro and macro levels—that can help chart the path to transformation.

Skillfully accepting and navigating the dynamics of relationships become part of the bedrock on which transformative leaders ground their choices and actions and eventually measure their impact.

Skills of Transformative Engagement and Leadership

There are many specific skills that can be developed and applied within the transformative engagement and leadership framework to improve one's ability to lead change in global health. Here, two indispensible skills are briefly presented for consideration and practice.

Leading with Vision and Values

Vision in this context is defined as the belief in or description of a future that an individual or collective would like to see. It is used as a guide for engagement and discernment of both current and future actions. The following are examples:

I dream of a world in which every child has enough food to eat and a safe place to call home.

I believe that I can be an agent of change in improving the quality of life for those in my community who have been marginalized or disenfranchised.

I will be a doctor who leaves a lasting impact on her patients, not just by providing access to the highest quality of health care but also by caring about the lives and livelihoods of patients as they seek to improve their health.

Values in this context are defined as a set of beliefs, ideals, and morals that an individual or collective considers important, if not essential. Values are influenced by and influential on culture and experience. They guide behavior and attitude whether we are conscious of them or not; therefore, when intentionally reflected on and carefully considered, they serve as guidelines for engagement and leadership in all things.

BOX 16.1

EXAMPLES OF VALUES DEFINED THROUGH ACTION

I will strive to lead with the following core values in all that I do to pursue my vision:

Creativity: I challenge myself to open up space for creative exploration in confronting challenges and in pursuing action, even when taking the time for creative exploration feels inefficient.

Respect: I seek and offer respect by meeting all people and situations with an open mind, reserving judgment, challenging my bias and assumptions, actively using my voice, and remaining open to feedback.

Collaboration: I commit to working with others by reaching out across boundaries, asking for support, letting go of control, remaining open to compromise, and investing time in iterative processes and thinking.

Faith: I engage the power of faith in something greater than myself that informs my vision, recognizing where I have agency and voice, surrendering to the unknown, staying present to life as it is, and engaging with hopefulness and joy.

Given transformative engagement and leadership's orientation to making positive, directed, and incremental change, any individual, group, or institution seeking to operate within a transformative leadership framework will embed, whether explicitly or not, the diagnosis of a problem as well as the idea of a desired future outcome based on an intervention or approach.

To diagnose a problem is to place a judgment, which is often rooted in some sense of moral value, on the current reality. This means that transformative engagement and leadership—whether pursued by an individual or an institution—is a moral endeavor rooted in values. To conceptualize a desired outcome that has not yet been fully realized is to have hope in the possibility of a future that is different from the current reality—this is vision. This said, in order to lead with vision and values, we cannot just be engaged passively in our vision and values; rather, we must actively articulate, enact, and engage them in our everyday lives, work, and relationships. By individually and collectively articulating the values that guide our diagnosis, intervention, and desired outcome (see Figure 16.1), we allow our vision and values to become dynamic and practical tools for decision making, collaboration, and action. Paulo Freire's description of praxis as "action and reflection of men and women upon their world in order to transform it" is an apt notion to apply to leading with vision and values (1968/2000, p. 79).

FIGURE 16.1   Action and Reflection

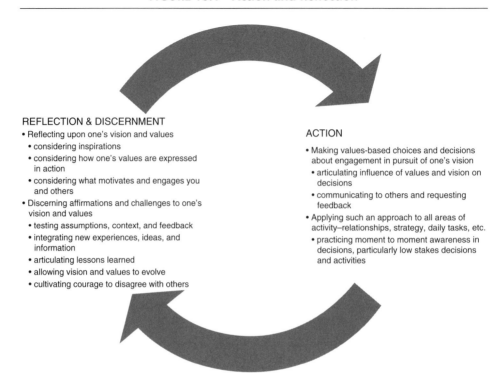

REFLECTION & DISCERNMENT
- Reflecting upon one's vision and values
  - considering inspirations
  - considering how one's values are expressed in action
  - considering what motivates and engages you and others
- Discerning affirmations and challenges to one's vision and values
  - testing assumptions, context, and feedback
  - integrating new experiences, ideas, and information
  - articulating lessons learned
  - allowing vision and values to evolve
  - cultivating courage to disagree with others

ACTION
- Making values-based choices and decisions about engagement in pursuit of one's vision
  - articulating influence of values and vision on decisions
  - communicating to others and requesting feedback
- Applying such an approach to all areas of activity—relationships, strategy, daily tasks, etc.
  - practicing moment to moment awareness in decisions, particularly low stakes decisions and activities

Developing a vision and set of values with which to pursue that vision involves taking stock of our life experience, noticing what is unfolding beyond our own immediate experience, discerning our hopes and dreams, and declaring how we want to see the world in the future.

This praxis takes courage and leads to inspiration. Our vision and values connect to the innermost parts of our being, and when communicated and acted on effectively, they connect others to the innermost parts of their own being. Courage is a practice—not a quality—in which we come to know, to honor, and to lead with that innermost part of self, and we develop faith in the relationship between our inner self and others. The word for "faith" in the Pali language, *saddha*, literally means "to place the heart upon," which is precisely what leading with vision and values asks transformative leaders to do in their words and work (Salzberg, 2003).

Pursuing Deep Listening and Meaningful Connection

To listen is very hard, because it asks of us so much interior stability that we no longer need to prove ourselves by speeches, arguments, statements, or declarations.

True listeners no longer have an inner need to make their presence known. They are free to receive, to welcome, to accept. (Nouwen, 1997, p. 71)

Deep listening is to be fully present to what is happening in any given moment so that you may hear with clarity the fullness of what is unfolding. It requires letting go of inner chatter, initial judgments, usual assumptions, and ideas for follow-up comments, in order to listen for what is actually being said or shared with you. To engage in deep listening, the mind must be intentionally and actively open, aware, attentive, and receptive. To practice, bring intention to the ways in which you listen. Become aware of your inner thoughts and feelings as you strive to hear the specific sounds and words that are being shared with you.

Meaningful connection is a way of connecting that abandons preconceived notions, agendas, or worries about how one is being seen, in order to be fully present in relationship. It requires letting go of inner chatter, initial judgments, usual assumptions, and ideas for how you would like to present yourself, in order to be fully present in the relationship with the person or people in front of you. Deep listening and hospitality are required to engage in meaningful connection. To practice, bring intention to the ways in which you connect with others. Become aware of your inner thoughts and feelings as you strive to connect with those you meet and are in relationship with, and work toward cultivating open presence in moments of connection.

BOX 16.2

TIPS FOR PURSUING DEEP LISTENING AND MEANINGFUL CONNECTION

- Stay aware of and present to all that is unfolding within you and outside of you.

- Recognize and attempt to release patterns of thought—particularly assumptions and judgments—that you hold in orientation to others.

- Focus your attention to the words being spoken and/or the person or people in your presence.

- Meet people where they are and invite people to engage.

- Leave space for silence.

- Ask open-ended questions.

- Reflect back what you have heard for clarity and understanding.

- Share thoughts and perspectives without attachment to an agenda.

- Remain open to engagement and feedback.

- Be aware of nonverbal communication (yours and that of others).

- Allow questions and tensions to be held and named without jumping to fix them.

Building the skills of deep listening and meaningful connection requires comfort with the unknown and begins with the self. How we listen to and connect with our self forms the basis on which we can do so with others. In the work of transformative leadership, such practices are often called self-care or work-life balance. Such activities are an integral part of pursuing deep listening and meaningful connection with others, in part because they are different applications of the same skill and largely because we need to have a degree of interior stability in order to listen and connect with others.

Vulnerability is fundamental to embracing the unknowns and fragility of life, and those who have realized their own inherent worthiness and dignity are best able to embrace the vulnerability of their lives, work, and relationships. To believe in the worthiness and dignity of one's self fundamentally requires listening to and connecting with one's self, just as believing in the worthiness and dignity of others requires listening to and connecting with those people (Brown, 2015).

The pursuit of deep listening and meaningful connection is a praxis of its own. It can be developed in the course of daily activity as one brings greater intention to how one hears and is heard, sees and is seen, and knows and is known in relationship. The skill is not about having answers but rather about discovering what unfolds when we approach ourselves, others, and life with the goal of listening and connecting to the self, the other, and the unknown.

Practicing Transformative Engagement and Leadership: A Three-Part Exercise

This three-part exercise will give you an opportunity to reflect on a hypothetical field experience, consider it in light of your vision and values, and use listening and connection to open up to other perspectives and shared learning. The same three-part exercise can also be easily adapted to help you reflect on your own experiences.

BOX 16.3

LIVING THE DREAM IN LIMBE

CONFRONTING COMPLEXITY AND CONFLICT

You are in the midst of a six-month assignment with an NGO called Hope for Youth, located in a small country in sub-Saharan Africa. When you first read the job description sent by Hope for Youth, it sounded like everything you dreamed of, working side by side with the community to address needs related to water and sanitation, food and nutrition, education, and health. You believe that your studies have prepared you well for your middle-management role, and you have made an effort to learn about the culture, read about the history of the region, practice the local language, and engage with the local news.

You moved from your current home and have been placed in the village of Limbe, where you live and work alongside the community. Your modest home in Limbe has electricity but no running water inside, so you find yourself engaged in collecting water at the shared source with your neighbors daily. You regularly engage with the mothers and children in the community as you get water every morning; many of your colleagues are also community members, so they are your neighbors.

You work directly for Mary T., the founder of the organization, who is based in Cincinnati, but travels to Limbe a handful of times each year, staying for two weeks at a time, providing direction, taking pictures that she can use for fundraising purposes, and supervising the midlevel management staff. Reading about Mary T.'s vision was one of the things that drew you to this work. The impact of the past 10 years can be seen: improvements to the school and teacher training have made a difference, and attendance rates are up; nearly every household has a latrine; and many of the local community members have a steady income thanks to Hope for Youth.

Mary T. made a visit to Limbe right after you arrived, and she is just about to complete her second visit. You feel you have come to know the community and cultural context well in recent months, and what you have learned has led you to see Mary T. in a new light. You notice that Mary T. makes quick decisions without much discussion or consideration of the ramifications on others. The organization seems to be dependent on Mary T. to make decisions because others don't feel they are trusted to take on leadership roles in her absence. Also, staff have begun to confide in you, expressing concerns about their wages, which are staggeringly low. Mary T. recently began to take taxes out of the wages, but did not increase the base pay, so wages have effectively gone down for all of the local staff in recent months. On her initial visit, Mary T. asked you to check on staff members to make sure they are not taking money or lying about their work. Her request was overhead by a staff member, who was both hurt and offended, and the news spread quickly. You tried to spend a lot of time building relationships in order to overcome that mishap.

The Hope for Youth vision, values, and mission suggest that collaboration, partnership, trust, and community empowerment are central to the work. These values are what drew you to the organization and the community. Despite the expressed organizational commitment to partnership and shared learning, however, Mary T. seems to believe that everyone in the village should be grateful for her charity and service.

You feel that Mary T.'s attitude and behavior during this visit work directly against the values needed to pursue the organization's mission. When you have tried to delicately broach these topics with Mary T., she has reminded you that she has been working in the community for 10 years, is married to someone who grew up in the community, and knows the people and culture very well by now. "Oh, don't worry about that," seems to be her answer for everything. You see things differently now as compared to when you first arrived. You want to respect the work that Mary T. has done, but it is difficult to ignore the real problems you see between Mary T., the organization, and the local community members.

Reflecting on the Experience

Consider the scenario in Box 16.2 in light of the following questions:

1. What would transformative engagement look like for you in this scenario? Free-write in your journal tackling this question through each of the lenses of reflection and discernment: self, other, and life.
2. How might historical and cultural context be present in the dynamics of the described scenario? Consider your own historical and cultural context and what your role and responsibility might be given the larger context. How you might approach that role and responsibility?
3. What relationships (collective and individual) are present in this scenario? How might they influence your choices and behaviors, and how might they be influenced by your choices and behaviors?

Given your responses to these questions, what would you do in this scenario? Be specific about your proposed approach. What more would you want to consider or learn before committing to your approach?

Vision and Values Activity

Take 10 minutes to create a sample one- to two-sentence vision statement and set of five core values with which you will pursue that vision (hold to the time limit for the purposes of the exercise). Your vision statement may begin with a phrase like "I believe …" or "I dream of a world where …" Attempt to create your list of values in a way that defines each value through action—for example, "Compassion: I will seek to be present to and not avoid the reality of pain and suffering while I attempt to alleviate it."

With your sample vision and values statement, examine the Hope for Youth scenario (Box 16.2) and the reflection questions. How do your vision and values give you grounding and insight into what might be an aligned approach to action for you? How are your vision and values tested in the scenario?

Listening and Connection Activity

Take three minutes to write out your proposed approach to practicing transformative leadership in the scenario. Following the approach, write down three to five thoughts or feelings you notice that you have about the scenario and your proposed approach.

Invite a classmate who has also conducted the reflective practice to sit with you. You will each read aloud or summarize what you have written—the approach as well as the thoughts and feelings (estimated time per person: two minutes). The listener will engage in deep listening, resisting the urge to respond, question, edit, define, clarify, or analyze what the other wrote. After the first person has shared, the listener will be asked to reflect back the essence of what has been shared without adding any commentary or analysis (estimated time for the reflect-back: one minute). Then switch roles.

Once you have finished the activity, together you can reflect on the experience of both sharing and listening in this way, and individually, you should journal with the following questions: How do I listen? What gets in the way of my listening? When do I feel listened to? How does listening relate to connection?

Chapter Summary

Applying the framework and skills of transformative engagement and leadership to the field of global health is an essential component of moving beyond the status quo in pursuit of innovation, collaboration, and impact. The pursuit of change asks a lot of the pursuer in terms of development of a personal and professional foundation of moral, reflective, and practical frames and skills. The ability to engage and lead change is not a given with the platform of a title, role, or specific kind authority—it is rather an approach and set of skills that are developed and practiced in all areas of engagement and action over time. The framework presented here offers the basis of the approach and the foundation on which many skills can be developed and honed. The skills of leading with vision and values and of pursuing deep listening and meaningful connection are perhaps two of the most essential skills to begin one's own development and practice.

Key Terms

Deep listening

Discernment

Meaningful connection

Reflection

Transformative engagement and leadership

Values

Vision

Review Questions

1. Apply the three lenses of self, other, and life to an engagement or leadership challenge you have encountered or witnessed in the field of global health.
   a. Describe the scenario.
   b. Explore the experience, thoughts, ideas, and orientations through each lens.
   c. Articulate learnings and/or questions for ongoing consideration.
2. What are the historical and cultural narratives that influence your engagement in global health? Consider your identity and experiences as an individual as well as with whom and where you seek to practice. How might your approach to engagement and leadership shift given this contextual awareness?
3. Think of a global health engagement or leadership challenge you have encountered or witnessed. List and explore all the relationships that are present in the case. Consider primary, secondary, and tertiary relationships. How might each relationship influence your choice and path of action?

Suggested Reading

Dudley, D. (2010, September). *Drew Dudley: Everyday leadership.* [Video file]. TED. Retrieved from https://www.ted.com/talks/drew_dudley_everyday_leadership?language=en

Kleinman, A. (2008). *What really matters: Living a moral life amidst uncertainty and danger.* New York, NY: Oxford University Press.

Lederach, J. P. (2005). *The moral imagination: The art and soul of building peace.* Oxford, England: Oxford University Press.

Lipsky, L. D., & Burk, C. (2009). *Trauma stewardship: An everyday guide to caring for self while caring for others.* San Francisco, CA: Berrett-Koehler.

Mathieu, W. A. (1991). *The listening book: Discovering your own music.* Boston, MA: Shambhala.

Sinek, S. (2009). *Start with why: How great leaders inspire everyone to take action.* New York, NY: Portfolio.

References

Berg, D. (1998). Resurrecting the muse: Followership in organizations. In E. B. Klein, F. Gabelnick, & P. Herr (Eds.), *The psychodynamics of leadership* (pp. 27–52). Madison, CT: Psychosocial Press.

Brown, B. (2015). *Daring greatly: How the courage to be vulnerable transforms the way we live, love, parent, and lead.* New York, NY: Gotham Books.

Freire, P. (2000). *Pedagogy of the oppressed.* New York, NY: Continuum. (Original work published 1968)

Lorde, A. (1977). Poetry is not a luxury. In *Sister outsider: Essays and speeches.* New York, NY: Crossing Press. (Original work published in *Chrysalis*)

Nouwen, H.J.M. (1997). *Bread for the journey: A daybook of wisdom and faith.* San Francisco, CA: HarperSanFrancisco.

Rushing, J. (2016, January 8). Bryan Stevenson wants to end racial injustice. *Al Jazeera America.* Retrieved from http://america.aljazeera.com/watch/shows/talk-to-al-jazeera/articles/2016/1/8/ending-injustice.html

Salzberg, S. (2003). *Faith: Trusting your own deepest experience.* New York, NY: Riverhead Books.

CHAPTER 17

GUIDELINES FOR PLANNING A GLOBAL HEALTH LEARNING EXPERIENCE

Sweta Shrestha, MPH

We shall not cease from exploration and the end of all our exploring will be to arrive where we started and know the place for the first time.

—T. S. Eliot

LEARNING OBJECTIVES

- Understand principles and some recommended best practices for global health engagement in the context of an instructor-led course
- Review the program of an actual interdisciplinary field course in Nepal and consider how the different activities (community visits, learning opportunities in health and social service programs, cultural excursions, and personal reflection) complement each other
- Identify insights and practices that you would like to apply to your own global health experience

With the rise of the popularity of global health among students, there has been an influx of programs and courses along the spectrum of "global health field opportunities." Students should seek out programs that are oriented toward community assets and voice and that apply a critical lens to the study of disease, disparities, and development. Ethical global public health engagement is based on respect, reciprocal sharing, and self-reflection. One must be cautious of programs that present communities as helpless and pitiable, perpetuate a savior mentality, or engage students in health care or other activities for which they are not qualified or

Foundations for Global Health Practice, First Edition. Lori DiPrete Brown.
© 2018 John Wiley & Sons, Inc. Published 2018 by John Wiley & Sons, Inc.

prepared. Whether these programs are motivated by financial gain or good intentions, they are potentially harmful and do disservice to both students and communities by perpetuating dynamics of dependency and missing opportunities for authentic relationship and sharing. So, how can students of global health select an instructor-led global health course that will engage them with other cultures and communities respectfully and authentically?

Elements of a Global Health Field Course

The following case study and guidance comes from my personal experience in developing and leading field courses in both Sri Lanka and Nepal. The insights and recommendations are meant to help students gauge the quality of an instructor-led field course. The chapter will cover essential elements of such courses, including the following:

1. Course leadership
2. Place-based knowledge and preparation
3. Pre-departure training on cultural competency
4. Learning before doing
5. Listening and reflecting
6. Respectful engagement driven by the community

Course Leadership

The success of a field course is largely dependent on the leadership. The course should be led by faculty and staff who

- Have extensive background in the community or country
- Have extensive partnerships in the country and the community
- Have experience teaching
- Have a demonstrated understanding and expertise in global/public health
- Understand the mission and objectives of the program and the field experience

Institutes of higher education should seek out and encourage course leaders who identify—through their ethnicity, background, and/or culture—with the communities they are working in. Course leaders who have a personal background in the country are able to make connections and discuss the nuances of culture and place with a depth that is often very difficult for leaders who have only a peripheral knowledge of the community. Being aware of the power and privilege that come with certain identities, nationality, race, and/or gender is central to the growth of students' understanding of the world; therefore, field course leaders who have thought critically about these spaces and topics are essential assets for the leadership team.

Place-Based Knowledge and Preparation

Instructor-led courses should emphasize pre-departure study of the social, political, and historical context of the community that students will visit. Students should be encouraged to take ownership of this learning. Completing the country profile outlined in chapter 13 can be a useful preparatory exercise (see also chapters 1 and 21).

Pre-Departure Training on Cultural Competency, Privilege, Power Dynamics, and Representation

Training in cultural competency is a key element of a comprehensive field course orientation. There are many definitions of cultural competency, and there has been discussion of this topic in chapters 1, 2, and 14. Here we will focus on the importance of being aware and appreciative of cultural differences, the importance of intentional perspective taking to learn about other points of view, and ongoing reflection about power and privilege.

Cultural competency starts with culture itself. In preparation for global health engagement, students need to consider the ways in which everything in our lives is shaped by culture (language, clothing, body language, songs, play, religious practices, time constructs, etc.). This is important for effective engagement overall, and especially where global health is a focus, as cultural factors are critical to understanding of health, wellness, illness, decision making, privacy, and hygiene. These understandings are foundational for effective global health practice.

Essential to the conversations about culture is a discussion about "dominant culture" and the role of power and privilege in global health. Often, students are going into places and spaces where populations have historically been marginalized, victimized, or oppressed. Community members may have had other experiences with educational institutions or global health and development actors who did not see their strengths, and instead treated them as an example of poverty, suffering, and need. It is essential that students and course leaders enter communities with respect for local knowledge and experience, and awareness of their own privileges and power.

Understanding power dynamics is key to understanding global health challenges. A field experience is incomplete without attention to the role of power in the community, both historically and at present. Who holds power? How does power manifest itself? What is, and has been, its role in government, land rights, religion, language, culture, knowledge, and economics? Exploring how different kinds of power impact access to health and wellness is essential for future global health leaders.

Students engage in global health experiences expecting to learn about another culture and community. Yet they often lack a full understanding of their *own* culture and power, and how it can manifest in their interactions with communities and in their perceptions and judgments about cultural differences. The dominant discourses associated with being in the cultural majority or having economic or social privilege can manifest in the attitude that my way is the "right way" or the "normal way" of doing things. Beliefs and practices that differ from that norm can be cast as somehow underdeveloped, primitive, or inferior. It is essential to help students realize the ways in which these kinds of unexamined attitudes can shape their interactions with community members.

Intertwined with considerations about power dynamics is the importance of recognizing privilege. Privilege can be defined as special rights or advantages that are granted to a particular person or group of people. It is important that participants be aware of the privileges associated with their identity and life experiences, such as education, resources, and good health. Each individual's relationship to privilege impacts how they interpret what is happening around them, both in relation to the community and within their own group. Through self-reflection and discussion, students can become more aware of these dynamics, gain new insights, and develop more authentic understandings about themselves and their world.

The conversation about cultural competency should begin prior to departure, and continue throughout the course and beyond. Appreciating differences, learning about what is hidden from us in our own worldviews, and growing in our understanding of the perspectives and experiences of others should be ongoing processes. It is essential for students and course leaders alike to understand that cultural competency is not a static acquisition of knowledge but rather a mind-set and a frame of reference through which to view the world and things foreign or different from what is in our own communities.

Another important aspect of cultural competency training as students get ready for a global health field course is the ethics of video-recording, taking photographs, and employing other methods of capturing images, stories, and voices. In today's era of smartphones, selfies, Instagram, Facebook, and Twitter, the things you say, capture, and post can travel around the world in less than a minute. Therefore, it is essential for students and course leaders to make a commitment to ethical practices. As a member of the global health community, you have a responsibility to present your experiences authentically, protect the privacy of your hosts when appropriate, and refrain from disseminating images or descriptions that reduce the people you meet to a stereotypical or offensive representation in a picture or tweet. Organizations such as Unite for Sight have established some policies related to photographs and videos, which are excerpted in Box 17.1.

BOX 17.1

ON TAKING PHOTOGRAPHS AND VIDEOS

In order to decide if a picture should be taken or later used, consider the following questions:

- Has the person/people whom you are capturing with the photo given consent?

- Are they able to give consent (children, elderly, disabled, sick patients)?

- Does the person whose image is captured have the power, autonomy, and knowledge about their rights to give proper consent?

- What is your goal in taking the picture?

- Is the picture a fair representation of the person? Culture? Country?

- Who will see the image or story? Is it something that the subject of the photo would want?

- Can the identity of the person in the photo be kept confidential?

Source: Adapted from "Ethics and Photography in Developing Countries," by Unite for Sight, 2015. Retrieved from http://www.uniteforsight.org/global-health-university/photography-ethics

---

Learning before Doing

A fundamental component of ethical global engagement for students comes from the realization that a student's primary objective while on a field course is to learn from the experts in country and from the community. Students are often motivated to go into global health with a desire to *help* and *do something*. This is where some global health field programs have drifted problematically to a model that, for example, allows underqualified students to perform and assist with medical procedures with limited or no training. Even if students are well supervised, it is essential for them to know that if they would not be allowed to do a certain activity at their home institutions in the United States, then they should not do them in their host community either. Wearing scrubs or white coats or carrying stethoscopes in communities, without the appropriate skills, degree, and licenses, is a deliberate effort to be seen as a medical professional from a high-resource setting with power, resources, medicine, and knowledge. These practices are harmful to the community if the students do not have the skills and context to provide the care needed.

Students must also critically examine their sense of confidence, competence, and readiness to "help" or "solve problems" when they are very new in situations as a learner. Even though their intentions may be good, they are reflecting an implicit attitude that they have superior knowledge and judgment and that the problems that have plagued communities are actually rather easy to solve. The appropriate stance for a learner is to listen, share ideas, develop relationships, and participate in activities with curiosity and openness. It is also important to refrain from judgment and from imposing your ideas and will on a community that you are just getting to know.

It is essential for students to consider the role of power, currently and historically, and how the history of colonialism and other forms of cultural domination have played a part in constructing ideas about the role of the benevolent doctor/ savior/hero. During the colonial era, the benefits of medicine were used to justify colonial presence, while often discrediting traditional cultures and indigenous health care. These power dynamics, though changing, are still part of our history and identity. The students and instructors' nationality, race, language, mannerisms, and access to education are all indicators of their affiliation to the Western world. When students recognize and deconstruct these power dynamics, they can begin to interpret culture and community life on its own terms and to understand their role in it in a different way.

Listening and Reflecting

As students work on learning about and from communities and spaces that they are given access to, it is essential to integrate reflection into the daily curriculum. Listening, absorbing, contextualizing, and reflecting are at the core of what makes field courses transformative. Listening is a seemingly simple skill that many have lost the ability to do well in the age of instant information, multitasking, and oversaturation. Listening involves students paying attention to who is saying what, and why, and—equally important—what is *not* being said and who is *not* part of the conversation. The language, cadence, delivery, and ways of expressing thoughts and ideas vary widely across domestic and international settings. It is essential that students listen with an open, friendly, and nonjudgmental attitude, and make a deliberate effort to be patient if they have trouble understanding a foreign language or unfamiliar accent. They should take care not to listen for their own preconceived narratives but rather to hear what is being said on its own terms. They should also remember that every encounter is a great learning opportunity. Whereas academia emphasizes learning from those with higher education and titles, conversations with community members can provide unique opportunities for learning that reflect great wisdom and the nuances of culture and community life.

Along with listening to people and communities, students need also to "listen" to the both the built and the natural environment in order to understand the full scope of the determinants of health and wellness. The following questions are offered as guidance to listening to the environment:

- What do you hear?
- Can you hear people talking to each other outside?
- Are children playing? Laughing?
- Can you hear animals? What kinds? What are they doing?
- Is there noise pollution?
- Can you hear machines? What kind? Where?
- What do you hear at night? First thing in the morning?

Listening well is how we gather information about the world. In order to process and understand the data gathered through listening, it is essential that students practice reflection as part of their daily wrap-up. Having a space and time to reflect allows students to contextualize the things they have seen and understand the purpose and reasoning behind the things they are hearing, especially in the context of health and wellness.

Reflection is a good time to continue consideration of some of the topics introduced earlier in this chapter. Students should be encouraged to notice and discuss community assets and strengths daily, especially if that day's experience has included exposure to hardships and suffering. They should also be encouraged to spend some time on perspective taking, seeing the world through the eyes of the community members. It is an excellent time to continue the conversation about privilege, power, and how discourses of dominance may be impacting their ability to understand what is truly happening. Reflection enables students to process the information that they rapidly encounter in the course of the day, share the highs and lows of the day, and deconstruct their narrative of "the other" in exchange for something that holds more truth and reflects the humanity that we all share.

Respectful Engagement Driven by the Community

Respect is the foundation on which a good global health field course experience is built. Field experiences can strain communities and academic institutions and take precious resources away from already burdened systems. So why do we continue to conduct field courses in low-resource settings?

Field course experiences are opportunities for mutually beneficial engagement. Communities can plan activities aligned with their own agendas, enjoy friendships across cultures, and have an opportunity to share their points of view with students. Field experiences offer students the opportunity for exploration and for critical analysis and understanding of global development, geopolitics, and health and wellness.

By examining and questioning the impact, implications, and consequences of global engagement, students prepare for global citizenship that is informed by social justice, respect, and deeper understanding of the complexity and diversity of our world.

To foster that mind-set in students, it is essential that respectful partnership be at the core of their learning experience. Students see the interactions and relationships of the field course leaders with the communities as the proximal role model in their own understanding and relationship with the community and people. Respectful partnership is part of the charge for global health field courses. If course leaders and students are going into a community, it is essential that the community *want* to host them and have a clear and accurate understanding of the activities that will be carried out and the ways in which the students will be part of community life. Critical also is the knowledge that hosting students and faculty from the United States and other Western nations will not negatively impact them in the long run, in terms of socioeconomics, safety, politics, culture, and mental health. If not navigated properly, hosting outsiders within the community can create jealousy and competition among community members. Having a regular open dialogue and respectful partnership with community members can allow for problems to be addressed as they arise.

Although we are invited into the community to learn and observe, sometimes sharing intimate aspects of life, it is important to treat community members with dignity and respect. They are not case studies, laboratory specimens, or material for interesting sound bites. They are people, with complicated lives just like ours, and with feelings and emotions similar to our own. Global health field courses engage students in communities where there are complex legacies in relation to international engagement. It is an honor to be welcomed there, and we have a responsibility to respond with respectful engagement.

Case Example: Nepal Global Field Course

As a guide to help faculty, staff, community members, and students develop and choose an appropriate field course, the University of Wisconsin–Madison's Nepal global health field course structure and curriculum, specifically from the 2014 iteration of the program, is discussed in detail here. The field course is conducted in partnership with Shisir Khanal, from Teach for Nepal and Sarvodaya USA.

Field Course Learning Objectives

To increase students' knowledge, understanding, and practical field skills related to asset-based community development and its application to holistic health and wellness in village life, and to how health and well-being are affected by social, environmental, political, spiritual, cultural, and economic conditions in rural Nepal.

To *increase students' cultural competency* to engage in the international context, appreciating and honoring cultural diversity and cross-cultural understanding, respect, and collaboration.

To *increase students' knowledge of organizations* involved in improving health and well-being, including governmental programs, international and local NGOs, faith-based programs, university-affiliated programs, and social entrepreneurs.

To *expose students to promising practices in sustainable, holistic development* and the need for cross-disciplinary partnerships to address issues of health and well-being in impoverished areas.

To *stimulate self-knowledge of the power of cultural norms* and encourage students to apply what they learn when they return to the United States.

To *help students assess their own interests and capacities* for international study and work, and to *increase awareness of opportunities* to engage in such ventures.

To *engage in service with local Nepali counterparts* in ways that contribute to the community's own vision and efforts to improve health and well-being.

Field Course Partnership Principles

Our partnership with Sarvodaya seeks to break the barriers and dependency created by the traditional aid model and focuses on empowering communities through human connections and collaboration. Seeing development activities thrive locally in communities showcases the value of collaboration and community-driven initiatives. It also gives our students much to think about in terms of how international aid works, what should be prioritized for change, and why. This critical questioning of norms and assumptions serves as the core of the Nepal field course. Students complete the field course with an appreciation for the local experts and organizations and the systems that we often take for granted in the United States, an ability to ask questions about the nature and impact of international aid, and an awareness of the intelligence and strength present in low-resource settings around the world.

Field Course Itinerary

Prior to departure, students are required to attend an orientation to Nepal and Sarvodaya focused on introducing students to a brief history and the social and political context of the country. Along with learning about the history, culture, and day-to-day life in Nepal, students learn about asset-based community development and the Sarvodaya approach via presentations and academic literature.

In country, students attend lectures and presentations prepared by NGOs, local stakeholders, and organizations focused on improving the health and wellness of the country. During the time that the students are present in the village, they take part in a *Shramadhana,* a gift of labor designed to improve the health and wellness of the community, as chosen by the community members. Field trips to various organizations and communities are discussed in small-group settings with questions designed to help students process and contextualize their experience in terms of global health.

BOX 17.2
ITINERARY, NEPAL GLOBAL HEALTH CLASS, 2017

Day	Time	Activity	Reflection Session Focus
1	am	Arrival in Kathmandu. Pick up from the airport	First impressions, arrival journeys, expectations, and orientation
	pm	Visit "Swayamvu Nath," a Buddhist stuppa	
2	8 am	Heritage walk through Patan with Mr. Anil Chitrakar	Intersectionality between culture and health, built environments, the commons, heritage & norms
		Lunch around Patan Dhoka	
	2 pm	Traditional medicine—Baudha	
		Learn about traditional Tibetan medicine from traditional doctors in Baudha	
3	am	Lecture on public health governance by Mr. S. P. Kalaunee, Director of Governance & Partnership at Possible Health	How is the recent election both in the US and in Nepal going to impact health in communities in Nepal? What is the role of technology in health?
	pm	Visit Kritipur Hospital, and discussions with Dr. Saroj Dhital on global health and telemedicine	
4	am	Visit Tilganga Institute of Ophthalmology Learn more: http://tilganga.org/	What did you learn from each of the orgs? What does sustainability mean? Nuances of culture—the protective factors and enabling and risk factors.
	pm	Visit Shakti Samuha, an organization established by survivors of human trafficking that works to prevent trafficking Learn more: http://shaktisamuha.org.np/	
5	am	Visit Dhulikhel Hospital (about 1 hour away from Kathmandu) Visit hospital and learn about the services provided in the hospital and its community heath extensions Learn more: http://www.dhulikhelhospital.org/	What did you see during the drive, what didn't you see—comparison between urban and peri-urban Nepal. What is community health?
	pm	Arrive at Charikot, Dolakha (about 4–5 hour drive)	

Day	Time	Activity	Reflection Session Focus
6		Visit district hospital managed by Possible Health & Dhulikhel Hospital's extension nearby Learn more: http://possiblehealth.org/ Hike to famed temple in the community in the morning	Post-earthquake Nepal—what happened right, what is going on now. Accessing quality health care.
7		Return to Kathmandu	
8	am	Meet with Sumana Shrestha, founder of Medication for Nepal Learn more: http://medicationfornepal.com	Marginalized communities, distance of policy & practice, realities behind numbers and sustainability
	pm	Visit Blue Diamond Society Learn more: http://www.bds.org.np/	
9	am	"Connecting Rural Communities through Wireless," presentation by Internet Hall of Fame recipient Mahabir Pun Learn more: https://en.wikipedia.org/wiki/Mahabir_Pun Nepal Wireless: http://www.nepalwireless.net/	Foreign aid, innovation, leapfrogging technology
	pm	USAID	
10	am	Presentation on Teach For Nepal by Shisir Khanal Learn more: www.teachfornepal.org	
		Travel to Shramadana & Homestay Community—Chaughare, Lalitpur	
11		Shramadana—at the school—paint ECD room with educational frescos	How are things different, why and what is right, normal, and acceptable
12		Morning health panel featuring a community health nurse, traditional shamans, recently elected member of the local government Shramadana—at the school—finish painting & help w/moving construction materials for school Late afternoon: "Cultural Performance"	Reflection session focused on: home stay, what did you learn about the families, about yourself, and what impacts health in this community
13		Return to Kathmandu	
14		Open day in Kathmandu	

Day	Time	Activity	Reflection Session Focus
15		Drive to Pokhara (about 7 hours from Kathmandu)	Rules and expectations of hiking in the Annapurna Conservation Area in the Himalayan range
16		Drive to Naya Pul (1–1.5 hours)	
		Trek to Ulleri (3–4 hours) on foot (Entirely uphill trek)	What has made you push back? Made you uncomfortable, and how did you deal with it?
17		Trek from Ulleri to Ghorepani (Mostly uphill trek)	How is climate change going to impact the communities that we are walking through?
18		Sunrise hike to Poon Hill if weather permits Ghorepani to Ghandruk hike (8–9 hrs downhill)	What does access mean for people in this area?
19		Morning walk through famed village of Ghandruk Hike down to Naya Pul from Ghandruk (6–7 hrs)	
20		Free day in Pokhara	
21		Drive back to Kathmandu (8+ hrs)	What makes a person healthy? What is health?
22		Open day in Kathmandu Final day of class	Final reflection session focused on why global health & reading of the Gostin article "Why Rich Countries Should Care about Poor Countries"
		Farewell dinner—Durbar Restaurant	
23		Depart from Kathmandu Airport drop-off	

Field Course Activities and Reflections

During the *village stay*, students participate in a service-learning project. A recent example of a project involved plastering two school buildings so that classes could continue in those buildings during the monsoon season and the teachers of the school had a finished building in which to work. Local materials and techniques were used to plaster the buildings. Students worked in conjunction with Teach for Nepal fellows (young Nepalese spending two years in rural communities teaching) and community members, and participated in a Shramadhana. Students contributed their labor to a project that the community chose and worked on with other students, their host families, communities, and often the children as well. Students adhered to learning about and using the local resources and working on the time schedule of the villagers when participating in the home stays and the Shramadhana to ensure that their presence did not overburden the villagers and to gain an understanding of daily life in rural Nepal.

Excursions and *cultural visits* play an important role in the overall academic agenda. Students learn about health disparities and wellness in Nepal, and celebrating the culture and history of the country is part of that. The field trips are strategically chosen to exemplify the role of the built environment (Patan city heritage walkthrough, Swayambunath Stupa, Boudha Stupa), to gain appreciation of the geography of the country (Bandipur, Pokhara), and to learn more about the heritage and culture of the diverse people of Nepal (Bandipur, Solombu).

One of the most important and popular lectures is the *heritage walk* of the old Patan city with renowned conservationist Anil Chitrakar. Students learn about the importance of culture and history as they explore health in communities with deeply entrenched values and beliefs. Students are reminded of how health and wellness do not occur in a vacuum but are rooted in cultural practices, social structures, and historical memory.

Another important visit is to the *Dhulikhel Hospital Extension–Community Health Center* in Solambu, which is in the Kavre district of Nepal. The steep and often treacherous car ride to Solambu is a learning experience for students as they gain a new perspective on health care accessibility. The tour of the community health center gives them a glimpse into what organizations are doing to better health and wellness in far-reaching clinics.

Reflection sessions, both formal and informal, are an important part of experiential learning. Formal refection occurs on a daily basis at the end of the day, and students are given time to reflect on a few questions along with their experiences of the day. Students are also given time to write in their journals (part of their grade), which are turned in to field course leaders at the end of the field experience. Small-group discussions and thought-provoking open-ended questions, such as, "Why do we go to this specific site?" and "What was the point of today's visit?" are good ways to draw all students into the discussion. In addition, we frequently conduct reflection sessions over tea, which allows for a warmer, less academic environment.

In order to maintain students' thought processes around global health even during their downtime, specific readings are used for reflection sessions in Bandipur. Students pick the topic they are going to focus on before the start of the trip and have assignments due before leaving. This background information gives them a platform on which to generate questions for guest lecturers and organizations.

BOX 17.3

EXAMPLE OF ASSIGNMENTS AND GRADING

10 pts **Pre-departure assignments** will be modeled to generate awareness and knowledge about the status of health and disease in Nepal.

Geo-journal. Students will receive a template of a geo-journal to gain place-based knowledge of Nepal.

Annotated bibliography on topic of choice for academic paper. Students will turn in an annotated bibliography of 5–7 articles from the academic literature on the topic chosen and approved by course leaders.

Position paper. Students will answer 3–4 questions about global health pre- and post-trip to help illustrate their growth and their comprehension of global health concepts.

10 pts **Trip orientations**

Pre-departure orientations with course leaders and the Undergraduate Certificate in Global Health team.

35 pts **Participation and discussion**

Small-group reflection will occur every day (depending on schedule), and full participation of students is expected.

Q&A. Students are expected to fully participate and ask questions during site and organization visits. Failure to ask questions and participate during visits to different organizations will result in a deduction of participation points for that day.

10 pts **Journal**

Students are expected to keep a travel journal throughout the field experience and will turn in *5 journal entries* to course instructors at the end of the field experience.

10 pts **Position paper**

Students will write a short (2–3 page) position paper *before and after* their field experience, based on specific questions or a scenario presented by the course leaders.

25 pts **Academic paper**

Students will *pick one topic of interest* [from a provided list of options]. Drawing on the overall field experience and academic literature, they will write a paper on the global burden of the topic, its impact in Nepal, and the determinants of the problem, and make recommendations on how to reduce the burden of the problem.

Chapter Summary

As global public health becomes ubiquitous on campuses around the country, so do instructor-led, or "field," experiences. The field experience can serve as the capstone for a student's comprehension of the complexity of global health. For field-based programs to be ethically sound, they must include a focus on the strengths of the local setting and provide a critical lens through which to view, teach, and reflect on the public health context of the community. The following is a list of five key elements to keep in mind when preparing for an instructor-led field experience either in your own community or in an international setting:

1. *Course leadership:* see community leaders as experts
2. *Place-based knowledge and preparation:* learn before you go
3. *Pre-departure training on cultural competency:* embrace the assets of the culture you are visiting, be open to sharing with those you meet, and study the history of power and privilege within the community and how your power and privilege may impact the visit
4. *Learning before doing:* understand that the main takeaway from the experience will be learning and developing relationships, rather than helping and doing
5. *Respectful engagement driven by the community:* before going, ask the course leader about the partnership history between the program and the community: Does the community *want* to welcome a field course? Do you see evidence of positive mutual relationships?

Key Terms

Community engagement
Cultural competency
Place-based knowledge

Suggested Reading

Association of American Medical Colleges. (2011). Guidelines for premedical and medical students providing patient care during clinical experiences abroad. Retrieved from https://www.aamc.org/download/181690/data/guidelinesforstudentsprovidingpatientcare.pdf

Fischer, K. (2013). Some health programs overseas let students do too much, too soon. *Chronicle of Higher Education, 11*(4). Available to subscribers at http://www.chronicle.com/article/Overseas-Health-Programs-Let/142777

Kushner, J. (2016, March 22). The voluntourist's dilemma. *New York Times.* Retrieved from http://nyti.ms/1RiXnBs

Lavery, J. V., Green, S. K., Bandewar, S.V.S., Bhan, A., Daar, A., Emerson, C. I., … Singer, P. A. (2013). Addressing ethical, social, and cultural issues in global health research. *PLoS Neglected Tropical Diseases, 7,* e2227. doi:10.1371/journal.pntd.0002227

Michelle C. (2016, September 25). The problem(s) with mission trips. *Intentional Travelers.* Retrieved from http://intentionaltravelers.com/problems-with-mission-trips/

Wallace, L. J. (2012, August 1). Does pre-medical "voluntourism" improve the health of communities abroad? *Journal of Global Health Perspectives.* Retrieved from http://jglobalhealth.org/article/does-pre-medical-voluntourism-improve-the-health-of-communities-abroad-3/

Wilkinson, L. (2015, July 28). Appropriating on Facebook: How to share during fieldwork. *Economics That Really Matters.* Retrieved from http://www.econthatmatters.com/2015/07/appropriating-on-facebook-how-to-share-during-fieldwork/

CHAPTER 18

NAVIGATING GLOBAL HEALTH FOR STUDENT ORGANIZATIONS

Alexis Barnes, MIPH

Alyssa Smaldino

I believe that through working together, the students and my staff both gain knowledge. I see them become more confident, brighter, and more knowledgeable.

—Sedtha Long, Build Your Future Today (Grassroot partner in Cambodia, partnered with GlobeMed at University of Virginia)

LEARNING OBJECTIVES

- Understand the historical context behind health equity work, and why it matters
- Explore how partnerships are a tool to understand the complex, systemic barriers to achieving health equity
- Identify guidelines to hold student organizations and their universities accountable to ethical global engagement standards

Student organizations offer important opportunities for students to engage in global health issues and connect with local leaders around the world. This chapter will explore lessons for students and educators on managing power dynamics in global health through equity-focused partnerships, as well as approaches for advocates to hold global health-focused student organizations and academic institutions accountable to those partnerships.

Foundations for Global Health Practice, First Edition. Lori DiPrete Brown.
© 2018 John Wiley & Sons, Inc. Published 2018 by John Wiley & Sons, Inc.

Students as Global Health Partners

In the United States, millennials are on their way to becoming the most educated and most ethnically and racially diverse generation in US history (Pew Research Center, 2010). Universities cater to the needs of their incoming classes by providing dynamic learning opportunities where students can practice leadership in real-world contexts. Student organizations provide a space for students to apply their classroom curricula through practical experiences. Backed by a supportive university structure, experienced faculty, and resources, student organizations are well positioned to explore the complexities of global health work. Students thus have a unique opportunity to simultaneously study those complexities while pushing for a more equitable model of partnership.

Before engaging in opportunities that frame **health equity**—defined as the absence of avoidable or remediable differences among groups of people, whether those groups are defined socially, economically, demographically, or geographically (World Health Organization, 2016)—as the goal, however, it is important to become a student of history. The following sections will briefly outline the historical context behind working in global health and how to recognize examples of short-term global health experiences that perpetuate harmful power dynamics, including some volunteer opportunities commonly promoted by student organizations.

First, it is vital to understand that poverty is at the root of global health disparities and inequities. Yet it is not poverty of ability or potential. Intelligence, talent, and leadership capacity are equally distributed around the world. Opportunities and resources are not. It is also not inevitable that resources are distributed as they are—the reasons are based on structures of power, and they are remediable. It is with this lens that we view global health history and current engagement.

Throughout the colonial period, people of European descent significantly altered the health care and other structures of the African, Asian, and American continents. Colonial rulers established the power to determine who has access to what services, how natural resources are extracted and used, and which languages would become dominant (Smaldino, Lasker, & Myser, 2016). The United States and other Global North countries continue this legacy by heavily influencing the health systems of countries in the **Global South** through both private and government-funded health programs. Local health organizations, nongovernmental organizations (NGOs), and clinics, often established to fill gaps in the local public health system, also frequently rely on foreign resources to fund their programs. One approach to raising programmatic funds includes offering pay-to-volunteer programs.

These volunteer programs, alongside the global **voluntourism** industry, which provides tourists with short-term volunteer opportunities, generates billions of dollars in revenue annually (Hartman, Paris, & Blache-Cohen, 2014). Some of this money returns to the organization in need of funding, some to overhead costs, and some to the entity organizing the experience. These programs can be particularly appealing to students, who may have only a few weeks in the summer to gain volunteer experience abroad; a global health experience is often required for both professional and academic advancement in global health work. Given the historical context in which these types of volunteer programs exist, power dynamics play out in many ways between Global North volunteers and their Global South counterparts. Student volunteers from Global North countries bring with them hundreds of years of history; ever since colonialism disturbed local structures, the Global North now often acts as "the donor," the Global South now "the recipient." Needs are often misaligned with funding and resources when one party (the Global North) has most of the power.

The case study in Box 18.1 is provided to help contextualize how a group of students came to understand and respond to these power dynamics.

BOX 18.1

THE STORY OF GLOBEMED

GlobeMed was started by students who saw a need to change the status quo.

It was 2006. Victor Roy was a freshman at Northwestern University and a member of the Global Medical Relief Program (GMRP). GMRP-Northwestern was working with an international NGO to send medical supplies to a clinic that this NGO had built in Ghana. During the summer before his sophomore year, Victor decided to visit the clinic to see how the students had influenced local progress.

Upon arrival, Victor found an empty building with bags of medical supplies in the closet. He discovered that there was already a hospital down the road and that the community didn't need GMRP's supplies.

After spending some time understanding the community, Victor asked a local leader, "Why didn't you tell us that this wasn't what you wanted?"

"Victor, we are African. We listen to our donors."

The members of GlobeMed, the organization that ultimately evolved from GMRP, see that as the moment GlobeMed was founded. Their goal is to flip that notion on its head by empowering young leaders who can say, "We are partners. We listen to grassroots leaders."

But achieving this goal is harder than it sounds. The power dynamics that Joseph shared with Victor pervade the global health and development system. Repeatedly, GlobeMed partner organizations share stories of donors mandating an approach that the partners know will not work in their community. But they often feel compelled to follow that approach in order to receive the funds needed to sustain their work. GlobeMed seeks to change that dynamic through long-term partnerships between grassroots organizations and university chapters.

Given these imbalanced power dynamics and the damage that can result, the global health community, including student organizations, has a responsibility to carefully understand and act in the interest of the Global South partner. One way to start a conversation is to collect data and stories from the Global South related to perceptions of power. For example, in a 2013 GlobeMed program evaluation, 23 African NGO leaders reported their biggest challenges in global health partnerships to include lack of accountability and respect from donors and volunteers, lack of inclusion of established community structures, duplication of efforts by donors, and misaligned expectations for how to measure success. As more organizations invest resources in understanding these dynamics and listening to local leaders, host communities and organizations can express ideas and strategies for how they would like to see power shift to their communities.

Student organizations play an important role in this shift away from traditional power dynamics. Students who want to make a meaningful, long-lasting impact should take the time to learn about the historical and sociocultural dynamics of global health through experiential learning. Organizations on college campuses have the opportunity to provide an engaging space for dialogue about the history and dynamics of global health work to complement students' traditional global health coursework. Transformational change is possible, and has happened when people from all backgrounds have united in partnership and solidarity to fight for equity and justice.

Student Organizations and Harnessing the Power of Partnership

Frames are mental structures that shape the way we see the world. As a result, they shape the goals we seek, the plans we make, the way we act, and what counts as a good or bad outcome of our actions. In politics our frames shape our social policies and the institutions we form to carry out policies. To change our frames is to change all of this. Reframing is social change.

—George Lakoff, professor of cognitive science and linguistics at the University of California, Berkeley

Despite the historical and cultural challenges related to power dynamics in global partnerships, students and other global health advocates can shift our framing and commit to working in partnership to create meaningful change. Partnerships between student organizations and host organizations (in the Global South) can be implemented to understand the complex, systemic barriers to health. Through these partnerships, students learn to engage by asking questions and challenging their own assumptions about the root causes of health inequity. This creates a learning pattern for students to identify **social injustice** in other parts of life, repeating the cycle and helping tip the scale toward justice and health wherever they might go. It begins with partnership, and results in a systemic transformation through the daily actions and behaviors of people.

Box 18.2 explores the learning process around partnership through the perspective of a member and now mentor of a student organization, Eric Hettler, who shares reflections about his evolving understanding of power and partnership with a community in Uganda. (More lessons from Hettler's experiences can be found in chapter 8.)

BOX 18.2

CASE STUDY: FROM STUDENT TO MENTOR—AN EVOLVING PERSPECTIVE

Eric Hettler has been actively involved with Engineers Without Borders USA (EWB-USA) since he was an undergraduate student at Colorado State University in 2005. When reflecting on why he became involved with EWB-USA, Eric says, "As a passionate young college student, I really wanted to make a positive change in the world. I saw Engineers Without Borders as a good opportunity for me to apply the skills I was learning in the classroom to improve the lives of others. This combination of gaining experience and applying my skills while working to meet the needs of underserved communities throughout the world aligned perfectly with the stated mission of EWB-USA."

The first project on which he worked was a water supply and distribution system for two small communities in El Salvador. Although the project had been initiated before his arrival, it was not implemented until he was almost ready to graduate—almost five years after the request of the community. The long delays in a relatively simple water distribution project were understandably discouraging for the community. From their perspective, a group of American students would arrive about once a year, make promises about a water distribution system, leave, and then return a year later having made little progress. Toward the end of the project, the growing frustration hit a boiling point. The Peace Corps volunteer who was living in the community and was serving as a liaison between the students and the community water board composed an email that essentially said, "You have to realize how much your words and promises impact this community. This project is about people's lives and livelihoods. You have to stop viewing it as just simply an interesting science project."

Ultimately the project was successfully implemented, but those powerful words stuck with Eric throughout his work with EWB-USA. After working in East Africa for two years and living and working alongside individuals who could be impacted by these types of student-led projects, he returned to the United States feeling rather conflicted. He was concerned about how EWB-USA's student-led projects could end up negatively impacting a community, but he also realized that the projects would continue to be implemented with or without his involvement. With that in mind, he decided to become a mentor for a student group of EWB-USA.

Eric currently serves as a mentor for a group at the University of Wisconsin–Madison, and he regularly reminds the students about the lessons he learned from his experiences and failures on previous international projects. In addition, he regularly provides articles and essays that challenge some of the common preconceptions some students may have. The readings challenge the idea that any project is better than nothing, that the communities are helpless without the aid of well-educated college students, and that working on these projects is an entirely noble and altruistic endeavor.

In addition, EWB-USA has made progress in addressing some of the issues that are common when a group of students embarks on an engineering project in the Global South. First, EWB-USA approves only projects that are proposed by the community in which the work will be done. Second, the organization requires a Memorandum of Understanding (MOU) to be signed by the group and the community before any work begins. The MOU outlines the roles and responsibilities of the different parties involved in the project: the students, the community members, and the partner organization. Third, EWB-USA requires a trained and experienced professional engineer to be actively involved in the design and implementation of the project. Finally, it requires the student group to work with the local community to establish a sustainable local financial structure to ensure the continuing success of the project.

Although these goals are admirable, much work still needs to be done. In Eric's experience, the majority of projects are not brought directly from the community but rather through another NGO working within the community. At times, the NGO is truly representing the needs and desires of the community, but these relationships have to be carefully evaluated to ensure that the community is actually driving the demand for the project. Smaller organizations with in-country staff and long-term ties to the community are more likely to represent the true needs and desires of the community. The MOU is also a great idea in concept, but it must be drafted with careful coordination between the student group and the community to foster a truly equitable relationship; unfortunately, the MOU is often written by the student group first and only approved by the community after it has been written. The incorporation of trained professional engineers is certainly welcome from a technical standpoint, but typically the engineers themselves fail to understand the intricacies and power dynamics that can develop over the course of a project. Engineers tend to focus primarily on the technical aspects of the project, and the involvement of public health students and practitioners or social scientists is vital to expand the perspective of the group. Finally, establishing a payment system to ensure sustainability of the project is vital, but doing so requires a deep knowledge of the history and dynamics of the community that is typically beyond the reach of students who only spend a few weeks visiting.

Despite the concerns, EWB-USA has established a positive framework that can continue to be improved. "The biggest barrier currently facing the students is their lack of understanding about the historical and sociocultural dynamics associated with these types of engineering projects," Eric says. "By incorporating a more holistic approach that goes far beyond just the technical aspects of the project, the students will be more capable of identifying problematic and harmful power dynamics that too often develop when one of these projects is implemented. By incorporating students and professionals with a background in social sciences and public health, who have more training in community-based projects and are more able to thoughtfully engage with the community, the projects can be implemented in a much more just, equitable, and appropriate manner."

Note: The views expressed in this case example do not necessarily represent the views of Engineers Without Borders.

Student organizations can harness the power of partnership to increase such **leadership competencies** as flexibility, collaboration, cross-cultural communication, and accountability (see chapter 14). Partnerships between student organizations and grassroots organizations can be mutually empowering if the framing and purpose are clear and led by local leaders. As mentioned in the previous case study, a student organization should be prepared to create a Memorandum of Understanding, which is a formal agreement between the organization and the community that outlines how students will contribute to the progress of a project identified by that community.

Documentation of a partnership can be used as a living framework to reference goals, outline expectations for how communication between partners will unfold, and recognize the partner organization as the project leader. This documentation can be a useful tool for accountability, particularly when there are consistent leadership transitions between students governing the student organization. To make the potential strengths and weaknesses of a partnership more tangible, a global education partnership exchange called Fair Trade Learning compiled a framework to describe what a strong partnership may look like (Hartman, 2015). This framework is a useful tool that student organizations can use to ask themselves regularly, "Are our practices with our partner organization ethical and equitable?"

By building a mutually agreed-on framework that forecasts potential power dynamics, all partners can have a clear understanding of how to successfully work together. For example, Hartman's (2015) rubric outlines when and how to include key stakeholders in decision-making processes. Other factors to consider including in a partnership framework may be the role of leaders in the host community to guide projects, or tactics for ensuring that the rights of the most vulnerable community members are upheld. Through collective reflection and intention in these partnership-building experiences, participants can successfully initiate interventions.

Structures of Accountability

Record numbers of undergraduate students are finding opportunities to engage in projects or programs abroad. The majority of US students who participate in programs abroad are engaging in short-term programs (between two and eight weeks), according to the Institute of International Education (2009). Although opportunities for short-term engagement are increasing, many universities have not developed **accountability** systems to ensure proper oversight of these experiences. Simultaneously, many global health employers and medical school programs cite direct international and/or medical experience as an expectation for applicants ("How to Make Your Medical School Application Stand Out," n.d.).

This has created a system that often incentivizes students to conduct tasks they are unqualified to do and could not legally conduct in the United States. This not only exacerbates power dynamics but also can lead to harmful clinical outcomes that host organizations and clinics are then responsible for addressing. Students, university administrators, and faculty are implicated in these dynamics and therefore have a responsibility to understand and prevent unethical health-related activities from occurring.

There are multiple global engagement evaluation tools being used by universities across the United States, but not in a regulated or consistent way. The Forum on Education Abroad (2013), a forum of universities and overseas organizations that advocates for high-quality education abroad programs, released guidelines for students participating in clinical and health-related programs abroad. These guidelines reiterate the need for students to participate in these experiences from a place of learning, rather than from one of doing/fixing/practicing in the context of clinical care.

There are student organizations, NGOs, and universities that have recognized their role and responsibility to create awareness around similar standards. For example, students at the University of Wisconsin–Madison have put together a set of pre- and post-departure guidelines to provide an accountability framework for themselves when participating in global health experiences abroad (Center for Pre-Health Advising, n.d.). The following are some of these considerations:

- Volunteering with well-established programs with strong local ties. Programs should have worked with undergraduate students in the past and be engaged in the sustained support of a community.
- Recognizing that students are going abroad to learn, not to transform another community based on the students' own cultural norms or expectations.
- Ensuring that every participant is able to communicate the following statements in the local language or languages (recognizing that the language may need to be

tweaked to address local cultural norms): "I am an American student and not a health care provider. I am here to learn about health care. Do I have your permission to be present at this time?"

Another important contributor to the development of accountability structures in university-sponsored global health experiences is faculty. As advisors to students who participate in global health experiences, faculty can elevate the voices and positions of students who are concerned about elements of university-sponsored global health experiences that are not equitable to host sites. Members of the Working Group on Global Activities of Students at Pre-health levels state, "Advisors are uniquely positioned to advocate for changes that will both result in appropriate pre-health student learning abroad and expose the unnecessary risks for patients and students alike in the current dynamic" (Evert, Todd, & Zitek, 2015). To make that shift a reality, pressure from passionate student leaders is required.

Universities Allied for Essential Medicines (UAEM), with chapters at over 46 research universities, is a student organization that has built mechanisms to effectively hold academic institutions accountable to ethical global health standards. Its specific mission is to do this in the context of ensuring that biomedical research discoveries are beneficial to those in the Global South. To put pressure on universities to set high ethical standards in this area, UAEM measures three things: how universities are investing in biomedical research that addresses neglected health needs of the Global South, whether medical breakthroughs are being made affordable to people in the Global South, and whether universities are including curriculum on the translation of biomedical research discoveries to the Global South. UAEM publishes its findings in a report card (http://globalhealthgrades.org/).

This report card is not without limitations and is continually evolving; multiple universities have published critiques of the UAEM report card. For example, *The Lancet* published a letter from employees at Boston University which highlighted that the report card's single focus on biomedical research is not representative of the global health work conducted through their university (Wirtz, Vian, Kaplan, & Simon, 2013). However, this kind of tool has generated dialogue among students, NGOs, and universities about how best to create and measure standards for students who wish to engage in global health work. UAEM is a tangible case study of how students can impact systems, particularly at their own universities, and create change.

UAEM began at Yale in 2001. One of the first AIDS treatment drugs was developed at Yale, and student advocates worked to pressure the pharmaceutical company, eventually achieving a 90% price drop. This successful case led students to explore how a university could do globally accessible or socially responsible licensing. "Instead of it being all about what royalties you're going to get from [drug companies] if [universities] license their promising medical research, it's a conversation about how can we have provisions for low-income markets, where you allow them to produce it for sale at a much lower cost for those areas. How will you find some kind of other carve-out or a tiered pricing system. Or even just not have a patent outside of the high-income world" (Lee, 2013).

Participation and transparency are essential components of any accountability system. Accountability traditionally implies one set of actors holding another to account. If we shift our framing to put at the center the communities we aim to serve, accountability should be primarily to host organizations and communities—not to the student engaging in the global health experience.

Chapter Summary

The global health community has a responsibility to understand and respond to power dynamics that continue to influence health outcomes. When this is done well, global partnerships can provide a unique opportunity for students to learn by asking questions and challenging their own assumptions about the root causes of health inequity. Centering the communities and beneficiaries served through health equity work can hold student organizations and their universities accountable to ethical global engagement standards.

Review Questions

1. Review and discuss the case studies with your classmates. What patterns did you observe in the case studies related to priorities and power? What do these patterns indicate about whose priorities most often shape global health projects?
2. Ideally, how can partner communities in which student organizations work be involved in decision making about projects or research carried out by students?
3. Think about the organizations mentioned in this chapter, such as UAEM and GlobeMed. What power do students have on campuses to influence global systems? What is happening, can happen, or should happen on your campus? What is the role of students in advocating for health as a human right?

Key Terms

Accountability
Global South
Health equity
Leadership competencies
Social injustice
Voluntourism

Recommended Reading

Farmer, P. (2003). *Pathologies of power: Health, human rights, and the new war on the poor.* Berkeley: University of California Press.

Global Health Fellows Program II. (2015, August). *Survey of major employers of global health personnel: Executive summary.* Retrieved from https://www.ghfp.net/sites/default/files/Executive_Summary_-_Survey_of_Major_GH_Employers.pdf

Illich, I. (1968). *To hell with good intentions.* Speech presented at the Conference on InterAmerican Student Projects, Cuernavaca, Mexico. Retrieved from http://www.swaraj.org/illich_hell.htm

Mann, J. M., Grodin, M. A., Gruskin, S., & Annas, G. J. (1999). *Health and human rights: A reader.* New York, NY: Routledge.

Roberts, M. (2006). Duffle bag medicine. *Journal of the American Medical Association, 295,* 1491. doi:10.1001/jama.295.13.1491

Palilonis, M. A. (n.d.). *An introduction to global health and global health ethics: A brief history of global health* (Unpublished master's thesis). Retrieved from http://bioethics.wfu.edu/wp-content/uploads/2015/09/Topic-3-A-Brief-History-of-Global-Health.pdf

References

Center for Pre-Health Advising. (n.d.). Ethical considerations for service trips abroad. Retrieved from http://prehealth.wisc.edu/ethical-guidelines-for-uw-madison-students-engaged-in-health-related-service-abroad/

Evert, J., Todd, T., & Zitek, P. (2015, December). Do you GASP? How pre-health students delivering babies in Africa is quickly becoming consequentially unacceptable. *Advisor.* Retrieved from http://www.naahp.org/Publications/TheAdvisorOnline.aspx

Forum on Education Abroad. (2013). Guidelines for undergraduate health-related programs abroad. Retrieved from https://www.for umea.org/guidelines-for-undergraduate-health-related-programs-abroad

Hartman, E. (2015). Fair trade learning: A framework for ethical global partnerships. In M. A. Larsen (Ed.), *International service learning: Engaging host communities* (pp. 215–234) (Routledge Research in International and Comparative Education). New York, NY: Routledge.

Hartman, E., Paris, C. M., & Blache-Cohen, B. (2014). Fair trade learning: Ethical standards for community-engaged international volunteer tourism. *Tourism and Hospitality Research, 14,* 108–116. doi:10.1177/1467358414529443

How to make your medical school application stand out. (n.d.). *Princeton Review.* Retrieved from http://www.princetonreview.com/med-school-advice/make-your-medical-school-application-stand-out

Institute of International Education. (2009, November 16). Americans study abroad in increasing numbers [Press release]. Retrieved from http://www.iie.org/who-we-Are/News-and-Events/Press-Center/Press-Releases/2009/2009-11-16-Americans-Study-Abroad-Increasing#.V65eXpMrK8V

Lee, T. B. (2013, November 22). University patents limit access to medicine: These students want to change that. *Washington Post.* Retrieved from https://www.washingtonpost.com/news/the-switch/wp/2013/11/22/university-patents-limit-access-to-medicine-these-students-want-to-change-that/

Pew Research Center. (2010). Millennials: Confident. Connected. Open to change. Retrieved from http://www.pewsocialtrends.org/files/2010/10/millennials-confident-connected-open-to-change.pdf

Smaldino, A., Lasker, J., & Myser, C. (2016). Clear as mud: Power dynamics in global health volunteerism. In A. N. Arya & J. Evert (Eds.), *Global health experiential education: From theory to practice* (pp. 105–113). Abingdon, United Kingdom, and New York, NY: Routledge.

Wirtz, V. J., Vian, T., Kaplan, W. A., & Simon, J. L. (2013, July 20). Measuring universities' commitments to global health. *The Lancet, 382,* 204–205. Retrieved from http://www.thelancet.com/journals/lancet/article/PIIS0140-6736(13)61595-0/fulltext

World Health Organization. (2016). Equity. Retrieved from http://www.who.int/healthsystems/topics/equity/en/

CHAPTER 19

PLANNING FOR HEALTH AND SAFETY

Katarina M. Grande, MPH

Wherever you go, go with all your heart.
—**Confucius**

LEARNING OBJECTIVES

- Become familiar with common travel precautions for global learning experiences
- Be aware of useful preparations to consider for fieldwork in different environments

An exciting element that drives many to the field of global health is the promise of learning via going, seeing, and doing. Although you're reading a textbook right now, you'll discover that the immensely broad field of global health is experiential. It's this characteristic that makes global health work transformative—that makes people want to dedicate their lives to improving health equity for *everyone*. Nonetheless, you need to prepare for your first global health experience, as preparation is essential for health and safety. Let us explore some commonsense considerations to keep in mind while you are preparing for your first journey to a new place, regardless of the destination.

Before You Go

Plenty of resources are available online for you to learn about your destination. (The US Department of State, Bureau of Consular Affairs is a good place to start.) In addition to researching your logistical questions, however, look for stories. Read travel guides, but also find literature and books written by authors from the region. Gain

Foundations for Global Health Practice, First Edition. Lori DiPrete Brown.
© 2018 John Wiley & Sons, Inc. Published 2018 by John Wiley & Sons, Inc.

an understanding of the place's history and its relationship with foreigners. If possible, meet with individuals *from* your destination—they will be more valuable than any Google search. In lieu of speaking to an individual from the area, try to find people who have recently traveled to your destination region—your university's study abroad office may be a good place to start. They can provide you with an up-to-date student perspective. This experience sharing can provide you with important nuanced information that may not be posted on official websites.

BOX 19.1

TEN QUESTIONS TO ASK ABOUT YOUR DESTINATION

Find someone who is familiar with your destination and ask the following questions:

- Were there any cultural barriers that you found particularly surprising or challenging?

- What is the best way to convey respect?

- What mode of transportation did you utilize most frequently?

- What were the top three items you brought that were most useful?

- Considering that I will be visiting in _____ [season/month], are there certain clothing items that are essential? What clothing would be considered inappropriate (e.g., shorts for men, short skirts for women)?

- What types of gifts for hosts should I bring?

- Did you exchange money when you got there? Are there specific currency denominations that get a better exchange rate? Are ATMs abundant?

- Is there a health facility nearby that you would recommend?

- Are there specific precautions for women or LGBTQ individuals? Are there attitudes about racial, ethnic, or religious identities that I should be aware of?

- Could you please practice the main greetings in the local language with me?

Passport and Visa

While you're researching your destination, don't forget to ensure that your passport has at least six months of validity from your travel date (US Department of State, n.d., "Traveler's Checklist"). Your passport also must have at least two blank pages for **passport stamps** (a stamp indicating entry or exit from a country) or **visas** (a document often attached to a passport page that grants you permission to enter a country for a designated amount of time). Make two copies of your passport—leave one copy at home with a trusted friend or family member, and bring the second copy (but store it separately from the original). Check the country's visa rules well in advance of departure, as some countries require a travel visa before arrival.

Travel Warnings

Do regularly monitor the US Department of State's travel alerts and warnings (US Department of State, n.d., "Alerts and Warnings") in advance of your departure. Travel alerts pertain to short-term events that could impact travel, such as an upcoming election season that is likely to attract demonstrations and strikes, an emerging health concern such as an infectious disease outbreak, or an elevated risk of terrorist attacks ("Alerts"). Travel warnings are more serious and can indicate ongoing violence, increased frequency of terrorist attacks, or civil war ("Alerts"). Although many university-sanctioned programs will not bring students to an area with a State Department travel warning, sometimes exceptions may be made through a formal review process, or the decision may be up to you. Travel can bring a degree of risk, so it is important to assess your comfort level and make informed, careful decisions about the current safety implications of your potential destination. Many travelers choose to register with their embassy (the Smart Traveler Enrollment Program, https://step.state.gov/step/) so that their whereabouts are known in case of political unrest, evacuation, and other rare events.

Travel Medicine

Schedule a travel medicine appointment with your health clinic well in advance of your departure. Bring your itinerary to the visit—the travel medicine health care provider will want to know the types of places you'll be staying (rural, urban, high-altitude, remote). The provider will advise you on vaccines, prophylactic medications, and precautions applicable to the country you will visit.

Arrive at your appointment with specific questions and make sure you've looked up vaccine requirements. Vaccines recommended for your destination may include yellow fever, polio booster, hepatitis A, meningitis booster, Japanese encephalitis, and/or typhoid. Many countries where yellow fever is endemic require documentation of a yellow fever vaccine (a **yellow card** issued by the US Department of Health and Human Services). Some vaccinations require more than one dose for full protection, so ensure that you have time to make a return visit to your provider if necessary. If it is relevant to your destination, learn how to protect yourself from infections that do not have highly effective vaccines, such as tuberculosis or schistosomiasis.

In order to familiarize yourself with travel alerts pertaining specifically to health advisories, visit the Centers for Disease Control and Prevention's (CDC) Travel Health Notices page (http://wwwnc.cdc.gov/travel/notices). Another useful resource is the HealthMap website (www.healthmap.org/), which tracks current circulating pathogens and disease outbreaks. If mosquito-borne pathogens are a risk, make sure you discuss options for anti-malarial medications. If food-borne pathogens are a concern, ask about a prescription for general antibiotics and when it is appropriate to use them. You should be sure to obtain antibiotics that do not have resistance circulating in the region. If you take other prescription medications, be sure to have an adequate supply for the duration of your stay.

Health Insurance

Prior to departure, make a plan with your emergency contact if a health emergency should arise. You should also understand your health insurance situation abroad. Are you traveling with a program that includes international health insurance coverage? Do you need to purchase your own? If so, will you be visiting an area where medical evacuation coverage would be recommended? Cultural Insurance Services International is a common insurance option for students—explore CISI's site (http://www.culturalinsurance.com/students/service_and_support.asp) to understand what types of coverage may be relevant. Learn where the health facilities and clinics are in your destination.

While You Are There

Staying healthy while abroad requires you to pay attention to both physical and mental health. Further, health and safety are linked—if you're feeling well, you're more likely to make safe choices. The following section outlines a few tips for optimizing your ability to stay healthy and safe during your time away from home.

Society and Community

In many societies, the greatest promoter of safety is relationship building. If you build respectful relationships with your community and interact with your neighbors, people will look out for you. Another important safety activity is reading the news. Be aware of the political climate and what issues are currently being debated. Understand election cycles and the societal mood. Know that political activism may not be as protected as it is in your home country—ask your peers in country if it is safe to participate in political rallies, appear in the news, or speak publicly regarding your political opinions. Finally, keep in mind the social norms related to dress, conversation, and use of public spaces that may be different from your own.

Mosquitoes and Animals

Arrive with a general awareness of mosquito-borne pathogens in tropical regions; malaria, dengue, chikungunya, or Zika may be endemic. Use mosquito repellant liberally and regularly! Bed nets may be recommended if you are sleeping in lodging that does not have sealed windows and doors. Avoid contact with stray animals and wild animals during your visit. Depending on the length of your visit and the location of your site, consider the rabies vaccine prior to departure.

Food and Water

Experiencing the local cuisine is one of the best ways to learn about the people and culture of your destination. Nonetheless, follow these precautions regarding food and drink to the fullest extent possible while also respecting social courtesies:

1. Drink bottled or boiled water.
2. Wash fruits and vegetables using bottled or boiled water—cooked and peelable fruits and vegetables are safer.
3. Have a plan to respectfully decline when someone offers you food or drink that you do not feel comfortable eating or drinking.
4. Even if you follow all of these steps, you should expect gastrointestinal issues/traveler's diarrhea at some point—it is incredibly common. Have antibiotics on hand, as most traveler's diarrhea is of bacterial origin.

Be aware that in many settings, it is considered very rude to eat food without sharing. If you carry your own food for food safety reasons, always share what you have with the people around you.

Sanitation

Handwashing is one of the best defenses against illness and should be practiced with soap and water or hand sanitizer before and after eating and using the bathroom. Be sensitive to limited water supply. Another sanitation consideration relates to the availability of menstrual hygiene products. For those who menstruate, it is advisable to bring a full supply of tampons, pads, or other products, as it may be difficult (or expensive) to obtain in country.

Transportation

The most dangerous activity you'll participate in during your trip will likely relate to transportation. In areas where roads are poorly maintained and policies are not well enforced, travel by car, bus, truck, motorbike, tuk-tuk, or bicycle must be done with caution. Avoid traveling at night if possible. Stick with trusted, well-maintained vehicles whenever possible. When using taxis or other hired transportation, get recommendations from your local contacts or others who have traveled previously. If motorbike is your only transportation option in your area, bring a helmet from the United States and make a habit of carrying it with you wherever you go. Depending on your destination, helmets may be available, but they may not provide adequate protection.

Students on a budget may be tempted to choose cheap transportation options when traveling. Spending a bit more for safe transit, cutting expenses in other ways, is a wise investment. This is particularly true when you are first arriving in a new environment. Discuss a plan with your country partners regarding how you will get from the airport to your lodging safely—and acknowledge host-arranged transportation assistance by offering to pay for fuel, if appropriate.

Nightlife

In terms of experiencing nightlife, apply a similar approach to campus safety or travel as you would in any large city: travel in groups at night, use alcohol responsibly, and carry only what you absolutely need—it's best to carry cash and ID in your pockets rather than in a purse or bag. As in the United States, sexually transmitted infections (STIs), including HIV, are a risk—safe sex is important! HIV prevalence in some regions is high. Sex workers are at higher risk of STIs and therefore at higher risk of passing on infections to you. Note that social mores related to sexual activity and alcohol can vary greatly, so you may want to practice caution about developing intimate relationships quickly. Learn about the social meaning of accepting invitations, consenting to be alone with a potential partner, and other behaviors. This is important for your own safety as well as the safety of your group and of the women and men and other people whom you meet.

If you have a mental health or substance use disorder, you may want to talk about self-care with your health care provider and seek advice about how to turn down alcohol and drugs in a way that will be understood in the culture, and how to create other social opportunities. It is often possible to find a support group (conducted in the local language or in English) like Alcoholics Anonymous in the city you are visiting.

Psychosocial Health and Wellness

Cultural adjustment—as you adjust both to your new environment and then to your life back home—can be stressful. In addition, the challenges faced by the people, places, and organizations with which you work are complex and deeply rooted. Approaching your experience with a degree of idealism can be helpful, but try also to cultivate a healthy dose of realism and practicality in order to manage your expectations. Intercultural skills that help with adjustment include being aware of one's limitations, learning from interacting, being nonjudgmental, avoiding stereotypes, listening and observing, and tolerating ambiguity (Center for Global Education, 2016). Build time for reflection and self-care—activities to promote and maintain personal well-being and health—into your day. Examples of self-care activities may include journaling, exercising, processing a tough situation with a friend, cooking, or playing a game. Burnout, or mental exhaustion to the point of apathy, can be very real in global health work. If you arrive at your workplace with realistic expectations; build genuine relationships with your hosts, coworkers, and neighbors; and make room for self-care, the risk of burnout will decrease.

Chapter Summary

Your global health field experience can be life changing. By learning as much as you can before you travel, preparing for your safety, and practicing healthy habits while abroad, you will be able to focus on doing productive work and cultivating positive relationships.

Key Terms

Passport stamp
Visa
Yellow card

Discussion and Practice Assignment

Scenario: In 12 weeks, you will be traveling to a country that you have never visited to conduct a health assessment with a global health program. You are preparing a memo as an appendix to a grant application that you are writing to procure funding for your travel. Explore information on the US Department of State website related to your destination country. Visit healthmap.org and the CDC's travel health website (http://wwwnc.cdc.gov/travel/) to understand current health alerts. Visit other sites with relevant current information. Include the following items in your memo:

- Summary of location of destination
- Visa requirements for entering the country as an American
- Vaccinations required
- Summary of any current travel warnings
- Brief historical context of relations between the United States and the destination country
- Address of the US embassy nearest to where you'll be staying

Suggested Reading

Center for Global Education. (2016). SAFETI adaptation of Peace Corps resources. Retrieved from http://globaled.us/peacecorps/index.asp

Centers for Disease Control and Prevention. (2016). *CDC health information for international travel 2016*. New York, NY: Oxford University Press.

Freedman, D. O., Chen, L. H., & Kozarsky, P. E. (2016). Medical considerations before international travel. *New England Journal of Medicine, 375*, 247–260. doi:10.1056/NEJMra1508815

Massachusetts General Hospital. (2016). Global TravEpiNet. Retrieved from www.healthful.travel

References

Center for Global Education. (2016). Maintaining strong mental and emotional health. Retrieved from http://globaled.us/peacecorps/maintaining-strong-mental-and-emotional-health.asp

Centers for Disease Control and Prevention. (n.d.). Travelers' health. Retrieved from http://wwwnc.cdc.gov/travel/

US Department of State, Bureau of Consular Affairs. (n.d.). Alerts and warnings. Retrieved from https://travel.state.gov/content/passports/en/alertswarnings.html

US Department of State, Bureau of Consular Affairs. (n.d.). Smart Traveler Enrollment Program. Retrieved from https://step.state.gov/step/

US Department of State, Bureau of Consular Affairs. (n.d.). Traveler's checklist. Retrieved from https://travel.state.gov/content/passports/en/go/checklist.html

CHAPTER 20

GLOBAL HEALTH PROFESSIONAL SKILLS AND CAREERS

Sharon Rudy, PhD, BCC
Angelina Gordon, MA

Do not judge me by my successes, judge me by how many times I fell down and got back up again.

—Nelson Mandela

LEARNING OBJECTIVES

- Describe four skill areas crucial to successful global health careers
- Understand what global health employers are looking for in their employees
- List at least four "to dos" that you think can help you build your global health career

This chapter focuses on the practical aspects of building a successful career in global health and is written by experienced global health employers responsible for the hiring and support of hundreds of global health professionals over the past 20 years. We are looking at this topic from the perspective of what the work *actually is* and who does well—and who does not succeed and why.

What Are the Various Careers in Global Health?

Global health careers fall into three main categories: direct service, research, and development. All of these paths are legitimate and can be fulfilling, but *when* you decide to go to graduate school and *what* you choose to study matters. These decisions will determine how easily you pivot and change career paths. Yes, you will need a graduate degree if you want to have a flexible career with increasing responsibilities. We will unpack this a bit later.

If you are interested in being a nurse, midwife, doctor, or counselor, or treating clients in developing countries, you will want to develop a career pathway toward direct service. (See Jacquet, Evert, and Wyne, chapter 14, and the chapters of part 3, which feature the perspectives of a variety of health science professionals.)

If you primarily want to create new knowledge and enjoy the scientific method, consider a career in research. Development-centered careers encompass creating, implementing, and evaluating interventions that may include policy, health systems, communications, or service provider training components. There are many possible interventions, but they all fit into a category of direct interventions for a purpose, thus the term "development."

So, what are the organizations that might hire you for any of these activities? Organizations working in global health evolve as funding shifts and new needs arise. Use the Internet to explore who is out there and whether what they are doing is of interest to you. Check out the United Nations system (www.un.org), which includes the World Health Organization (www.who.org) and its many partnerships, such as Roll Back Malaria (www.rollbackmalaria.org) and Stop TB (www.stoptb.org). There are multilateral development banks like the World Bank (www.worldbank.org), the African Development Bank (www.afdb.org/en/), the Asian Development Bank (www.adb.org), and the Inter-American Development Bank (www.iadb.org). There are government assistance agencies, including the US Agency for International Development (USAID, www.usaid.gov), the largest international development donor in the world. Other US government entities involved in global health include the Centers for Disease Control and Prevention (CDC, www.cdc.gov), agencies implementing PEPFAR (www.pepfar.gov), and the US Peace Corps (www.peacecorps.gov).

What is most important is that you identify what you feel you are meant to do, and what career pathway you want. In this chapter, we will be reviewing key global health career competencies and some specific action steps that you can take to get from where you are now to where you want to be over time.

BOX 20.1

TYPES OF GLOBAL HEALTH ORGANIZATIONS

Foundation: a nonprofit organization that donates funds to support other organizations or resources for its own charitable purposes. (Example: the Bill & Melinda Gates Foundation)

Bilateral organization: development assistance given from one country directly to another. (Example: US Agency for International Development (USA) and the Government of Rwanda)

Multilateral organization: aid given by a donor country to an international organization. (Example: the World Bank)

Implementing organization: a nongovernmental organization (NGO) or company that is independent of a state or country and that receives donor funding to execute a development program or initiative. (Examples: Chemonics, John Snow Inc., Abt Associates Inc.)

Foundations, including the Bill & Melinda Gates Foundation (www.gatesfoundation.org) and the Rockefeller Foundation (www.rockerfellerfoundation.org), are increasingly involved in the global health space. An efficient way to check which foundations are currently focusing on global health is to do a "global health" search at www.foundations.org. There are also a number of private sector organizations that provide direct service, development, and research, including Doctors Without Borders (www.doctorswithoutborders.org), CARE (www.care.org), and Save the Children (www.savethechildren.org). An interesting way to see who is doing what is to access USAID's Global Health Bureau online listing of projects and what organizations are implementing them (User's Guide to USAID/Washington Health Programs, https://www.usaid.gov/what-we-do/global-health/global-health-users-guide).

What Does Success Look Like?

What does it take to be a successful global health professional? Representatives from the Consortium of Universities for Global Health outlined a large number of competencies in the interprofessional sphere (Jogerst et al., 2015). The published list was winnowed down from hundreds of skills and can be summarized into four categories: (1) health/technical expertise, (2) knowledge management, (3) business skills, and (4) interpersonal effectiveness.

Health/technical expertise. This skill cluster is defined as specific health/medical/ scientific specialties and disciplines and is ever changing. Academia focuses on this area and produces graduates with knowledge of specific topics, such as HIV/AIDS, malaria, tuberculosis, family planning and reproductive health, health systems, or health and environment. But an expanded definition of health and the types of professions that relate to health is increasingly important. Other technical areas that can connect to health include environment, engineering, information technology, business, veterinary science, and many others. For example, a professional with information technology experience may help develop an app that tracks the developmental milestones of a growing baby in utero for an expectant mother. The list of related technical knowledge and skills that have become relevant to global health over the years is expansive.

Knowledge management. You are preparing yourself for a fast-paced professional environment. Richard Riley, former US Secretary of Education, has said, "The top 10 in-demand jobs in the future don't exist today. We are currently preparing students for jobs that don't yet exist . . . using technologies that haven't been invented . . . in order to solve problems we don't even know are problems yet" (Gunderson, Jones, & Scanland, 2004, p. 506). Managing knowledge means that you know how to sort through a mountain of data; can distinguish information from knowledge (information is immediate, whereas knowledge has been evaluated and proven over time); and can discern the solid evidence from the poorly designed research or program. It also means you have strategies and tools to access megatrends—large, long-term shifts in global health that may affect governments, societies, and economies—and can keep up with fast-changing literature. Seek out organizations that sift through mountains of material to consolidate the current knowledge base on global health topics. These include universities that publish meta-analyses, and "think tanks" like the Aspen Institute, Rand Corporation, and the Center for Strategic and International Studies, who often publish big-picture documents.

Business skills. These skills include knowing the donors—foundations, bilaterals, and governments—who fund the areas in which you are interested. In international development, donors profoundly influence the priorities and timelines because they provide the resources to do the work. Knowing who they are and what is important to them is crucial. Being skillful in business also means knowing who the implementing organizations are—those companies most likely to hire you. Finally, it means knowing who the end user is—not only the governments, NGOs, and communities in foreign countries where you are likely to work but also the community you are aiming to support. Even systems and policies are meant to, in the end, effect change in the health of individuals. This skill cluster also includes the ability to write proposals and to manage, monitor, and evaluate programs. Much of development entails short-term interventions, usually in three- to five-year increments, and there are a lot of expectations regarding meeting measureable results.

Interpersonal effectiveness. The ability to build and maintain relationships and to master balancing priorities versus demands, or wants versus needs, speaks to a person's interpersonal effectiveness. Our experience as longtime employers of global health professionals has shown that this skill cluster is the most essential to a successful global health career.

What Are Employers Looking For?

There is an ongoing discussion in US global health that centers on the future of the American global health workforce and how best to prepare professionals. In 2015, the Public Health Institute (PHI) surveyed a representative population of seasoned global health (GH) project directors (Rudy, Wanchek, Godsted, Blackburn, & Mann, 2016). Here are some of the eye-opening results. Although clinical skills (specific health/medical/scientific specialties and disciplines) are important, and there were no big complaints about the academic preparation of these technical areas, 85% of respondents thought that academia could better prepare students with nonclinical skills. The most important nonclinical skills (see Figure 20.1) were in two competency areas. The first area emphasized business skills, including program management (57%), monitoring and evaluation (39%), and strategy and project design (33%). The second area focused

FIGURE 20.1   Top Nonclinical Skills

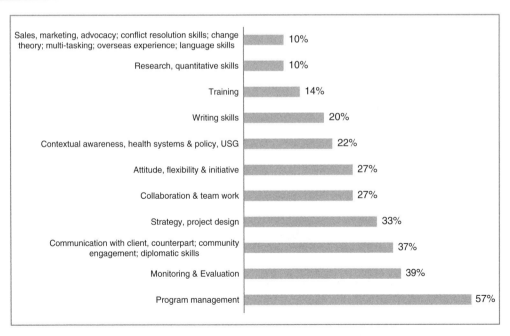

Source: Data from "The PHI/GHFP-II Employers' Study: The Hidden Barriers between Domestic and Global Health Careers and Crucial Competencies for Success," by S. Rudy, N. Wanchek, D. Godsted, M. Blackburn, and E. Mann, 2016, *Annals of Global Health, 82,* 1001–1009. doi:10.1016/j.aogh.2016.10.012

on interpersonal effectiveness: communication with the client, counterpart, and community (37%); and collaboration and teamwork (27%).

Do you need international experience to get a global health job? Another important message from employers is that although 64% said they had hired health professionals with only domestic experience for global health jobs, only 4% said this was a regular practice. GH employers generally do not hire candidates without international GH experience because they think candidates with only domestic experience lack the following: (1) understanding of the context and realities of GH (43%); (2) such characteristics as flexibility, adaptability, and creativity (30%); (3) cultural sensitivity (30%); (4) cross-cultural communication skills (20%); and (5) knowledge of key players and of systems and processes (13%). When asked why they had hired candidates with only domestic experience in spite of these drawbacks, they cited relevant technical skills, good organizational fit, and motivation. (See Figure 20.2.)

FIGURE 20.2   Why Are Candidates without Global Experience Selected?

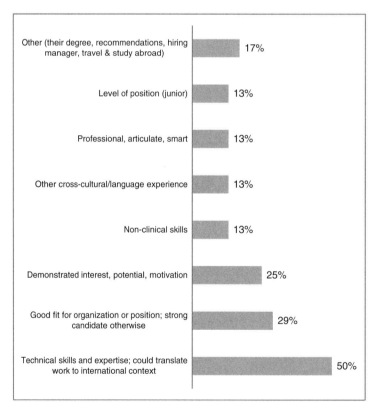

Source: Data from "The PHI/GHFP-II Employers' Study: The Hidden Barriers between Domestic and Global Health Careers and Crucial Competencies for Success," by S. Rudy, N. Wanchek, D. Godsted, M. Blackburn, and E. Mann, 2016, *Annals of Global Health, 82,* 1001–1009. doi:10.1016/j.aogh.2016.10.012

FIGURE 20.3   What Do Employers Look for in Domestic Job Applicants?

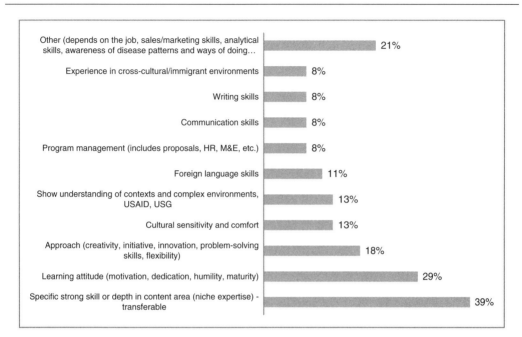

Source: Data from "The PHI/GHFP-II Employers' Study: The Hidden Barriers between Domestic and Global Health Careers and Crucial Competencies for Success," by S. Rudy, N. Wanchek, D. Godsted, M. Blackburn, and E. Mann, 2016, *Annals of Global Health*, *82,* 1001–1009. doi:10.1016/j.aogh.2016.10.012

How can you make up for the lack of international experience? Employers shared that depth of expertise in a critical area, a learning attitude, and demonstration of such traits as flexibility and cross-cultural skills would make them more likely to consider candidates without international experience. (See also Figure 20.3.)

How to Build Your Skills for the Road Ahead

You may be wondering how to apply the information from the previous section to your career. The keys to successful career planning are creating the habit of self-reflection, building a good social network, doing your research about job market trends, ensuring that your graduate program is a good fit, getting community-level overseas experience early, and staying connected virtually with the global community. In addition:

- A second language is critical: Arabic, French, or Spanish will serve you well.
- You need a professional network of people more senior *and* more junior than you.
- The immediacy of information requires that you have a well-curated virtual presence.
- An insatiable thirst for new career resources and data is important.

Your undergraduate classrooms are filled with students thinking about their future careers, but most are likely to be wondering how to take the next step. Engaging in critical thinking about not only what you want to do but also what you need to do to get there is worthwhile. Each 101 class for your bachelor's degree has prepared you for the next level of courses—stacking new knowledge, research, skills, and tools on top of each other like building blocks. Planning your career is no different and will require the same level of discipline, analysis, and creativity.

Create the habit of personal inquiry now. One of the best ways to avoid bad career choices is to continually ask yourself, *What do I love to do? What am I good at? Where do I need to be geographically?* Your answers will change over time, but start practicing now how to be self-reflective about your passions and talents. None of us loves everything we do, but if we are awake to what we are passionate about and why, we can find our best fit. Self-knowledge is the best guide to wise career choices.

Think about graduate school at some point. Undergraduate study is an important step in developing a successful career, but it is only the first. We recommend strongly that you seek out an overseas community-level living and working experience early. Organizations like the Peace Corps, the Global Health Corps, and others will provide you a path to a transformative experience that will serve you the rest of your life. This is the time for the grassroots, community-level work. Befriending and learning from community members will inform the rest of your career. However, at some point you will want to have a different kind of impact—or will need to make more money—and in that case you will need a postgraduate education. A master's degree is an essential building block to move you forward in your global health career. This is especially important at larger and medium-sized implementing partners and governmental agencies like USAID, the World Health Organization (WHO), and Catholic Relief Services. Your graduate classes will be smaller than your undergraduate ones, but more competitive as well. These are the students who will both compete with you for jobs and be your lifelong colleagues, so learn to work hard and be a team player. Employers such as the world's largest development donor (USAID) require a graduate degree for entry-level professional GH positions. This might seem like a steep ask for a job just starting out, but more and more employers are following suit because of the strong foreign talent looking for jobs in the United States.

You will eventually need an advanced degree if you do not want to hit a career or salary ceiling in your 30s. For those looking toward direct-service or development-centered careers, a medical degree, a master's in public health, a master's degree in a related technical field, or a master's in business administration is reasonable. If you are interested in a scientific or research career path, a PhD is likely needed.

When you are looking at graduate programs, figure out whether the program's strengths are in direct service, research, or development. One way to do this is to ask how the faculty is funded. If they get mostly federal National Institutes of Health (NIH) grants, do research overseas and then publish, chances are their strength is research and not development. If they are funded by foundations and USAID and have one- to five-year programs, chances are you will graduate with significant experience in development. All of these program and career paths are legitimate, but your priority is to find the one that is a good fit for you.

Seek out programs that include significant overseas living and working opportunities. Seek to establish relationships with organizations and people that will provide options for you to return to fieldwork later, and for longer. Internships matter, and the more a program can provide support for overseas work experience, the more valuable it will be to you.

Think about *with whom* to get overseas global health experience and *where* you need to be afterwards. Early career is the best time to gain significant community-level experience. If you've checked out the websites previously mentioned, you will see that currently there is one major geographic hub of global health work for development assistance—Washington, DC—but New York City; Boston, Massachusetts; Raleigh-Durham, North Carolina; Seattle, Washington; and San Francisco, California, are also areas where major global health organizations such as Global Health Corps (www.ghcorps.org), Abt Associates (www.abtassociates.com), IntraHealth International (www.intrahealth.org), Global Fund for Women (www.globalfundforwomen.org), and Asia Foundation (www .asiafoundation.org) work. There are also universities like those in the Triangle Global Health Consortium (www.triangleglobalhealth.org) in North Carolina, including Duke University and the University of North Carolina at Chapel Hill, that not only have robust global health programs but also are adept at the business of global health, meaning writing proposals for NIH and CDC grants (mostly research) or USAID and foundation grants (mostly development). These can be noted in the USAID User's Guide previously mentioned (https://www.usaid.gov/what-we-do/global-health/global-health-users -guide). Here are some other options for immersive global health overseas experience:

- Peace Corps is an opportunity to integrate fully into a host-country community, contribute to a local project, practice or learn a new language, and meet an incredible new network of like-minded, diverse professionals.
- You might also consider volunteering with a local NGO in a country of your choice. Although you would be responsible for transportation and housing, many NGOs, because they cannot afford to recruit internationally, often hire US citizens already in country looking for temporary work.
- Talk with your school's global health or public health program and see whether they have international connections with other organizations or schools that offer short-term employment. Good questions to ask: Location—city or rural setting? Current programming? Size? Funding source?

Invest time in curating your network. Your professional network is a fancy term for a collection of relationships. It is a living, breathing entity that requires maintenance. Give each part of your network—each relationship—respect, sincerity, and time. Make the effort to keep your relationships strong. Learning to balance work and activities that will benefit you professionally and personally takes practice. School is a near-perfect microcosm of what the opportunities and challenges to maintaining your network will be like when you enter the workforce. Schedule regular meetings with your network and keep them informal, high energy, and concise. As you climb the professional ladder, take care to keep your network diverse, of a manageable size, and active. The more senior you become, the more you will need to both regularly feed and curate your network. In this way, it is the opposite of Facebook or Instagram—you cannot be a spectator of your network; you must be a participant. The strength of your network will determine how able you are to compete with the next generation of GH professionals.

How you create and curate your professional network will determine how able you are to pivot and react to a changing GH workforce. No one person is able to scour the job boards, resource centers, and blogs as well as a group of people. Lean on your network to support your efforts. Is it up to the task? Begin by asking yourself what the current composition of your professional network is, and what is missing:

1. Have you befriended only people with similar academic, extracurricular, or professional interests?
2. How many people in your network are from different parts of the country or world, or are nonnative English speakers?
3. Are there both undergraduates *and* graduates with whom you discuss career plans?
4. How open are you with your parents and teachers—and therefore able to access their connections—about your professional pathway?

If you are able to spot some gaps in your network, here are a few places to begin filling them.

Social media often gets a bad rap for being the platforms and spaces where millennials talk about reality TV and the latest fashion trends. You know that more and more of your peers are using social media to connect, engage, and access news, information, and trends as never before. Use these tools' search functions—hashtags, trends, and related content links—to broaden and deepen your network over time. See who else on your campus is interested in global health and what organizations and people they follow. Twitter and LinkedIn are important platforms to showcase the most passionate and informed parts of your personality and career goals. Follow, like, and retweet sparingly until you have established a public persona that you are completely comfortable sharing with a future employer. Share publically only what is useful, and restrict access to your unguarded thoughts and reactions. If you have already made some missteps, don't panic, just delete and start again—you may find this liberating and useful in crafting a better professional network.

Seminars, webinars, and workshops can be an untapped resource to engage with like-minded and unlike-minded people. Select a workshop that is related to, but not directly organized by, your school or department; scan the room and sit next to the first person who makes eye contact. This is both practice for being uncomfortable in a new setting— a transferrable skill when you are the newbie at a job—and an opportunity to flex your interpersonal skills. Listen more than you speak, and follow up with your new professional acquaintance to demonstrate your sincerity and active participation in getting to know them. In a virtual setting, enter the web space early and introduce yourself to the group. Ask the first person who responds to chat privately and ask more about them and why they are participating. Follow up in person—coffee or lunch—to forge a more personal connection.

Extracurricular and school-sponsored clubs can be leveraged for more than just fun. If you are a group regular, introduce yourself to an unfamiliar person. If you are new to the group, go early and seek out a friendly face. Or consider meeting with the club's chair or de facto leader before the next meeting to get a better sense of its composition, affiliations, and ways to make it work for your career goals. It may not work, and that is okay too. Forge ahead.

Do your research on job market trends. The US Global Development Lab (www.usaid.gov/GlobalDevLab) lists Arabic, French, and Spanish as growing in-demand languages needed to work successfully in global health. Both *Forbes* and Bloomberg have taken into consideration economic outputs for the past 40 or more years, as well as population and migration figures in fast-growing areas of the world including sub-Saharan Africa and Asia. There is growing evidence that long-term field positions will be filled by more foreign nationals—professionals with a deeper understanding of the local infrastructure, politics, and policies, and the experience to really get things done. What does that mean for everyone else? The Lab predicts that American GH professionals will support in-country work on more short-term assignments. Any in-country work will require basic language skills. Those with both speaking and writing proficiency will be best positioned to secure the field jobs still open to nonlocals. We also predict that jobs in monitoring and evaluation and in capacity building—which include sustainability and scaling up—will continue to see significant growth; and anyone with deep expertise in a technical area or special population will have consistent marketability.

Stay connected with the global community. With your growing network ready to go, remember to do your part and stay abreast of career resources and websites that may help you or someone you know. Global health careers are as advertised—global. Recruitment has also gone global. Leverage your social media profiles, especially LinkedIn, to tap into the opportunities for work-study, study abroad, direct enrollment, or volunteer opportunities.

Prepare a resume. Excited to take the next step? Start with developing a strong resume that highlights your career interests and demonstrates your academic and extracurricular preparation thus far. Box 20.2 lists 10 tips to ensuring that your resume stands out from the pile.

BOX 20.2
RESUME TIPS

1. Include your degrees with your name at the top of your resume. Example: Sharon Rudy, PhD, BCC
2. Summarize your professional qualifications at the top of your resume.
3. Tailor your professional summary to the position to which you are applying.
4. Length does not matter; content does. Include all information related to your experience and qualifications.
5. PSR: Problem. Solution. Result. Use the PSR approach to discuss your role and accomplishments.
6. Spell-check and proofread. Twice.
7. You've matured, and so have your dreams. Review your resume for outdated information and remove it.
8. Do not include references in your resume.
9. Include professional affiliations—but not personal ones.
10. Do not include certain personal biodata in your resume, such as photos, social security number, religion, marital status, date of birth, nationality, or hobbies.

Start your job search. Once your resume is complete and up-to-date, begin searching the job boards and blog spots for organizations that can help you make a start toward the career of your dreams. Listed in Box 20.3 are a few resources and websites, culled by global health employers and experienced GH practitioners, that offer jobs, volunteer opportunities, fellowships and internships, and tools and industry information to support your global health career goals.

BOX 20.3
START YOUR SEARCH FOR A JOB OR INTERNSHIP

These websites are some of the most current leading resources for more information on development aid jobs and career preparation.

- Devex.com
- FedBizOps.org
- GHFP.net
- GlobalJobs.org

- Idealist.org

- InsideNGO.org

- OFDAJobs.net

- OTIJobs.et

- Peacecorps.gov

- ReliefWeb.com

- USAJobs.gov

Be ready for the unexpected. There will be plenty of pivots and surprises along the way, but you will find your place in the global health community if you have discerned carefully and prepared well. Wishing you all the best on the journey!

Chapter Summary

Most global health careers fall into three main categories: direct service, research, and implementation. You can identify which of these areas you may want to pursue by taking inventory of your skills and interests. Self-knowledge is the best guide to wise career choices. Therefore, it is critical that you practice frequent self-reflection in order to ensure that your decisions are informed by what motivates you. To be successful in your global health career, you will need to be able to demonstrate to future employers competency in four critical areas:

- Health/technical expertise: having specific health, medical, and scientific specialties
- Knowledge management: sorting through, consolidating, and effectively communicating large amounts of information
- Business skills: being savvy in the realm of international development and knowing what is important to the donors funding the work that you want to do
- Interpersonal effectiveness: building and maintaining relationships and balancing priorities

Global health employers have indicated that they would like to see greater preparation among graduates in the areas of business skills, interpersonal effectiveness, and international experience. Although most global health employers prefer that candidates have experience living and working abroad, many hire candidates without it, citing relevant technical skills, good organizational fit, and high motivation among these candidates. Having critical area expertise, a learning attitude, flexibility, and cross-cultural skills can all make up for a lack of international work experience.

It is important to begin planning for your global health career as early as possible. Keys to successful career planning include obtaining second-language skills (Arabic, Spanish, or French are good choices), developing a professional network of people who can help move your career forward, having a well-curated virtual presence, and maintaining a thirst for new career resources and data. Take advantage of opportunities that you may have access to while you are in school, such as language courses and opportunities for work or study abroad. Getting early community-level living and working experience overseas will position you well for job placement. Consider joining the Peace Corps or volunteering with a local NGO. Talk to your school's global/public health program and inquire about potential international connections with other schools or organizations offering short-term employment. Other ways to prepare for your global health career include curating your professional network, staying abreast of global health trends, and developing a strong resume that highlights your career interests and demonstrates your academic and extracurricular preparation.

Discussion Questions

1. Write down three to five key messages you are taking from this chapter.
2. Develop a description of your dream job. What would you be doing? What is the setting? Be specific about the image. Whom are you working with? Alone with a computer? Books all around? In a medical setting? Small town or big city? What is making you happy about this image? About this work?
3. Considering the advice in this chapter, create a path from where you are now to your dream job. Visualize each step and how one decision follows another. Write it down or draw it.
4. Talk with the person you trust most to know about global health professions.
5. Create a short list of technical areas or careers of interest and use social media to find people or organizations that fill or support these roles. Ask questions.

Activity: Skills Inventory

The rubric in Box 20.4 is adapted from the Association of Schools & Programs of Public Health Global Health Competency Model. Use it to assess your current and desired skills. Discern which skills you have attained, which need more preparation, and which may not be relevant to your particular global health track. You can do this exercise periodically to assess your accomplishments and plan for future growth. You can use it to select courses, direct your independent reading, or help you decide what kind of internships or volunteer work you might undertake to put your skills to use and learn new ones.

BOX 20.4

ASSESS YOUR GLOBAL HEALTH SKILLS AND INTERESTS

1 = Minimal interest/relevance; 2 = Desired skill; 3 = Some experience; 4 = Competent

	1	2	3	4
Competency: Capacity Strengthening The broad sharing of knowledge, skills, and resources for enhancement of global public health programs, infrastructure, and workforce to address current and future global public health needs.				
Design sustainable workforce development strategies for resource-limited settings.				
Identify methods for ensuring health program sustainability.				
Assist host entity in assessing existing capacity.				
Develop strategies that strengthen community capabilities for overcoming barriers to health and well-being.				
Collaborating and Partnering The ability to select, recruit, and work with a diverse range of global health stakeholders to advance research, policy, and practice goals, and to foster open dialogue and effective communication.	1	2	3	4
Develop procedures for managing health partnerships.				
Promote inclusion of representatives of diverse constituencies in partnerships.				
Value commitment to building trust in partnerships.				
Use diplomacy and conflict resolution strategies with partners.				
Communicate lessons learned to community partners and global constituencies.				
Exhibit interpersonal communication skills that demonstrate respect for other perspectives and cultures.				
Ethical Reasoning and Professional Practice The ability to identify and respond with integrity to ethical issues in diverse economic, political, and cultural contexts, and promote accountability for the impact of policy decisions upon public health practice at local, national, and international levels.	1	2	3	4
Apply the fundamental principles of international standards for the protection of human subjects in diverse cultural settings.				

Analyze ethical and professional issues that arise in responding to public health emergencies.				
Explain the mechanisms used to hold international organizations accountable for public health practice standards.				
Promote integrity in professional practice.				
Health Equity and Social Justice The framework for the analysis of strategies to address health disparities across socially, demographically, or geographically defined populations.	1	2	3	4
Apply social justice and human rights principles in public health policies and programs.				
Implement strategies to engage marginalized and vulnerable populations in making decisions that affect their health and well-being.				
Critique policies with respect to impact on health equity and social justice.				
Analyze distribution of resources to meet the health needs of marginalized and vulnerable populations.				
Program Management The ability to design, implement, and evaluate global health programs to maximize contributions to effective policy, enhanced practice, and improved and sustainable health outcomes.	1	2	3	4
Conduct formative research.				
Apply scientific evidence throughout program planning, implementation, and evaluation.				
Design program work plans based on logic models.				
Develop proposals to secure donor and stakeholder support.				
Plan evidence-based interventions to meet internationally established health targets.				
Develop monitoring and evaluation frameworks to assess programs.				
Utilize project management techniques throughout program planning, implementation, and evaluation.				
Develop context-specific implementation strategies for scaling up best practice.				
Sociocultural and political awareness The conceptual basis with which to work effectively within diverse cultural settings and across local, regional, national, and international political landscapes.	1	2	3	4

	1	2	3	4
Describe the roles and relationships of the entities influencing global health.				
Analyze the impact of transnational movements on population health.				
Analyze context-specific policymaking processes that impact health.				
Design health advocacy strategies.				
Describe multi-agency policymaking in response to complex health emergencies.				
Describe the interrelationship of foreign policy and health diplomacy.				
Strategic Analysis The ability to use systems thinking to analyze a diverse range of complex and interrelated factors shaping health trends to formulate programs at the local, national, and international levels.	1	2	3	4
Conduct a situation analysis across a range of cultural, economic, and health contexts.				
Identify the relationships among patterns of morbidity, mortality, and disability with demographic and other factors in shaping the circumstances of the population of a specified community, country, or region.				
Implement a community health needs assessment.				
Conduct comparative analyses of health systems.				
Explain economic analyses drawn from socioeconomic and health data.				
Design context-specific health interventions based on situation analysis.				

Source: Adapted from "Global Health Competency Model," by the Association of Schools & Programs of Public Health, October 2011. Retrieved from http://www.aspph.org/educate/models/masters-global-health/

Key Terms

Health/technical expertise

Interpersonal effectiveness

Knowledge management

Suggested Reading

Devex International Development. *Meet the next generation development professional.* Retrieved from https://pages.devex.com/rs/685-KBL-765/images/Meet_the_next_generation_development_professional_Devex_ebook.pdf

References

Association of Schools & Programs of Public Health. (2011, October). Global health competency model, version *1*.1. Retrieved from http://www.aspph.org/educate/models/masters-global-health/

DiPrete Brown, L. (2014). Towards defining inter-professional competencies for global health education: Drawing on educational frameworks and the experience of the UW–Madison Global Health Institute. *Journal of Law and Medical Ethics, 42*(Suppl. 2), 32–37. doi:10.1111/jlme.12185

Gunderson, S., Jones, R., & Scanland, K. (2004). *The jobs revolution: Changing how America works.* Chicago, IL: Copywriters.

Jogerst, K., Callender, B., Adams, V., Evert, J., Fields, E., Hall, T., Olsen, J., . . . Wilson, L. L. (2015). Identifying interprofessional global health competencies for 21st-century health professionals. *Annals of Global Health, 81*, 239–247. doi:10.1016/j.aogh.2015.03.006

Rudy, S., Wanchek, N., Godsted, D., Blackburn, M., & Mann, E. (2016). The PHI/GHFP-II employers' study: The hidden barriers between domestic and global health careers and crucial competencies for success. *Annals of Global Health, 82*, 1001–1009. doi:10.1016/j.aogh.2016.10.012

PART THREE

GLOBAL HEALTH PERSPECTIVES

CHAPTER 21

SO YOU WANT TO SAVE THE WORLD? FIRST, YOU'VE GOT TO KNOW IT

Brian W. Simpson, MPH, MA

It began in the forests of Guinea.

The country's southern border with Liberia and Sierra Leone made an ideal home for viruses that afflict humans. It offered an impoverished people often on the move seeking work, a changing ecology caused by deforestation and mining, and a weak, ineffective health system. In late December 2013, these forces collided when a two-year-old boy in the remote village of Meliandou fell sick. He suffered fever, black stools, and vomiting, and died within days, according to a 2014 World Health Organization history of the outbreak. Then his mother died. Then his three-year-old sister. Then his grandmother and the nurse who had treated him.

The World Health Organization's experts believe the boy was Patient Zero—the first person to fall sick—in West Africa's devastating Ebola outbreak. (He was likely infected by an animal.) The Ebola virus, which had never before caused a significant outbreak in the region, would sweep across the three countries, infecting more than 28,000 people and killing more than 11,000.

Take a look at the threads in the previous paragraphs: the poverty, the mobile population, environmental degradation, and a virus new to the region. When tests in March 2014 finally confirmed that the Ebola virus was killing people in Guinea, the alarm bells of an unprecedented outbreak should have sounded not only for epidemiologists but also for anyone familiar with global health. Indeed, the international NGO Médecins Sans Frontières (MSF) called for an immediate and robust global response. Instead, we let the virus outpace us and cause thousands of deaths.

Knowledge, as is often said, is power. And that's never more true than in global health. With knowledge, we can stop disease outbreaks in their tracks. We can prevent

Foundations for Global Health Practice, First Edition. Lori DiPrete Brown.
© 2018 John Wiley & Sons, Inc. Published 2018 by John Wiley & Sons, Inc.

child and maternal deaths. We can reduce malnutrition, and so on. But we can do those things only if we can dive into a sea of information (and misinformation) and surface with knowledge.

Sounds good. But how do we do that?

You're reading this chapter because of your interest in global health. You may be dipping your toe in the field, or you may have already have worked abroad or close to home on a critical health issue. Regardless of where you are in your global health journey, you've probably got an inkling of what's out there, and you want to make a difference. A few words of advice before you head out to change the world:

First, you have to know it.

Your studies, of course, are a good start. And there's no substitute for seeing things firsthand. Once while interviewing a Ugandan researcher about poor compliance with HIV medications, I said I couldn't understand why people wouldn't regularly take a medication that would keep them alive. As I was saying this, it dawned on me that I hadn't taken my lifesaving, preventive malaria medication that very morning. I felt foolish, but learned a big lesson. And while traveling to a malaria research site in Zambia, a colleague and I stopped to talk with some local people fishing in a river. A friend pointed to a man fishing with a net and said, "That's a mosquito bed net." An NGO or a government agency might have proudly counted that net as successfully delivered, but it certainly wasn't preventing malaria. Moments like these offer invaluable insights into how things work in the real world.

Aside from coursework and firsthand experience, what's the best way to learn what's happening in the world? The news media is an obvious answer, but literally hundreds of global health–related news articles and blog posts are published every day. There's no way for one person to keep up. (Don't try a Red Bull–fueled global health news reading binge—it would only leave you jittery and brain-fried.) In today's media environment, we risk being paralyzed by too much information. William Powers (2010) described the conundrum well in his book *Hamlet's Blackberry*: "The great paradox of information: the more of it that's available, the harder it is to be truly knowledgeable" (p. 112).

Since I was first introduced to global health while reporting in Uttar Pradesh, India, in 1999, I've always wanted to learn more about outbreaks, discoveries, innovative interventions, and so on. But I quickly ran into information overload like everyone else.

Global health has two defining characteristics. First, it is an incredibly diverse field, encompassing everything from road traffic injuries and substance abuse to family planning, infectious and chronic disease, refugees, vaccines, and health systems. The multitude of important topics necessarily creates a deluge of information.

Second, people in global health tend to work in silos. This means they don't often share ideas with others. Rare is the vaccine access specialist who compares notes with the contraceptive expert or tobacco control researcher. If they peek out of their silos, global health practitioners might learn some valuable lessons from others.

With both of these issues in mind, I suggested to colleagues at the Johns Hopkins Bloomberg School of Public Health that we start a magazine to serve the global health community, but was told that the idea was too costly. Then we got some good advice: start an email newsletter that would curate the most important news of the day. So on January 2, 2014, I scoured the global media and cobbled together brief summaries of the most important stories. I pasted these into an email and sent it to folks in my office. They liked it. Word of this easy-to-scan digest spread to other departments. Faculty and students signed on. Realizing its value, we opened it up to the larger global health community. *Global Health NOW* (globalhealthnow.org) has enjoyed terrific growth since then and now reaches tens of thousands of readers.

My colleague Dayna Kerecman Myers and I curate the news, picking the most important stories so that our readers don't have to "sip from the fire hose" of news articles published each day. We rely on scores of Google alerts, news sites, blogs, tips from our readers, and social media, as well as news feeds from the World Health Organization, the Centers for Disease Control and Prevention, UNICEF, universities and research institutions, and NGOs like MSF. We also follow the key journals, such as *The Lancet, Nature,* the *New England Journal of Medicine,* and many others.

As we look at all of these sources, we evaluate what stories to include based on standard news judgment: impact (how many people are affected), timeliness, future threat, prominence (what global leaders are doing about it), and human interest (what's surprising or odd about the issue). We make the best decisions we can, but we're far from infallible. As you would with any curated content, you'll want to make sure to keep your eyes open for other news and consider other sources as well.

At *Global Health NOW,* we also develop original articles on issues that the mainstream media aren't covering. In news articles and commentaries, our writers have covered everything from e-cigarettes to kala azar (leishmaniasis), TB in India, and oil spills in the Amazon. In 2015, we joined with the Consortium of Universities for Global Health to launch an Untold Global Health Stories contest to bring attention to important global health issues. We had 170 entries in our first contest and selected mycetoma as the Untold Global Health Story of the year. The flesh-eating, bone-destroying disease, caused by bacteria or fungi, afflicts the very poor in 23 countries and has spread misery for centuries. However, its prevalence and etiology are largely unknown even today. Mycetoma may not make the news in the United States or Europe, but that doesn't mean it's not an important global health issue. In fact, our coverage helped encourage the World Health Assembly to formally add mycetoma to the official list of neglected diseases—making it more likely to get research funding. Since then, we've also documented untold global health stories such as the paralytic disease konzo in the Democratic Republic of Congo and the issue of accidental burns in Nepal.

■ ■ ■

That's what we do. What can you do? Pay attention. Learn about global health issues. Follow the news. Find your own reliable sources. Follow experts on social media. Ask your faculty and fellow students about their news sources. Carve out specific topics and areas that you're interested in and follow them closely. You can easily set up Google alerts to ping you when stories about heart disease, global surgery, or another issue dear to you are published.

And you can do more than just passively follow the news. The news media are far from perfect. Sometimes stories get bungled. Sometimes they're flat-out wrong. You can evaluate a story's credibility by asking yourself some questions:

- Is it reported on the ground by a journalist who viewed events firsthand?
- Do other articles on the issue impart similar information?
- Is it based on reliable sources and/or scientific evidence?
- Did it interpret the science accurately?
- Is the news site or publication reputable—or is it a blog that's mostly known for opinion writing?
- Does the site have an obvious bias?

You'll soon have opportunities to do more, such as talk with people who have been in the field and gather your own information in classes or conferences. You can also connect with NGOs working in an area or an issue that interests you. You can follow the latest scientific journal articles in your area. And then you can join the conversation by sharing your views on social media. With an informed perspective, you can add to the global conversation and help educate others.

As you move forward with your career, you no doubt will have many opportunities for work and travel. With them comes a responsibility. By now, I hope you agree about the importance of knowing what's going on in global health. As a researcher, a practitioner, and even as a global citizen, you will find that acquiring knowledge is just the first step. For the global health enterprise to succeed, we all need to share our knowledge and then act on it.

References

Powers, W. (2010). *Hamlet's Blackberry*. New York, NY: HarperCollins.

World Health Organization. (2014). Ground zero in Guinea: The Ebola outbreak smoulders—undetected—for more than 3 months. Retrieved from http://www.who.int/csr/disease/ebola/ebola-6-months/guinea/en/

CHAPTER 22

SINCE YOU ASKED
REFLECTIONS ON MY FIRST GLOBAL HEALTH EXPERIENCES

Lori DiPrete Brown, MS, MTS

This chapter is adapted from a TEDx Talk at UW–Madison, November 23, 2013.

Students often come to me for advice about their global health experiences. They want help with discerning and articulating their interests and passions, they want practical advice, and very often they want to know about how I began my own global health journey: Where did I go? What did I do? What did I learn? Here I will share some stories and insights from my early global health experiences, drawn from fieldwork in Central America that I did when I was in my 20s.

In 1983, when I was 22, I left the United States for the first time. I was a first-generation college graduate, and had managed the financing of my education with help and support from my wonderful family and with generous financial aid from Yale and the Pell Grant program. I had devoted all my earned income to tuition and housing, and did not have the privilege of international travel until after I graduated.

Honduras

Armed with undergraduate training in psychology and philosophy, a used guitar, and a manual typewriter, I joined the Peace Corps. I worked with a youth program at Aldea S.O.S, a home for abandoned and orphaned children in the Honduran capital, Tegucigalpa. I provided counseling and support to a group of about 20 teenage girls. I had taken a global health class—there was only one course offering at the time—I had become proficient in Spanish, and I did a summer internship that provided me with counseling skills and experience working with teenagers who were homeless or who had experienced abuse.

Foundations for Global Health Practice, First Edition. Lori DiPrete Brown.
© 2018 John Wiley & Sons, Inc. Published 2018 by John Wiley & Sons, Inc.

I felt very humble about what I could offer the girls with whom I lived, but I sought the guidance of the long-term staff at Aldea S.O.S., made my share of mistakes, and found ways to make the journey to adulthood a little easier, with job counseling, help with homework, personal counseling, and simple presence. Although I had the option of a room in one of the main buildings, I chose to live in the residence with the girls. In addition to offering day-to-day support, I also traveled with them to the villages where they were born to help them get their birth certificates, which they needed in order to gain access to school, working papers, and other social benefits. These journeys took me all around the country, on buses, in the back of pickup trucks, and on foot.

When I think about the lessons from that time that might be useful for my students, one particular series of events comes to mind. I was having coffee one day with a Peace Corps friend who expressed concern that I was getting burned out as a live-in counselor and that I wasn't really doing development work. There was no sustainability to what I was doing, she said. No multiplier effect, as when you train trainers or provide seed to farmers, who in turn provide seed to others. I was mainly counseling, comforting, and refereeing the girls on chores.

I was a kind of glorified babysitter, really. It doesn't sound world changing, does it?

A few weeks later, I was involved in a fair at the orphanage. We filled the dusty, colorless field near the children's home with games and fun for a day. The girls and I dressed up like clowns to entertain the younger children. By the end of the day, I was answering to the call "*Payasa, venga,*" which means "Come here, Clown." We had a *piñata* and candy. It was simple. A day at the fair. A magic day that we hoped the children would remember.

That night one of the girls, Carolina, came to my room to talk. She sat down on my bed and said nothing, clearly on the verge of tears. I was sure it was boyfriend trouble again, and began to fill the silence with words of advice, solidarity, and support, asking questions that might help her tell me what happened. "It's not that," she said finally. "I just miss her." At 17 years old, after living in the orphanage for most of her life, she finally wanted to talk about her abandonment, and she had come to me. I felt so sorry to have gotten things so wrong, to have missed the obvious sorrow. I put my arms around her, and she cried for a while, and I cried also. She did not expect me to do anything more, and I didn't.

After she left, I sat alone in my room and thought about the words "multiplier effect" again. Suddenly I realized how arrogant and wrong that whole idea was. It implied that comforting Carolina, being a buffer against her sorrow for a few hours, was not important enough for someone like me to bother with. That a one-to-one return on investment was not acceptable when it came to the people like Carolina. According to the multiplier logic of international development work, the fun fair didn't measure up either. Making joyful memories for children who had suffered so much? That was, at best, a loss leader.

That day, I let go just a little bit of wanting to do great things. I realized I was willing to be a person who has the time and heart to do small things, the small things that justice, friendship, and compassion demand. In this case, I had not done the small thing particularly well, but I could work on that; I could keep trying. I hoped that meaningful change could somehow come from this kind of engagement. I took some comfort in arithmetic. After all, one and one does make two. That was certain, multiplication aside.

Nicaragua

During graduate school, I went to Nicaragua as part of a health and human rights research team from the Harvard School of Public Health. We were visiting a town in Chontales, which was as far into the war zone as we could go and still be relatively "safe." We conducted a household survey to document the impact of the war on civilians—issues such as disruptions to the health care system, damage to schools, internal migration, and various negative health impacts. The results told the story that we expected, an important one, and we published them as planned.

For me, though, the greatest learning occurred at the end of the interview, when I put down my clipboard and asked, "Is there anything else you would like me to know?" Then I leaned forward and listened. I listened to what people said when they were free from the confines of structured questions and coded answers. When the clipboard was not creating a small barrier between us. They told me stories about how the war had affected them. They talked about their fears and their hopes. They talked about how they might solve problems in relation to food, shelter, and getting the kids back in school somehow.

During the course of the interviewing, we came to a house that had all the windows and doors shut, even though it was the middle of the day. I wasn't sure whether I should knock, but I did, and Juana and Fidelia, two sisters who lived together there, let me in. After the survey, they told me their stories. Juana spoke briefly and calmly. She was married to a Misquito Indian. He'd been a miner, but was now working as a day laborer. They had been relocated because their town was considered unsafe for civilians. Her home was in a war zone. Violence or the threat of it was everywhere. She looked over her shoulder when she washed clothes or when she walked upright in the quiet fields. She heard gunshots in the morning. Her sister, Fidelia, had a thin face and urgent speech. She began to speak each time Juana paused for a moment. It was sometimes hard to keep track of who was saying what. Fidelia, a widow with eight children, had lost her husband when he was killed at a family party on their farm, along with nine other men and a woman who tried to defend them. Fidelia began to list the widows and count the orphans—34 children in that small village had lost their fathers; a whole generation of men were lost, she said. Because of what they had been through, Juana and Fidelia were often afraid to speak out, but they wanted to tell me these things. They wanted me to know, and they wanted me to tell someone else.

Research is an important tool for changing the world. I knew that before I went to Chontales. But what I didn't expect was that the fact-finding survey that we had worked so hard to design was just a starting point. I learned about the importance of story, witness, solidarity, and hope.

Guatemala

A few years later, I found myself in Guatemala working with CARE (Cooperative Assistance and Relief Everywhere) to develop a monitoring system for a water and sanitation program. This took me to a remote village in Quetzaletango to see a newly installed well and water system.

We set out at sunrise and drove until the road ended. A simple meal awaited us there—blue corn tortillas, beans, and sour cream, and sweet coffee in a tin cup. I am not sure if it was the early morning air, the hospitality, or the food itself, but I still remember this as one of the best meals of my life. Then we hiked up to the village through the beautiful, sparsely inhabited terrain. We came to a river that had to be crossed on a walking bridge. It was just a plank really, the width of a log with no rails. Everyone in our party crossed with ease. But I made the mistake of looking down; I hesitated and then my anxiety spiraled. I was sure I would fall from this balance beam bridge down to the water below. I stood there frozen on one side of the bridge, with the rest of the team on the other. A local woman happened to be coming up the path on the other side. She smiled at me reassuringly—she did not speak English or Spanish, and I did not speak her language, Mam. She looked to be about five months pregnant, but she crossed over the bridge and extended her hand to help me cross. Her kindness enabled me to look straight ahead and cross the bridge. I am not sure what I would have done without her help.

When we arrived, the villagers were assembled, waiting for us. We sat in a circle, and they told us about the water project. Until that moment I only knew that CARE had provided materials and assistance with building the water tank. As the head of the water committee told us the history of the project, I realized the extent and intensity of the community effort. What the NGOs called "the local contribution" included working with government over months to procure land rights to the site of the well. It involved carrying every brick, and all other materials, up to the village along the route we had just hiked. It included building the water system, building the latrines, and deciding who would do extra work on behalf of the widows and the elderly who could not do their share.

The lessons of that day in rural Guatemala have echoed again and again in my work. Communities are full of energy and desire for change. Outside assistance can be useful, but if we look honestly at our successes, our contributions are always small when compared to the efforts and contributions of partners, local leaders, and community members. We who have the privilege of crossing worlds are constant recipients of hospitality and assistance, we are accommodated in ways that we don't even see, and, mostly, we are treated with great kindness.

Your First Global Health Experience

There are big challenges in our world, and there will be many opportunities to be part of collective action to make large-scale changes in how we use resources and care for each other and our planet. In the meantime, though, small changes are big. The small lessons and achievements associated with your first global health experiences are important. They can move the frontiers of what is possible, and they are seeds of hope and the galvanizing force behind big important changes. Taking action for modest changes in the personal realm is how you begin to align your professed values with who you are as a citizen of the world. With commitment and time and collective effort, you will end up being part of change in bigger ways than you ever imagined.

CHAPTER 23

LEADERSHIP LESSONS FROM THE LAST MILE
A PEACE CORPS STORY

Carrie Hessler-Radelet, MS

Never doubt that a small group of thoughtful committed citizens can change the world. Indeed, it is the only thing that ever has.
—**Margaret Mead, cultural anthropologist**

The Peace Corps model is one of complete integration. Volunteers live and work among the people they serve. They are there to do a job, but they do so much more. They play soccer with the primary school kids; they swap stories over meals with their neighbors; they drink tea with the village headmen. Their presence at the "last mile" of development and the strong relationships of trust they build within their communities give them unique insights into local development challenges, and credibility when introducing new approaches. They inspire others to discover their potential and to be their best.

Walking "the Last Mile" with Daisy Duarte in Mozambique

Daisy Duarte is a Peace Corps volunteer in Mozambique, where she works on HIV/AIDS and sexual and reproductive health, with a focus on adolescent girls and young women. She works closely with her local host country counterpart, a woman named Armenia. Together, Daisy and Armenia support a Peace Corps–founded local organization called REDES (Raparigas em Desenvolvimento, Educação, e Saúde), which in English means Girls in Development, Education, and Health. REDES is a national network of girls' clubs in Mozambique that promote girls' empowerment and HIV prevention through gender awareness, reproductive health, and life skills training.

Foundations for Global Health Practice, First Edition. Lori DiPrete Brown.
© 2018 John Wiley & Sons, Inc. Published 2018 by John Wiley & Sons, Inc.

When Daisy arrived in her host village, she was equipped and ready to deliver evidence-based HIV/AIDS and reproductive health interventions targeting young women. But it quickly became obvious that for adolescent girls in the village, the most credible source of reproductive health information came from the initiation ritual that each girl participated in after her first menses.

In Daisy's community, initiation rituals are important rites of passage for boys and girls—and they are guarded as a sacred secret. The initiation for girls is led by a woman named Paciencia, a village elder who has conducted the secret ritual for as long as anyone could remember.

Armenia told Daisy about her own initiation, and how some of the things they were taught to do during the initiation ritual were painful and unhealthy. For example, girls were taught to always boil condoms—and to use them hot—to prevent HIV/AIDS. Another practice was ritual scarification and tattooing on the girls' hips, where a single razor blade was used on all the initiates.

Daisy and Armenia attended an HIV/AIDS Training of Trainers led by REDES, where they developed a strategy for working within their local culture, building on some of the practices that are effective and addressing others that are harmful and painful, such as condom boiling and shared razor blade use.

Daisy and Armenia knew that Paciencia was an important stakeholder in the community and that she was critical to reaching that key population with accurate information. In order to make a difference in the reproductive health and HIV/AIDS behaviors among adolescent girls in their community, they needed to gain Paciencia's trust and acceptance.

Armenia's family helped arrange a meeting with Paciencia, who was initially very resistant to questions related to the content of her initiation ritual. But Daisy and Armenia did not give up. They met with Paciencia frequently and got to know her personally. They spoke to her in her own local dialect and spent many hours listening to and learning from Paciencia. Over time, Paciencia became open to learning more about evidence-based reproductive health, family planning, and HIV/AIDS interventions, and they slowly gained her trust.

Eventually, they were able to talk about alternative initiation rituals based on local culture that were consistent with good health practice. Paciencia finally agreed to work with Armenia and Daisy in adapting the initiation ritual to make it healthier and more evidence based. Armenia and Daisy didn't rewrite the centuries-old ritual, but instead modified aspects of it to correct myths and misinformation around reproductive health and HIV/AIDS.

A few months later, Daisy was invited to the initiation of Armenia's sister, Claudina, and the change was noticeable. The reproductive health and HIV/AIDS information was accurate and thorough and did not include harmful practices. Later, other women in the community came forward and told Daisy that they had wanted to speak to

Paciencia about her initiation practices, but had not wanted to question tradition or be seen as disrespectful. They were very grateful that Daisy and Armenia had followed an evidence-based approach that took into consideration their knowledge of local traditions and culture—one that resulted in the removal of the inaccurate and harmful elements of the initiation without compromising the important rite of passage and cohesion that the girls' initiation ritual brought to their community.

Daisy says that she is now better able to connect with the girls and their culture. The initiation ceremonies continue every two months or so, and the good health practices have been maintained at the insistence of the women in the community. Daisy and Armenia are currently working with Paciencia and the nurses at the local hospital to set up a network of adolescent reproductive health services that will link girls in their community to needed reproductive health services after they complete their initiation. Paciencia's welcome by providers in the formal health system has increased her sense of worth and has piqued her interest in continuing to learn more about effective reproductive health and HIV/AIDS; and the nurses are happy to have a connection with an influential traditional leader. Armenia and Daisy are seen as catalysts of community-led change, and they have made a difference in the lives of many young women in their community.

Leadership Lessons

As Peace Corps director, I have visited thousands of Peace Corps volunteers and their counterparts, and I have tried, throughout my tenure, to model some of the leadership lessons I have learned from them. Here are five of my most important takeaways, gained from volunteers and counterparts like Daisy and Armenia:

1. **Build relationships of trust.** Whether we're talking about family or diplomacy or business, the most important moments in life are defined by relationships. Being able to walk in someone else's shoes, to see the world through their eyes and to empathize with their hopes and fears—these are indispensable skills for shaping progress in today's interconnected world. Daisy and Armenia spent many, many hours getting to know Paciencia—and gaining her trust—before they even began to talk about the initiation ritual and the reproductive health and HIV/AIDS practices that were being taught there. Building relationships of trust with key stakeholders is a critical first step to making lasting change at the community level almost anywhere in the world.

2. **Understand cultural context.** Daisy and Armenia worked collaboratively with and within the context of the existing culture to identify and build on positive practices, rather than trying to impose change on the culture. Although culture itself is typically difficult to change, it can also be a great bridge between current problems and potential solutions, if a leader is able to find the commonalities that exist between

the current practices and the desired practices. When leaders are able to work with, not against, the local culture, change is not only more likely but also more likely to last.

3. **Exercise patience.** In our results-driven world, most leaders are under a great deal of pressure to deliver impact in record time. But the path to sustainable change is rarely straight, and the best leaders are willing to put in the time and energy to yield real long-term results. Rather than just blazing ahead with a new initiation curriculum that they designed, Daisy and Armenia took the time to seek Paciencia's input and buy-in. Real change takes time. Great leaders know that, and honor the process by letting it unfold at a pace that is sustainable.

4. **Lead with passion.** Extraordinary leaders love their work and care about the people with whom they collaborate. Their passion drives them forward, helping them regard barriers as opportunities and nurture creativity in finding solutions. Their enthusiasm is infectious, and it motivates others around them to support their cause. In this way, passionate leadership is authentic, because it emanates from the heart. Daisy and Armenia's passion for helping adolescent girls not only sustained them when they faced Paciencia's initial objections but also helped them engage and mobilize others in their community to extend reproductive health services to adolescent girls beyond the initiation ritual.

5. **Be trustworthy.** Extraordinary leaders understand the importance of earning trust. In order for a leader to be accepted, followers must be confident that a leader has their best interests at heart. Leaders who are trusted are able to enhance performance and engender commitment to common goals. Followers feel safe expressing themselves, which improves communication, creativity, and productivity. Trustworthy leaders are nonthreatening—they govern by compassion. By reaching out to Paciencia and gaining her trust, Daisy and Armenia were able to bring best practices to a centuries-old initiation ritual and improve reproductive health for adolescent girls in their community for years to come.

Recommended Reading

Gates, M. (2016). Advancing the adolescent health agenda. *The Lancet, 387,* 2358–2359. doi:10.1016/s0140-6736(16)30298-7

Helping women in Africa avoid H.I.V. (2016, February 26). [Editorial]. *New York Times.* Retrieved from https://www.nytimes.com/2016/02/26/opinion/helping-women-in-africa-avoid-hiv.html?_r=2

Patton, G. C., Sawyer, S. M., Ross, D. A., Viner, R. M., & Santelli, J. S. (2016). From advocacy to action in global adolescent health. *Journal of Adolescent Health, 59,* 375–377. doi:10.1016/j.jadohealth.2016.08.002

Patton, G. C., Sawyer, S. M., Santelli, J. S., Ross, D. A., Afifi, R., Allen, N. B., . . . Viner, R. M. (2016). Our future: A Lancet commission on adolescent health and wellbeing. *The Lancet, 387,* 2423–2478. doi:10.1016/s0140-6736(16)00579-1

UNAIDS. (2015). Empower young women and adolescent girls: Fast-track the end of the AIDS epidemic in Africa. Retrieved from http://www.unaids.org/en/resources/documents/2015/JC2746

UNAIDS. (2016). HIV prevention among adolescent girls and young women. Retrieved from http://www.unaids.org/en/resources/documents/2016/20160715_Prevention_girls

Wamoyi, J., Stoebenau, K., Bobrova, N., Abramsky, T., & Watts, C. (2016). Transactional sex and risk for HIV infection in Sub-Saharan Africa: A systematic review and meta-analysis. *Journal of the International AIDS Society, 19*(1). doi:10.7448/ias.19.1.20992

CHAPTER 24

HOW GLOBAL HEALTH IDENTITY POLITICS HARMS LOCAL COMMUNITIES

EXPERIENCE FROM AN "AIDS ORPHAN" IN UGANDA

James Kassaga Arinaitwe, MPH, MA

If I were given one hour to save the world, I would spend 59 minutes defining the problem, and one minute solving it.

—Albert Einstein

I was born in a rural village in Western Uganda in 1982—a year when my country was embattled in a civil war. By the time I was four years old, Uganda had experienced only 25 years of freedom from British colonial rule and had never experienced a successful regime change since its independence. Between 1971 and 1979, the country had been ruled by a brutal dictator—Idi Amin—notorious for the massacre of almost half a million people.

My family, cattle farmers by trade, had lost both their ancestral lands and their cattle to one of the dictator's military commanders, who threatened to take their lives if they did not surrender their resources. Given the context and environment of the internally displaced family into which I was born, juxtaposed with the failing political and economic systems after the ousting of the dictator, it is fair to say that my life was almost predestined to be challenging, if not impossible, to survive.

Uganda's public health and economy in the 1980s had been destroyed. The civil war led to the establishment of a militant political party and a president who still rules to this day. In 1986, my two younger sisters died of measles, and another following them

Foundations for Global Health Practice, First Edition. Lori DiPrete Brown.
© 2018 John Wiley & Sons, Inc. Published 2018 by John Wiley & Sons, Inc.

with a diarrheal illness. Four years later, my mother succumbed to breast cancer. Soon after, my father contracted HIV and tuberculosis, and died right before celebrating my 10th birthday. My brother died years later, due to a disease that physicians were unable to diagnose. Today, I'm the lone survivor of a family of seven; my six family members died due to the failed public health and economic systems.

In the 1990s, the HIV/AIDS epidemic was beginning to take root in Uganda. An unnatural "orphanage industry" subsequently developed as a result of misguided aid efforts that were ignorant of the local context. I witnessed this firsthand. What follows here are adapted excerpts of an op-ed essay I wrote (Arinaitwe, 2016) regarding how cultural incompetence and the "labeling" of orphans can harm those whom global health and aid are intended to help.

Ebola Orphans in Africa Do Not Need Saviors

West Africa's Ebola epidemic has produced no shortage of heartrending stories. Recently, a number of these have focused on the so-called Ebola orphans—the *New York Times*'s pitiful account of four-year-old "Sweetie Sweetie" in Sierra Leone (Gettleman, 2014) is one striking example—who are presented as the littlest victims of a global public health emergency. The Western media's portrayal of Sweetie and her brethren as abandoned waifs reinforces the persistent "Save Africa" narrative (Akhila, 2012) of a hopeless continent. These are the types of stories that spur handout contributions or that prompt well-meaning couples to hop on a plane to Sierra Leone in hopes of saving "Sweetie" and her wretched siblings from their West African misery, one orphan at a time.

What It Means to Be an Orphan

This type of coverage excels at generating pity for the victim to gain the interest of westerners, but gives little dignity to the child and the community in which she has been raised.

It's important to recognize that there is a cultural difference at play when we discuss orphans. More often than not, children in Africa are raised by extended families and their village communities, unlike in Western societies where child rearing is the sole responsibility of the parents. I know of two young men who lost both their parents to AIDS in a small impoverished Kenyan village close to the Ugandan border. The village, having been part of these children's upbringing, knew their dreams just as well as their own parents. The young men had set out to be doctors. After receiving college scholarships from Brown University, they had no money to afford their tickets to the United States. The village organized, and sold everything from goats and chickens to agricultural produce to send the young men to school.

The "Sons of Lwala," named after their village, have returned after their medical education and built the first medical clinic in their village, a testament to a community raising its own future leaders. The story of the Sons of Lwala is not unique to this village; similar stories exist across Africa. In my case, it was my extended family and a few local organizations, not aid organizations, that served me most powerfully. I witnessed a flood of well-intentioned, but often misguided Western NGOs and volunteers infiltrate the town closest to my village in the 1990s, just as my family began to die off.

At the time, home-grown Ugandan organizations, such as The AIDS Support Organization (TASO), were the sole reason my father was able to live two years beyond his HIV diagnosis. My mornings were often spent walking miles to TASO headquarters to pick up his antiretroviral medications and food rations. But organizations like TASO were few, and soon they were overwhelmed by international aid. The organizations quickly surrounded "AIDS orphans" like me, and used us to tell their own narratives and advance their own agendas. Instead of supporting local communities and relatives, like my grandmother, to care for orphans like me, international organizations and donors poured resources into orphanages that were often poorly staffed and ill-equipped.

Rethinking How to Provide Aid

An unintended consequence of this situation—which we see time and again—was a flood of eager and well-intentioned international volunteers who fueled the rise of the orphanages. This orphanage industry soon became a tourist attraction (Zakaria, 2014a).

These volunteers often raise the hopes of the orphans and then, after quickly departing, leave the orphans even more vulnerable in the emotional aftermath of abandonment. The children left behind after their peers are whisked off by adoption wonder if they were not chosen because there is something inherently wrong with them. Their self-confidence is battered.

The United Nations Convention on the Rights of the Child highlights that institutionalized care should never replace home-based care, and studies have shown the promise of child villages instead (Office of the United Nations High Commissioner for Human Rights, 2011). In the worst cases, the unregulated orphanage industry has sometimes led to child trafficking and illegal adoptions. Abundant Western aid has actually made these child protection crises profitable for some.

Ironically, too much aid can actually make things worse. The countries in West Africa that best responded to containing Ebola were those with the least aid. Sierra Leone, Liberia, and Guinea—the countries that have failed to stop Ebola—receive Western aid to the tune of 73% of their GDP (Msimang, 2014) and house thousands of NGO workers in their capital cities.

This counterintuitive relationship between aid and good health care systems and governance is an example of the deeply troubling wider narrative of aid failures in Africa, where depending heavily on Western aid and patronage for sustenance leads to corruption, cronyism, and failed governance structures. William Easterly (2015), a professor of economics at NYU, has shown that countries that receive copious aid are less likely to be democratic and more likely to nurture autocrats and have weak institutions.

The answer to these crises is home-grown African solutions (Lemma, 2014), with the right strategic support from the international community to ensure that children are not left waiting for a benevolent, and often elusive, Western savior. Most important, this help does not have to uproot these children from their community or transform them into "victims."

To be sure, no orphan can survive in a place without family, psychological, and social support. Without my own grandmother and countless other individuals both at home and abroad who have supported me, I probably wouldn't be where I am today.

Community versus Institution

Part of what helped me was having a great and affordable elementary education. What these children need is early childhood education centers with supportive caretakers, nutrition, and stimulation. These resources can develop only if aid programs focus on institution building and on structural changes rather than one-time solutions or saving children one at a time.

For every Sweetie, there are countless children left wondering why they weren't plucked away. I dream of an Africa where all Africans, both on the continent and in the diaspora, seek accountability and transparency from our governments, aid agencies, and corporations with our votes and our voices. We have already started to unite to work together across ideological and geographical backgrounds to invest our resources, skills, and ideas to drive our own economic and social agenda.

Only then can we ensure that the child survivors of Ebola are born in an Africa where they are seen not as victims or beggars but as captains of their own fate and the next generation of drivers for our social and economic development.

Implications for the Future

The wide coverage of the "Ebola orphans" epidemic by Western media that focused entirely on outward or foreign interventions as solutions to Africa's vulnerable children stripped both the dignity of these children and the dignity of the communities and families that supported them before the arrival of Western media. It is important for future generations of global public health practitioners and journalists to implement the suggestions I lay out in this section.

Given the context I've described in this chapter, it is important that both aspiring global health leaders and their respective organizations make informed decisions about the unintended consequences that arise from the way we label, define, and identify global health beneficiaries. Although the global development industry is a little more aware of the harms of these labels than it was 10 or 20 years ago, it is vital that global health students and volunteers understand the importance of community-driven solutions in order to avoid the mistakes of past organizations and policies.

Here are my top three recommendations for the future generation of global health leaders on how to ethically and sensitively work in local communities:

Research before action. It is important for leaders of organizations as well as volunteers to do thorough research, not just about the issue they are passionate about solving but about the historical, geopolitical, social, economic, and ethical ramifications of why the particular challenge exists. There are several organizations and leaders who do this well; Partners in Health (PIH), led by renowned medical anthropologist Dr. Paul Farmer, is one of them.

Privilege is not expertise. It is important to understand one's power and privilege, rooted in historical contexts—such as the history of colonialism and slavery—and how they can easily harm communities. Voluntourism has been championed by those with privilege, who assume they possess a sort of experience that gives them the right to "educate" or "save" those in the "developing world" (Zakaria, 2014b). Privilege does not grant one expertise to solve a global health issue.

Community before institution and intervention. In order to understand how an intervention might harm rather than help the community you intend to serve, ask questions, learn, and spend time with the people you aim to serve before crafting interventions. Community-evolved—or locally led—interventions take time. This type of community engagement involves studying and living with communities, as well as identifying those local leaders who can best solve their community's challenges. Take that extra time and do it right.

References

Akhila. (2012, February 11). Mr. Kristof and the narrative of "Americans saving Africans." Retrieved from http://akhilak.com/blog/2012/02/11/mr-kristof-and-the-narrative -of-americans-saving-africans/

Arinaitwe, J. K. (2016, February 27). Ebola orphans in Africa do not need saviours: Western aid needs to support home-grown solutions to create a new generation of African leaders. *Al Jazeera*. Retrieved from http://www.aljazeera.com/indepth/opinion/2015/01/ebola -orphans-africa-saviours-201511264250427392.html

Easterly, W. (2015). *The tyranny of experts: Economists, dictators, and the forgotten rights of the poor.* New York, NY: Basic Books.

Gettleman, J. (2014, December 13). An Ebola orphan's plea in Africa: "Do you want me?" *New York Times.* Retrieved from http://www.nytimes.com/2014/12/14/world/africa/an-ebola-orphans-plea-in-africa-do-you-want-me.html?_r=1

Lemma, S. (2014, November 13). Africa doesn't want any more western band aids. *Al Jazeera.* Retrieved from http://www.aljazeera.com/indepth/opinion/2014/11/africa-doesn-want-any-more-we-20141112103245331194.html

Msimang, S. (2014, October 19). "There is no Ebola here": What Liberia teaches us about the failures of aid. Retrieved from http://africasacountry.com/2014/10/there-is-no-ebola-here-what-liberia-teaches-us-about-the-failures-of-aid/

Office of the United Nations High Commissioner for Human Rights. (2011). *The rights of vulnerable children under the age of three: Ending their placement in institutional care.* Retrieved from http://www.europe.ohchr.org/Documents/Publications/Children_under_3__webversion.pdf

Zakaria, R. (2014a, August 14). The travel book gives the orphanage four stars. *Al Jazeera America.* Retrieved from http://america.aljazeera.com/opinions/2014/8/cambodia-orphanagetourismwatopotwesternvolunteerism.html

Zakaria, R. (2014b, April 21). The white tourist's burden. *Al Jazeera America.* Retrieved from http://america.aljazeera.com/opinions/2014/4/volunter-tourismwhitevoluntouristsafricaaidsorphans.html

CHAPTER 25

GENDER AND COMMUNITY WELL-BEING

WOMEN REVERSING GLOBAL HEALTH CHALLENGES AND GENDER INEQUALITIES

Araceli Alonso, PhD
Teresa Langle de Paz, PhD

The fuller development of a culture of peace is integrally linked to . . . [e]liminating all forms of discrimination against women through their empowerment and equal representation at all levels of decision-making.

—UN Declaration on a Culture of Peace and Programme of Action, September 13, 1999

Why does gender matter for global health work?

- Because gender norms have implications for health
- Because many of the challenges of global health have a disproportionate impact on women and girls
- Because girls and women face barriers that increase their vulnerability to ill health
- Because gender analysis is powerful and helps us engage in global health differently
- Because women's health also has a significant impact in the health of others

Foundations for Global Health Practice, First Edition. Lori DiPrete Brown.
© 2018 John Wiley & Sons, Inc. Published 2018 by John Wiley & Sons, Inc.

Come on a Journey to Lunga Lunga

Lunga Lunga is a rural village in Kwale County, the most southeastern county of the Kenyan Coast Province. So are other villages, such as Jirani, Mpakani, Maasailand, Perani, Umoja, and Godo. Things have changed profoundly since Araceli Alonso first arrived in Lunga Lunga in 2009. Through this narrative, we are taking you on a journey to explore with us the reasons why.

In 2009, Lunga Lunga had a population of 15,276, of which 10,015 were estimated to be living in poverty, defined as a monthly adult income of Ksh 2,913 or less (approximately US$30) (Ministry of Lands Department of Physical Planning [MLDPP], 2011; Kenya National Bureau of Statistics [KNBS] & Society for International Development [SID], 2013). The villages of the Kenyan Coast Province in general struggle with poverty-related health concerns and higher than average rates of child mortality when compared to the national average (MLDPP, 5). Malaria in particular has been ranked the number one cause of death and morbidity in Kwale County (MLDPP, 2011).

What do you think may have caused this situation, and what may be some of the factors that make it worse?

Consider this: 39% of the county residents (and 45% of the population of Lunga Lunga) have no formal education, and only 10% of the county population has received a secondary education or higher (KNBS & SID, 2013). Such an extensive lack of formal education is directly related to poor health, disease, and morbidity rates. But there is more to learn about Lunga Lunga before making assumptions about the causes of poor health and about possible strategies for change.

The social composition in Kwale County is a reflection of the diversity of the county in which it is located. Kwale County is populated by two main ethnic groups: the Digo (60%) and the Duruma (25%) (MLDPP, 2011). Other ethnic groups include Kamba, Luo, Taita, Luhya, Shirazi, Maasai, and non-Africans. Social organization is centered on family unity, with males generally accepted as the head of the family (MLDPP, 2011). Unity among families centers on respected village elders, who are tasked with making important community decisions. Some of these ethnic groups used to clash with each other over property, land, or other sustenance-related matters. They do not clash anymore, and women have a lot to do with it.

The Situation upon Arrival

As a medical anthropologist, Professor Alonso detects a number of health-related issues upon arrival. A global health expert would immediately deduce that there are two major problems to address: infectious diseases spread rapidly in the community, and common illnesses that could be easily prevented become endemic. There are many specific matters to be concerned with:

1. Life expectancy is low by Western standards. Many people do not live longer than 40 years.
2. Child marriage of girls and adolescents is quite common, a situation that is linked to a number of health-related matters, such as early pregnancy, high maternal and infant mortality, vesico-vaginal fistula, severe anemia, miscarriage, stillborn babies, premature and low-birth-weight babies, and increased exposure to diseases (malaria and HIV).
3. Female genital circumcision is practiced there to different degrees—extensively among some ethnic groups—with severe risk of hemorrhage, sepsis, tetanus, trauma to adjacent structures, urinary tract infection, and HIV. Please note that we have referred to this practice the way the women do, as "circumcision." However, the World Health Organization uses the term *female genital mutilation* (FGM) and defines this as all procedures that involve partial or total removal of the external female genitalia, or other injury to the female genital organs for nonmedical reasons.
4. Myths, legends, and culturally based beliefs may have dangerous consequences for health; for instance, the belief in a disease caused by bad spirits or *degedege,* which can only be treated by a traditional healer, may stop people from receiving timely medical treatment for other illnesses.
5. The lack of basic resources, such as medicines, drinking water, and latrines, clearly has a negative impact on people's health.
6. Lack of public services, or services that are out of reach for the majority of the population, especially the rural population, makes access to health services and hospitals very difficult for patients and for health professionals; sometimes there is no means of transportation at all, and the roads are in very poor condition.

How to address all these problems and health-related issues so that positive change lasts?

The initial response for outsiders often is to believe that funds would solve everything: "If there were a charitable foundation or a large international NGO to support all the things that need to be done . . ." As you read the list, you may have thought this as well. But we want to show you that although funds are important, sustainable development can also be promoted with small funds by making use of creativity, imagination, sensibility, and, most of all, with the involvement of women and girls at all levels of decision making.

Women as Agents

As you imagine yourself in Lunga Lunga, do you notice that women and girls are disproportionately affected by every single one of the problems listed earlier?

A gender approach, or, said in a different way, a **gender and feminist analysis** of the situation, is necessary to determine why and how this is so. An analysis through a feminist lens will provide the insight to establish **gender equality** and **gender equity** as goals. Gender equity in sustainable health and development does not imply an equal distribution of resources; rather, it requires a differential distribution according to the needs of girls and boys, women and men, to achieve the maximum level of health and well-being—physical, psychological, and social.

Within a gender approach, some feminists warn us, it is important not to essentialize people—that is, not to reduce them to a single essential trait, such as biological categorization as "men" and "women." This can contribute to perpetuating strict socially and culturally determined roles that limit people from expressing who they are and what they want to be. Among other things, gender roles should be taken not as fixed and naturally given to each biological sex but rather as something that can be contested and reshaped by people themselves.

What does a gender approach and a feminist analysis mean when addressing global health issues, besides the fact that gender equity and women and girls are the main concerns? They recognize that women are the agents of social change. The women of the Kwale district are the ones envisioning, initiating, and carrying out changes that improve their health and general well-being, and promote development in their communities. But still, why women? What else does it mean to put women in the spotlight of our analysis?

Women tend to be the carriers of culture, the ones who pass beliefs, myths, and legends from one generation to the next; women tend to be "touched" by cultural norms and prescriptions more than men—for example, by requiring them to preserve their honor and the honor of the family and entire communities. Women often carry a heavy weight—sometimes far too heavy—on their shoulders because it is difficult to contest or reverse traditional roles. Women are the carriers of many cultural values that are symbolically projected onto them. Women's bodies are deeply affected by culture; their health deteriorates due to diverse cultural factors that are perpetuated generation after generation but that could be amended; culture is malleable because culture is human made. Often, women must comply with social roles and demands that they have not chosen, that they dislike, and that negatively affect their lives, their health.

But women also have much power in their hands: they can be the transformers of culture, beliefs, myths, and legends. Women are the keepers of health, too. By virtue of culture, they are the caretakers of children, families, and communities; they have direct access to the health of others and can play a determinant role in preserving it. Women can take care of their bodies, too; they can control the impact of the environment on their bodies, but also certain cultural circumstances, as they fulfill expected social roles and demands.

If you understand and agree with these observations, you are ready to continue our journey throughout the Kenyan Kwale district. As a feminist, you are ready to approach the actions and realities of the women who inhabit Lunga Lunga and the other six villages. You are ready to analyze the context and problems to and work on global health issues with a gender lens.

What Can Be Done?

How can outsiders contribute to ameliorating the health and well-being of the 120,000 people who live in the seven villages of Kwale district that we are visiting with you—Lunga Lunga, Jirani, Mpakani, Maasailand, Perani, Umoja, and Godo?

Too often, outsiders are tempted to make decisions and suggest changes quickly, or to start from scratch, failing to recognize that there is local knowledge and experience, a history to guide them. Somehow, and rather problematically, outsiders are guided by the conscious or subconscious belief that they have all the answers and solutions. But we are determined to do things differently.

As the first foot is set down in the Kwale district, it is clear that collaboration with the local government is urgent and necessary in order to develop a program of disease prevention, health promotion, and well-being in these isolated and difficult-to-reach communities. There are local resources that can be tapped for the sake of the local people, alliances and synergies that can be fostered. The goal is to develop a model of integral and sustainable health at low cost that could be easily transferable to other communities; the model should specifically engage girls and women and be beneficial to them.

Overcoming people's prejudices will not be easy; for instance, some people resist seeking care at the government regional clinic despite being able to afford it. Yes, there may be regional clinics available, but due to complex circumstances, sometimes they might not work for everybody as they could or should; this is what happens in Lunga Lunga and the other nearby villages.

Promoting and sustaining health and well-being are not just about providing quality medical services. Although access to health services is a human right, there are also other needs that can be considered human rights—for instance, education, nutrition, and even play. Basic needs and basic rights are directly related to development, but they must be addressed in conjunction with less tangible or less visible and yet equally determinant matters to health and well-being. Development must enhance people's opportunities to grow and flourish as human beings; it must provide a context for development in which visible and invisible impediments can be overcome. Well-being is what happens when the outcomes of development reflect the diverse experiences and singular expressions of people as they enjoy opportunity and choice.

In Lunga Lunga, the first village where programs were developed, the local women taught us a great deal about what could be done. We thought we knew what well-being was, but they showed us aspects of well-being that are not found in academic sources. Strategically and scientifically informed programs are important for global health success, but success also has to do with the human qualities and capacities of those who participate in the programs. In Lunga Lunga, women were sensitive enough to listen to other community members and work with local leaders and facilitators to understand the local needs, wishes, abilities, and capacities for change and leadership of their peers. As outsiders who came to the villages to live with the local women for some time, we were able to form relationships and share vulnerabilities, experiences, and knowledge in ways that enriched one another as human beings. Communication and receptivity were ameliorated and enhanced. The success of the programs had something to do with the fact that, during all the interactions, knowledge-related hierarchies were eased out among everybody involved: the women from the villages and the local and foreign facilitators.

The following actions were chosen as the starting point to address urgent matters in Lunga Lunga:

1. Offering health services through two new venues: the *Nikumbuke* Health Center and the *Mama-Toto* mobile clinic, which included disease prevention, health promotion, basic treatment of disease, and a referral mechanism for major illness
2. Creating a system of health literacy for a vast number of people through summer health camps
3. Developing a system of education and sustainable health from within through a "train-the-trainers" program
4. Implementing a program of service-learning at the university level to serve as a regular support system for action

But this was just the beginning! These intervention actions were the catalysts, the background to enable many other positive things to occur in the context of our engagement and beyond.

What Happened: The Surface and the Layers

Approximately seven years into the program, the achievements are real and important. They are the local women's achievements, supported by Araceli Alonso and the other outsiders and institutions that have collaborated with them along the way. The success of the programs depended largely on a collective community effort prompted by women, along with the very special leadership and facilitative role of one of the local women, Bendettah Muthina Thomas. Madam Bendettah, as the other women referred to her, believed that the community had the ability to make things better for themselves and to boost the well-being of its people. When we asked Bendettah what she thought well-being was, she said: "Well-being is when you have what you need. You have the resources that you need to face challenges. It does not mean that you have no challenges. But you can face them."

When, after a rigorous evaluation process, the project was honored in 2013 with the prestigious United Nations Public Service Award, we had a good opportunity to list some of its main features and achievements:

Health Care

- *Nikumbuke* Community Health Center—a permanent center in Lunga Lunga
- *Nikumbuke* Health Post—general family medical services for disease prevention, basic diagnosis, basic treatment, child health, family planning, health literacy
- *Nikumbuke* Dental Unit—prevention, treatment, dental hygiene literacy
- *Mama-Toto* mobile clinic—medicine and health literacy on wheels

Public Health and Health Promotion

- Installation of rainwater tanks of 20,000–40,000 liters. Approximately 100 tanks have been installed since 2010.
- Under the Net Antimalaria Campaign. Between 2011 and 2012, approximately 1,000 insecticide-treated nets (ITN) were distributed to women beyond child-bearing age.
- Ongoing training of health promoters. In four years, 52 health promoters have been trained with a "train-the-trainers" program; for each training, the health topics were selected by the village leaders and by the trainees.
- *Afya Ukumbi* street theater. A group of women regularly perform health skits in their own communities, in the streets, at schools, and so on. The skits address cholera, malaria, HIV, maternal health, nutrition, family planning, FGM, domestic violence, and myths and beliefs, among other themes.

Sustainable Development Programs

- Weekly computer classes. Both girls and boys join in equal numbers. The *Nikumbuke* Community Center owns around 14 computers.
- Tailoring school for girls. Twenty sewing machines have allowed around 200 girls to become nationally certified to open private tailoring businesses in their own villages or in the city and to use their skills to make clothes to sell, and build their livelihoods.
- Business incubator. This microfinance system controlled by the women enables them to start small businesses in the market with fruits, vegetables, poultry, goats, fabrics, and so on.
- Scholarships for girls in primary, secondary, and postsecondary education. Since 2010, three girls have completed college, and others are currently enrolled. The Maasai girls from Maasai land that borders Tanzania are attending school for the first

time; these girls are the first in their community ever to have a birth certificate that allows them to enroll in government-run schools.

- Reforestation initiative and sustainable nutrition program: planting of *Moringa oleifera* trees (Ashfaq, Basra, & Ashfaq, 2012). Hundreds of trees have been planted by the women with the intention of complementing nutrition, purifying the water, and giving shade to their houses and to animal shelters.

- *Moringa Oleifera* Trees and Maize Co-operative. Twenty-seven women from Lunga Lunga control a cooperative and have hired men to work for them. The cooperative is serving a wide number of people in Lunga Lunga, who benefit from its service at a low cost. Other communities have requested the installation of cooperatives in their territory.

- Community library. In 2013, a small community library was opened in Lunga Lunga with books for children in English and Swahili. The number of books rapidly increased as more donations arrived from Europe and the United States, and also from some organizations in Kenya. The same year, a Little Free Library* was built in the *Nikumbuke* Community Center, where women and girls could take one book and return another.

- Women's soccer league. In 2014, the first two soccer teams were created upon specific request of the women from two villages: Jirani and Mpakani. Later, in 2015, the seven villages had their own soccer teams, and the first large competition was celebrated.

It goes without saying that there were many challenges along the way. Some were related to material goods and funds—for example, the need to pay the local people and medical personnel working in the programs; others had to do with logistics—for instance, lack of public transportation, difficult orography and accessibility, and lack of clean water and facilities. Other challenges were related to cultural beliefs about the origins of illness or the traditional healing methods used to treat diseases. But the most difficult challenges had to do with gender roles—that is, the deeply rooted inequalities, violence, and lack of autonomy that the women of Lunga Lunga and the nearby villages endured.

It takes some distance and much reflection to realize that besides the visible achievements listed here, there are other deep changes that have occurred in these communities. It takes a feminist gender analysis to understand and explain what the positive transformations in the Kwale district are really about, and the depth of their reach. It takes scientific knowledge and skills to appreciate the nuances of change. But it also takes close contact and direct knowledge of the people to understand how and why

---

*The model of the Little Free Library, based on the idea of "Take a book; leave a book," began in Wisconsin in 2009, and soon became a global phenomenon. As of 2017, there were more than 50,000 Little Free Libraries registered worldwide. In Lunga Lunga, the Little Free Library became a repository for health information (hand-painted health brochures and small books made with recycled cardboard).

the local women have so productively built sustainable individual and collective well-being in their communities, how and why they have made the most out of the grassroots health-related programs fostered by outsiders.

A Model to Replicate: Health by All Means

We believe there is a model for change to be extrapolated from the happenings in Lunga Lunga and the six other villages; we call it Health by All Means (Alonso & Langle de Paz, in press). We believe that some aspects of this model can be adapted or mirrored elsewhere to bring about long-lasting well-being in development.

The local women whom you met in your figurative journey to the Kwale district live within social structures and cultural gender prescriptions that restrict or impede their well-being. But, as you witnessed, they are very capable of rebelling against and surpassing such limitations. They just need some help to enhance their daily well-being for them to push forth a cascade of positive actions.

We believe there is a force that lies beneath the changes that took place in the Kwale district. In Lunga Lunga and the six other villages, much of women's ability to make the most of the programs began in emotionality. Their behavior was guided by emotional processes fed by well-being. Well-being created the right context for positive emotions to emerge and thus gave way to their latent capacity to (emotionally) rebel against gender-related restrictions. Emotions are processes of many interacting emotional components. One of these components is what we call "feminist emotion," a sort of nonreasoning awareness that gender discrimination should be contested, and a primary agency to do so. Put differently, the daily encounter with gender-related prescriptions or gender-induced hardships prompts women's capacity for change.

In Lunga Lunga and the nearby villages, there is much struggle and suffering caused by the global disparities and injustices of the world; and, as we mentioned at the beginning of this narrative, women get the worst part of it. But women do not accept gender discrimination, at least at the emotional level. We use the concept of "feminist emotion" to explain why and how the women from Lunga Lunga and the other villages had the strength to survive, thrive, become leaders, and subvert traditional roles (Langle de Paz, 2016). On a daily basis, women rebel in many ways, conscious and nonconscious, visible and invisible, against the limitations and suffering caused by gender discrimination.

There is always joy, hope, love, and happiness in spite of adversity. The Health by All Means model triggers and nurtures positive emotions and feelings by enhancing well-being. In Lunga Lunga and the other six villages, women had the chance to realize their potential as human beings, beyond social expectations or cultural restrictions related to gender. The programs created a context for gender-related rebelliousness to emerge inevitably and naturally because women's capacity for change was enhanced by well-being. But it was mainly women who made change possible in Lunga Lunga; it was the local women who decided what well-being meant and how to go about achieving it. It was the women's own ability to take advantage of what outsiders offered, their capacity to get attuned to the emotions and to the positive synergies of all the programs.

Although health was the venue to well-being, the tool for inter- and intracommunity harmony and peace, the catalyst was, ultimately, women's agency. Women were the agents of well-being for themselves and their entire communities, the key to development and social harmony, the missing piece for change and peace.

■ ■ ■

This is how a model for realizing positive change through health was born in Lunga Lunga: it was fostered by the local women's agency and leadership. You have witnessed its birth by reading this chapter. We have interpreted it and named it Health by All Means. We have guided you through your own intellectual process of discovering it.

We currently write about and analyze Health by All Means. Through our scientific lenses, we theorize about the model and plan to replicate it. We teach about it. Many outsiders now support the programs in Kenya; Araceli Alonso oversees them all. The programs are scaling up to other settings and are the cornerstone of the UNESCO Chair on Gender, Well-Being, and a Culture of Peace at the University of Wisconsin–Madison. But the women from the Kwale district of southeastern Kenya stand proud and strong, projecting themselves, their strength, their agency, their leadership, and their joy onto their own people. They exceed all of us, our analyses and conclusions. They exceed themselves because they are a mirror to other women elsewhere, the soul of a global health model.

The United Nations defines a *culture of peace* as "a set of values, attitudes, modes of behavior and ways of life that reject violence and prevent conflicts by tackling their root causes to solve problems through dialogue and negotiation among individuals, groups and nations. The culture of peace and non-violence is a commitment to peace-building, mediation, conflict prevention and resolution, peace education, education for non-violence, tolerance, acceptance, mutual respect, intercultural and interfaith dialogue and reconciliation" (United Nations, 1999).

Health by All Means embodies a concrete materialization of a culture of peace: a set of components and programs, an approach toward emotionality and knowledge that enables peace and harmony through health, development, and gender justice. Health by All Means is about hopes realized and sustainable well-being. It is about "feminist emotion," the present expanding into a brighter future for women and for all, a painful past rewritten. Women themselves do it all.

Key Terms

Gender and feminist analysis
Gender equality
Gender equity

Recommended Reading

Langley, R. L. (2013). Gender-based biology. In *Sex and gender differences in health and disease* (pp. ix–xiv). Durham, NC: Carolina Academic Press.

Rosenfield, A., Min, C., & Baardfield, J. (2010). Global women's health and human rights. In P. Murthy & C. L. Smith (Eds.), *Women's global health and human rights* (pp. 3–7). Sudbury, MA: Jones & Bartlett Learning.

Vlassoff, C., & Moreno, C. G. (2002). Placing gender at the center of health programming: Challenges and limitations. *Social Science and Medicine, 54,* 1713–1723.

World Health Organization. (2009). *Women and health: Today's evidence, tomorrow's agenda.* Retrieved from http://apps.who.int/iris/bitstream/10665/44168/1/9789241563857_eng.pdf

References

Alonso, A., & Langle de Paz, T. (in press). *Health by all means: Women turning structural violence into health and wellbeing, philosophy and action.* Madison, WI: Deep University Press.

Ashfaq, M., Basra, S.M.A., & Ashfaq, U. (2012). Moringa: A miracle plant for agro-forestry. *Journal of Agriculture and Social Sciences, 8*(3), 115–122.

Kenya National Bureau of Statistics and Society for International Development. (2013). *Exploring Kenya's Inequality: Pulling Apart or Pooling Together?* Retrieved from http://inequalities.sidint. net/kenya/wp-content/uploads/sites/3/2013/10/Preliminary%20pages.pdf

Langle de Paz, T. (2016, Winter). A golden lever for politics: Feminist emotion and women's agency. *Hypatia: A Journal of Feminist Philosophy, 31*(1), 188–203.

Ministry of Lands Department of Physical Planning. (2011). *Kwale District and Mombasa Mainland South regional physical development plan: 2004–2034.* Retrieved from http://cae.uonbi.ac.ke/ sites/default/files/cae/artsdesign/urbanplanning/UNCRD%20KWALE-MOMBASA%20 REPORT.pdf

United Nations. (1999). *Declaration on a culture of peace.* Retrieved from http://www.un-documents .net/a53r243a.htm

CHAPTER 26

STRENGTHENING IMMUNIZATION PROGRAMS
LESSONS LEARNED ON ENGAGING STAKEHOLDERS

James Conway, MD

You miss 100 percent of the shots you never take.
—**Wayne Gretzky, professional hockey player**
The only difference between a good shot and a bad shot is if it goes in or not.
—**Charles Barkley, professional basketball player**

One of the most important public health advances in the history of human society has been the development and widespread availability of vaccines. As recently as the early 1900s in the United States, infectious diseases were widely prevalent, and were responsible for significant morbidity and mortality. With limited options for treatment, preventive measures were the only effective available means for management (Centers for Disease Control and Prevention [CDC], 1999).

Although the first vaccine had been developed in 1796 against smallpox, and vaccines against rabies, typhoid, cholera, and plague were discovered over the course of the 19th century, immunization only came into widespread routine practice in the United States during the 20th century. There are now vaccines available for humans to protect against more than 20 different infectious diseases that once routinely devastated communities. And, despite the complexity and high costs involved in the process, many more are still being developed, some in response to the emergence of newly recognized diseases.

Foundations for Global Health Practice, First Edition. Lori DiPrete Brown.
© 2018 John Wiley & Sons, Inc. Published 2018 by John Wiley & Sons, Inc.

Yet despite the incredible progress in developing vaccines against these infections, many of these same diseases continue to affect individuals and populations in less resourced regions, as access to immunizations is still a challenge in many areas. In reviewing progress toward achieving the Millennium Development Goal for preventing mortality in children under five years of age, it is therefore not surprising that the countries unable to achieve the desired goals were those where immunizations were not routinely administered to substantial proportions of children. Even more alarming, as the frequency of these preventable infections declines in highly immunized populations, there is increasing vaccine hesitancy due to concerns about vaccine safety in more developed countries. As a result of these issues, vaccine-preventable diseases continue to circulate, and in some regions are making a return.

Herd Immunity and Immunization Goals

Control of vaccine-preventable diseases depends on "herd immunity." If a sufficiently high proportion of the population is immune to disease, it prevents the spread of contagious diseases, even for those who are not immune—essentially protecting the entire "herd." Every infectious disease has different communicability and attack rates, but in general, outbreaks of disease are prevented when more than 80% of a population are immune, and elimination of disease is possible when greater than 90% of individuals are no longer susceptible. This epidemiologic information then translates into the WHO Expanded Programme on Immunization and U.S. Healthy People 2020 immunization goals: at least 80% coverage for new vaccines, and eventually more than 90% coverage as use becomes well established (Conway & Green, 2011).

Because of this need to achieve high rates of immunity, efforts to improve routine immunization administration need to simultaneously focus on convincing parents and families to immunize in order to protect individuals, and on advocating for systemic improvements in order to make vaccines routinely available to all. Advocacy activities therefore need to be wide in scope—addressing both the ground-level activities in communities, in order to address individual concerns, and the organizations that develop, produce, distribute, and manage immunization programs, in order to provide cost-effective protection for the greatest number of people (Sabnis & Conway, 2015).

Decision Making and Vaccine Hesitancy

In addressing individuals and their health care decisions, there are many more similarities than there are differences when comparing domestic and international sites. When diseases are circulating widely and there is awareness of the potential severity of these infections, there is generally more tolerance for side effects. However, as diseases become more rare, any vaccine side effects, whether real or perceived, become of disproportionate concern, as collective memory of these diseases fades (Conway & Green, 2011).

With any pharmaceutical product, there are two critical issues: safety and efficacy. From a regulatory standpoint, vaccines are actually scrutinized much more closely, and held to much higher standards, than other pharmaceutical products. For most medicines, a condition is being treated, and as long as there is substantial benefit, some side effects are tolerated. However, vaccines are different. They are given to healthy individuals with the goal of keeping them healthy. Therefore, there is less tolerance for side effects, as well as a need to perform careful vigilance for unexpected adverse events occurring after immunization. Yet despite this vigilance, rumors and concerns about the safety of vaccines continue to circulate (Conway & Green, 2011).

Social media and the Internet have clearly played a role in escalating these fears, at least in more-resourced areas. When families who refuse to vaccinate their children are asked about their primary sources for making these decisions, only one third indicate that they obtained their information from medical providers. Two thirds report that their decisions were based on material from friends, family, Internet sites, or alternative health providers (Salmon et al., 2009). Essentially, misinformation leads some people to believe that vaccines may cause harm and that the natural disease is not as dangerous. After recognizing this, public health groups have responded by developing educational materials that use a variety of media to attempt to correct misconceptions. At the individual level, providers try to advocate for the protection of each individual in their interactions with each family.

In understanding individual decision making in regard to immunizations, there are clear determinants of communication that result in acceptance. Trust in the health provider and the relationship with that provider are critical. Parents are much more likely to immunize if they feel satisfied by discussion with the provider, if vaccination is a cultural norm in their community, and if such behavior is part of a social contract in which protection from disease requires group cooperation (Benin, Wisler-Scher, Colson, Shapiro, & Holmboe, 2006). In essence, each encounter between a health provider and a potential vaccinee represents an act of advocacy.

In less-developed countries, there are parallels to this vaccine hesitancy, where concerns are prompted and rumors spread within a community, often after adverse events occur following immunization. These concerns may begin due to cultural, religious, or even political issues and misunderstanding (Larson, Cooper, Eskola, Katz, & Ratzan, 2011). Unless these are addressed immediately, they risk becoming widespread and significantly impacting acceptance of vaccine programs, and therefore immunization coverage (Streefland, Chowdhury, & Ramos-Jimenez, 1999). Examples of these phenomena include the resistance to polio immunization in Nigeria due to both political and religious opposition, with resulting resurgence of flaccid paralysis in the northern areas of the country, and more recently issues in Pakistan after the CIA used vaccine programs as cover during the search for Osama bin Laden, leading to widespread distrust and subsequent attacks on vaccine workers.

If public health programs do not address these rumors appropriately, sustained concerns can lead to widespread resistance to vaccination activities. The core principles that help restore public confidence in vaccines include identification and engagement with *all* potential stakeholders, allowing these partners to express the concerns of their constituents and providing legitimacy to the responses. In addition, vaccine programs worldwide have realized the benefits of transparent decision making and honest disclosure of uncertainty and risks (Larson et al., 2011).

Vaccine Access

Addressing access issues at the population level is obviously a greater challenge, again with many parallels between domestic and international sites. Advocacy activities play a crucial role in optimizing protection against vaccine-preventable disease at this level as well.

In the United States, school entry requirements have been developed as a means to encourage vaccination of individuals, though most states allow exemptions for medical or religious reasons. Although this strategy has been successful in many areas, almost half the states allow "personal belief waivers," which enable families to opt out due to their personal convictions (Conway & Green, 2011). As you would expect, these states have the lowest immunization rates in the United States. Due to recent disease outbreaks, including an outbreak of measles originating at Disneyland in California, there has been some movement to tighten these regulations, largely in response to community and medical advocacy (Sabnis & Conway, 2015).

Removal of financial barriers is also an important aspect of improving immunization programs. During the Kennedy administration in the United States, it was recognized that uninsured families had a financial disincentive to immunize their children. The Vaccines for Children (VFC) program was designed to provide free vaccines for poor families (CDC, 1999). Over 50 years ago, Section 317 of the Public Service Act was passed in response to lobbying and advocacy activities, providing additional resources for immunizing priority populations, including underinsured children and adults not eligible for VFC support (Conway & Green, 2011). More recently, the Affordable Care Act created statutes ensuring that insurers covered vaccines for children across the United States.

Most countries around the world have chosen a different approach, and instead try to offer basic vaccines as an entitlement—essentially free for all individuals at the appropriate age. However, there are challenges to this approach, as many offer vaccines against only a limited number of diseases—largely dictated by the cost of these vaccines and the perception of their importance. Obviously, there can be a perceived financial disincentive to investing in vaccines if there is not recognition of the savings that result from immunizing. Calculation of the benefits in both direct medical costs saved (not caring for sick people) as well as the indirect costs (lost time from school or work, and the inability to contribute to the economy), as shown by Ozawa and colleagues, continues to provide advocates with convincing material to argue for expanded access at the national level (Ozawa, Clark, Portnoy, Grewal, Brenzel, & Walker, 2016).

Vaccine Development

Obviously, development of new vaccines by academic researchers and members of the pharmaceutical industry represents a response to a need; but how that need is defined often represents the outcome of public health advocacy. There are thousands of preventable diseases, caused by viruses, bacteria, fungi, and parasites. Each of these diseases causes some morbidity and perhaps mortality, and the populations affected, as well as the associated financial costs, largely determine how new projects are prioritized. However, there is clearly also the corporate motivation for financial profit that needs to be recognized. For many years, new vaccines have been primarily developed for diseases that affect Western populations, where research and development costs could be recouped from sales. Prevention against neglected tropical diseases, or illnesses that affect poorer countries and populations, has only recently received the attention it deserves. Some of this activism has actually occurred due to improved disease surveillance and epidemiologic data that has helped raise awareness. Resources to support development of these newer vaccines have helped reshape the vaccine landscape. Examples include the Meningitis Vaccine Project, which resulted in development of MenAfriVac in 2010, recent progress toward improved tuberculosis vaccines and new efforts related to malaria vaccination.

However, there are also many expensive vaccines that were originally designed for Western markets, for which there is incredible need in resource-challenged areas as well. Vaccines against pneumococcal infections, rotavirus diarrhea, and human-papillomavirus-related cancers, to name a few, are only recently being introduced in the countries where the highest burden of disease exists. Nongovernmental organizations such as the Global Alliance for Vaccine Initiatives (GAVI) offer a novel approach to making such vaccines available and affordable. This collaboration among philanthropic groups, the vaccine industry, WHO, UNICEF, the World Bank, the Gates Foundation, and others provide a means to both support and advocate for countries to assume responsibility for program improvements. By creating a public-private partnership in 2000, GAVI enabled poorer countries to apply for support, but also required them to provide cofinancing to support system strengthening while receiving deeply discounted vaccines (Ozawa et al., 2016). Many years of advocacy from an array of organizations resulted in this unique collaborative approach to improving access.

International cooperation to empower local medical organizations and professional societies to serve as vaccine advocates is an evolving area of attention as well. Although information and pressure from outside organizations can be helpful, internal demands and requests to add new vaccines or expand services are powerful. The real understanding of the needs of a community and of the disease prevention priorities should be derived from local expertise. Political and health care leaders respond to their own constituencies, because there is legitimacy in the requests that are based on both a deeper understanding of the circumstances and an investment in the outcomes (Larson et al., 2011). Although advocacy can span from the local to the international level, the responses to these activities is largely determined by the perceived credibility of the activist's primary purpose.

■ ■ ■

Vaccines offer a unique study for the role of advocacy in public health. Understanding the benefits to individuals (prevention of illness) as well as the community (prevention of outbreaks, with the resulting disruptions and financial implications) provides incentive to press for widespread access for all members of a society. However, individual fears and concerns are a constant threat to maintaining immunization coverage. Similarly, managing larger societal barriers that hinder the development and introduction of new vaccines, and maintaining support for immunization programs given other competing health needs as certain diseases become less common, are always a challenge. As a global society, we see the consequences when diseases re-emerge that were once rare. Although there are economic and cultural differences throughout the world, the challenges are very similar—and the need for advocacy never ending.

Suggested Reading

Conway, J. H., Green, T. L. (2011). "Childhood Immunization Policies and the Prevention of Communicable Diseases." *Pediatric Annals, 40*(3):136–43. doi:10.3928/00904481-20110217-07

Global Alliance for Vaccines and Immunizations. (2001). *Advocacy for Immunizations.* www.path .org/vaccineresources/files/GAVI-AdvocacyHandbook.pdf

Sabnis S. S., Conway, J. H. (2015). "Overcoming Challenges of Childhood Immunization." *Pediatric Clinics of North America, 62*(5):1093–1109. doi:10.1016/j.pcl.2015.05.004

References

Benin, A. L., Wisler-Scher, D. J., Colson, E., Shapiro, E. D., Holmboe, E. S. (2006). "Qualitative Analysis of Mothers' Decision Making about Vaccines for Infants: The Importance of Trust." *Pediatrics, 117*(5):1532–41. doi:10.1542/peds.2005-1728

Centers for Disease Control and Prevention. (1999). "Achievements in Public Health, 1900–1999: Impact of Vaccines Universally Recommended for Children." *Morbidity and Mortality Weekly Report, 48*(12):243–48.

Conway, J. H., Green, T. L. (2011). "Childhood Immunization Policies and the Prevention of Communicable Diseases." *Pediatric Annals, 40*(3):136–43. doi:10.3928/00904481-20110217-07

Larson, H. J., Cooper, L. Z., Eskola, J., Katz, S. L., Ratzan, S. (2011). "Addressing the Vaccine Confidence Gap." *The Lancet, 378*(9790):526–35. doi:10.1016/S0140-6736(11)60678-8

Ozawa, S., Clark, S., Portnoy, A., Grewal, S., Brenzel, L., Walker, D. G. (2016). "Return on Investment from Childhood Immunization in Low- and Middle-Income Countries." *Health Affairs, 35*(2):199–207. doi:10.1377/hlthaff.2015.1086

Sabnis S. S., Conway, J. H. (2015). "Overcoming Challenges of Childhood Immunization." *Pediatric Clinics of North America, 62*(5):1093–1109. doi:10.1016/j.pcl.2015.05.004

Salmon, D. A., Sotir, M. J., Pan, W. K., Berg, J. L., Omer, S. B., Stokley, S., Hopfensperger, D. J., Davis, J. P., Halsey, N. A. (2009). "Parental Vaccine Refusal in Wisconsin: A Case-Control Study." *Wisconsin Medical Journal, 108*(1):17–23.

Streefland, P., Chowdhury, A.M.R., Ramos-Jimenez, P. (1999). "Patterns of Vaccination Acceptance." *Social Science & Medicine, 49*(12):1705–16.

CHAPTER 27

HIV: US TO GLOBAL PERSPECTIVES

Katarina M. Grande, MPH

The global HIV/AIDS epidemic is an unprecedented crisis that requires an unprecedented response. In particular it requires solidarity—between the healthy and the sick, between rich and poor, and above all, between richer and poorer nations. We have 30 million orphans already. How many more do we have to get, to wake up?

—Kofi Annan, secretary-general of the United Nations, 1997–2006

If you embark on a global health career, at some point you will likely work on a project related to HIV or be funded by dollars earmarked for HIV. Why is this? Plenty of serious global health issues exist—poverty, auto accidents, malaria, other mosquito-transmitted infections, diarrheal illness, health care infrastructure gaps, famine, tuberculosis, chronic diseases, reproductive health issues—the list goes on. But as of 2017, HIV accounts for over half ($4.65 billion) of total global health funding ($8.5 billion) allotted by the US government (Valentine, Wexler, & Kates, 2016)—a pattern that has remained steady for years. The history of US government prioritization of HIV as a global health initiative began in 2003, when President George W. Bush announced the genesis of PEPFAR—the President's Emergency Plan for AIDS Relief. At $15 billion over five years, PEPFAR emerged as the largest-ever global health initiative to target a single disease.

The initial focus of PEPFAR was truly an emergency response. Highly effective antiretroviral treatment for people living with HIV appeared in the 1990s, but the high costs made the treatment unavailable to much of the Global South. UNAIDS (2016b) estimates that nearly 17 million people in East and Southern Africa were living with HIV in 2003, yet only 50,000 were on treatment (White House, 2008). PEPFAR and its coordinated response changed those numbers dramatically—within a few years, two million people in the region were accessing treatment. By 2016, about half of people living with HIV globally were accessing the lifesaving medications (UNAIDS, 2016a).

HIV Background

HIV is an infection that spilled over from chimpanzees into humans (likely via blood exchange during bush meat hunting and butchering) in the early 1900s, but it did not reach epidemic levels until the late 1970s (Avert, 2016a). It was not named until 1982, when the Centers for Disease Control and Prevention (CDC) coined the term "acquired immune deficiency syndrome (AIDS)." In 1986, the virus that causes AIDS—human immunodeficiency virus (HIV)—was named. HIV is transmitted via blood, breast milk, and sexual fluids. Globally, most infections are transmitted between heterosexual partners, but other key populations impacted—such as men who have sex with men, sex workers, transgender people, young women, and people who inject drugs—vary regionally. Nearly 70% of people living with HIV reside in sub-Saharan Africa (UNAIDS, 2016d), which is where much of PEPFAR-funded efforts are focused.

Strategies for Ending HIV

Although PEPFAR spurred significant additional financial focus on HIV, thousands of global institutions, grassroots organizations, and private companies also play a role in the efforts to end the HIV epidemic. For example, the Joint United Nations Programme on HIV and AIDS (UNAIDS) focuses on global coordination and data collection related to the epidemic; The AIDS Support Organization (TASO) in Uganda, a grassroots organization, works especially hard on advocacy and on-the-ground community service delivery; and private pharmaceutical companies play an important part in developing new HIV medications and lowering drug prices.

The methods of combating HIV in both the Global North and the Global South have evolved rapidly over the past three decades. The mid-1980s to 1990s were characterized by treatment, limited mostly to people in the Global North, with harsh drugs that had many negative side effects. In the early 2000s, PEPFAR coined the prevention strategy "ABCs"—practice Abstinence, Be faithful, use a Condom consistently and correctly. As the evidence base grew and US government administrations changed, funded prevention strategies after 2008 shifted away from focusing on promoting abstinence (Lo, Lowe, & Bendavid, 2016) and other behavior changes. Condoms remained a key prevention tool, but after studies showed that consistent treatment with antiretroviral (ARV) medication essentially eliminated sexual transmission risk due to lowering the viral load, "treatment as prevention" became a major focus. Consistent ARV medication also works extremely well for the prevention of mother-to-child transmission of HIV, so efforts focusing on treatment for women remained a critical approach. Medical male circumcision was shown to reduce the risk of heterosexually acquired HIV for men by 60%, so large-scale voluntary adult male circumcision campaigns worked to reach over 10 million men in sub-Saharan Africa by 2016 (Avert, 2016c). Needle and syringe exchange programs and harm reduction methods are an effective and important prevention strategy pertinent to people who inject drugs. The next global prevention tool, already widely in use in the Global North, is pre-exposure prophylaxis (PrEP)—people who are HIV-negative take one ARV pill, once a day, for HIV prevention. After that will likely be long-acting injectable ARVs, currently undergoing clinical trials.

Although massive progress has been made—AIDS-related deaths have fallen by 48% since the peak in 2005 (UNAIDS, 2016c)—many barriers remain to effectively combat the global HIV epidemic. As PEPFAR transitions from an emergency response phase to a supportive phase, funders have an expectation that countries will become less dependent on foreign funds to pay for HIV treatment and prevention efforts. For many countries, this is a great challenge. In addition, HIV often exists in a context of stigma: cultural and religious beliefs around sexuality and HIV can lead to stigma; and stigma can lead to discrimination, poor access to health services, and violence (Avert, 2016b).

Working in HIV Globally and Locally

The complex context and global reach of HIV is part of what drove me to work in the public health field focusing on HIV. I have worked on the receiving end of PEPFAR funding on a governance-focused project in Uganda, on the disseminating end of PEPFAR funding as a program management fellow at Centers for Disease Control–Tanzania, and on the domestic end as an HIV epidemiologist at a state health department in the United States. Although the epidemic looked different in terms of demographics impacted, the parallels between my work in East Africa and my work in the United States are many.

First, amazing and passionate individuals are working in the field of HIV. For so many people I met in East Africa and the United States, working in HIV was more than a job focus—it was personal. Many workers' loved ones, friends, family, and community members had died due to complications resulting from HIV. Many workers are part of the LGBTQ community or are LGBTQ allies. The energy that a personal connection brings was key in keeping people focused in their work and preventing burnout.

Second, as much as politics and administrations drive HIV-related funding and policies, the field is paved with advocacy generated by extraordinary grassroots organizations. The AIDS Coalition to Unleash Power (ACT UP), founded in New York, became known for its awareness-generating protests of pharmaceutical companies for charging prohibitively high prices for lifesaving ARVs, federal administrations for prohibiting needle and syringe exchange programs when the science supports their efficacy, and insurance companies for having spotty coverage of HIV drugs. The policy that funds HIV care and treatment in the United States—the Ryan White Comprehensive AIDS Resource Emergency (CARE) Act—was championed, in part, by the San Francisco AIDS Foundation (2016). South Africa's Treatment Action Campaign advocated for guaranteed ARVs for pregnant women living with HIV by suing its government. TASO in Uganda began in

1987 as a grassroots care organization after people living with HIV experienced discrimination in the public health care system. It now serves as a model HIV care and prevention organization.

Third, innovations in HIV prevention come from around the world. For example, South Africa and numerous countries have established HIV interventions related to football (soccer). Football tournaments host voluntary counseling and testing events to decrease stigma, coaches deliver HIV prevention messaging and education to increase players' knowledge and communication skills around HIV, and football celebrities lend a voice to outreach programs (Khan, 2010; Hershow et al., 2015). Cash transfer programs in southeast Africa provide participants with a simple monthly cash payment of $1–$5, which has shown an HIV prevention effect among school-age girls (Baird, Garfein, McIntosh, & Ozler, 2012). In the United States, the District of Columbia Department of Health (2016) offers free mail-order condoms through its Rubber Revolution campaign. An exciting aspect of working in HIV prevention is learning from other countries' innovation and success.

Like any public health work, working in HIV has its challenges—regardless of location. Depending on politics and funding, it can be difficult to implement some evidence-based interventions. For example, some social marketing messages that promote condom use are widely displayed in East Africa, but similar messages are less accepted in conservative areas in the United States. In Tanzania and Zanzibar, I worked with HIV prevention professionals who set up a very successful methadone clinic, which promotes decreased injection drug use; in the United States, many communities do not allow such clinics. In East Africa and elsewhere, HIV prevention interventions targeted at men who have sex with men are sometimes challenged or banned; in the United States, this is not as often the case. One final challenge I observed is the burden of reporting on HIV. Funders, especially the US government, rightly demand accountability. However, the amount of time workers spend collecting data and writing reports can be a real problem and sometimes comes at the expense of on-the-ground programming.

As is the case with most public health topics, HIV is a systems issue. Reversing the epidemic requires collaboration among science, policy, social justice, diplomacy, education, advocacy, media, and dozens of connector fields. Wherever your global health career takes you, I hope you have the chance to work with people as passionate as those I have encountered in the HIV field.

Suggested Reading

Matthews, D. D., Smith, J. C., Brown, A. L., & Malebranche, D. J. (2016). Reconciling epidemiology and social justice in the public health discourse around the sexual networks of black men who have sex with men. *American Journal of Public Health, 106,* 808–814.

Piot, P., Bartos, M., Ghys, P. D., Walker, N., & Schwartlaender, B. (2001). Global impact of HIV/AIDS. *The Lancet, 410*, 968–973.

Winge, K. (2006). *Never give up: Vignettes from sub-Saharan Africa in the age of AIDS*. Minneapolis, MN: Syren Book Company.

References

Avert. (2016a). History of HIV and AIDS overview. Retrieved from http://www.avert.org/professionals/history-hiv-aids/overview

Avert. (2016b). Stigma, discrimination, and HIV. Retrieved from http://www.avert.org/professionals/hiv-social-issues/stigma-discrimination

Avert. (2016c). Voluntary medical male circumcision for HIV prevention. Retrieved from http://www.avert.org/professionals/hiv-programming/prevention/voluntary-medical-male-circumcision

Baird, S., Garfein, R., McIntosh, C., & Ozler, B. (2012). Effect of a cash transfer programme for schooling on prevalence of HIV and herpes simplex type 2 in Malawi: A cluster randomised trial. *The Lancet, 379*, 1320–1329.

District of Columbia Department of Health. (2016). Condoms and condom information. Retrieved from http://doh.dc.gov/service/condoms-and-condom-information

Hershow, R., Gannett, K., Merrill, J., Kaufman, B. E., Barkley, C., DeCelles, J., & Harrison, A. (2015). Using soccer to build confidence and increase HCT uptake among adolescent girls: A mixed-methods study of an HIV prevention programme in South Africa. *Sport in Society, 18*, 1009–1022.

Khan, N. (2010). Using football for HIV/AIDS prevention in Africa. Retrieved from http://www.grassrootsoccer.org/wp-content/uploads/F4_HIV_Report.pdf

Lo, N. C., Lowe, A., & Bendavid, E. (2016). Abstinence funding was not associated with reductions in HIV risk behavior in sub-Saharan Africa. *Health Affairs, 35*, 856–863. doi:10.1377/hlthaff.2015.0828

San Francisco AIDS Foundation. (2016). Our history. Retrieved from http://sfaf.org/about-us/our-history/

UNAIDS. (2016a). *AIDS by the numbers: Ending the AIDS epidemic by 2013 as part of the Sustainable Development Goals*. Retrieved from http://www.unaids.org/sites/default/files/media_asset/AIDS-by-the-numbers-2016_en.pdf

UNAIDS. (2016b). AIDSinfo. Retrieved from http://aidsinfo.unaids.org/

UNAIDS. (2016c). Fact sheet 2016. Retrieved from http://www.unaids.org/en/resources/fact-sheet

UNAIDS. (2016d). *Global AIDS update 2016*. Retrieved from http://www.unaids.org/sites/default/files/media_asset/global-AIDS-update-2016_en.pdf

Valentine, A., Wexler, A., & Kates, J. (2016). The U.S. global health budget: Analysis of the fiscal year 2017 budget request. Kaiser Family Foundation. Retrieved from http://kff.org/global-health-policy/issue-brief/the-u-s-global-health-budget-analysis-of-the-fiscal-year-2017-budget-request/

The White House. (2008). President Bush's global health initiatives are saving lives around the world. Retrieved from https://georgewbush-whitehouse.archives.gov/infocus/bushrecord/factsheets/globalhealth.html

CHAPTER 28

TUBERCULOSIS AND THE LONG AND WINDING ROAD TOWARD A GLOBAL HEALTH CAREER
A FOCUS ON ACCESS TO SERVICES

Carolina Kwok, BSc (PT), MPH

Human ordeals thrive on ignorance. To understand a problem with clarity is already half way towards solving it.

—**Amartya Sen**

Global health has long held my fascination; I am intrigued by the challenges to attaining basic health needs, such as proper nutrition and access to medicines. Health seemed to me to be a clear human right, and the inability to access this right was a great injustice. My initial path to address these injustices was to learn more about the clinical perspective, and I focused on inner-city populations in Toronto. The biggest barriers I encountered in trying to rehabilitate patients were mostly social, further exacerbated by lack of community-based care. Even within Canada, there were evident systemic issues such as poor affordable housing options, access to proper nutrition, mental health support, and community-based care that were preventing these patients from accessing a high quality of life including good health. Working with these populations broadened my conception of "access" to good health beyond geographic considerations.

Although these were issues that hindered access in Canada, I saw them manifest in larger proportions when I started working with rehabilitation teams in Nepal. The access-to-care issues were more acute in these settings where infrastructure and resources were limited, where gender inequities predisposed women to increased risk

Foundations for Global Health Practice, First Edition. Lori DiPrete Brown.
© 2018 John Wiley & Sons, Inc. Published 2018 by John Wiley & Sons, Inc.

of disability, where tools and educational support for providers and patients were minimal, and where there were shortages of skilled providers. Confronted with the stark realities and interconnectedness of health with environment, economic development, and social structures, I understood there was a field larger than the clinical realm where I had started my work.

Since departing from clinical work, I have had fortunate opportunities to be exposed to different contexts and disease areas, furthering my understanding of global health in low-resource settings. Most recently, I have been working in the area of multi-drug-resistant tuberculosis (MDR-TB) in low- and middle-income countries in Asia where over 50% of all TB cases now arise. TB is an ancient disease that is predominantly a disease of the poor, affecting those who are least able to afford proper diagnosis and long appropriate treatments. Growing concerns about antimicrobial resistance have emerged in the last few years, and the increasing difficulty in diagnosing and treating the related diseases further challenges health systems. Many of these countries also have large private health sectors that can both further exacerbate the epidemic through provision of inappropriate diagnosis and treatments and also enhance social inequities to quality health care. For example, over 50% of all TB cases are detected in the private sector in India (World Health Organization [WHO], 2015), presenting a challenge for effective TB control for national TB programs, where public sector programs are already strained. Expanding regulation and support to the private sector is a necessary but difficult task.

In the TB space, drug development has slowed, and many potential candidates are only at early basic research stages (WHO, 2014). Drug-resistant TB has become an increasing concern globally as existing drugs are now being exhausted, and treatments are toxic, long, and arduous and can be catastrophic to patients and their families. In addition, a growing proportion of TB control budgets are now dedicated to MDR-TB diagnosis and treatment, which affect only a small proportion of the entire TB population. Funding gaps pose challenges to implementing intended interventions, from national strategic plans to actual resources available, and as donor funding continues to shift in priorities, national governments will face critical decisions on how to sustain and expand current programs should external funding cease or decrease. Previous disease control efforts could be reversed if control programs are ineffectively transitioned to countries (Cohen et al., 2012).

Access in the TB space involves getting drugs and diagnostics to patients at the right time, in the right place, and at sustainable prices. This is directly linked to the market for TB drugs and diagnostics, where the main considerations are availability, affordability, quality, acceptability and adaptability, and delivery (Unitaid, 2014). The TB drugs market, particularly the MDR-TB market, is small and fragmented; complicated and differing tendering and procurement practices exist between countries due to a high variation of drug regimens across countries. There are limited numbers of suppliers developing active pharmaceutical ingredients and formulations, and limited market incentives to grow supplier bases and develop new products. For example, WHO treatment recommendations do not prescribe a set MDR-TB regimen, which can translate to different variations of regimen compositions, along with different packaging preferences. This fragmentation splits the market, rendering small volumes, such that the demand is unattractive for new suppliers to enter the market, therefore threatening supply security globally. As a result, prices are high and volatile, which can affect the availability and affordability of these drugs. Current drugs for MDR-TB can be toxic and burdensome for patients, reducing their acceptability; however, for the first time in decades, there are promising drugs in the pipeline, but TB programs have been slow to adopt these drugs at a broader level, slowing uptake globally.

In the countries where I work, the goals are to optimize regimens, help countries plan new product introductions as they come to market, and reduce fragmentation of procurement globally by increasing visibility of the market through streamlining the countries' procurement practices. Many of the bottlenecks and challenges in accessing correct diagnostics and drugs at the country level are related to process inefficiencies that can lead to stock-outs of medicines, inappropriate dispensation of drugs, decreased trust in the system, and, ultimately, poor health outcomes. A cross-cutting element in the work to improve drug access and health outcomes is using data effectively for policy and programmatic decisions. Making data easier to understand and interpret will help country program managers develop targeted solutions for the diagnosis and treatment of TB patients. Concurrently, a holistic approach and close collaboration with partners at the country and global levels are needed to ensure that the market dynamics are appropriately monitored with suppliers and procurers so that patients have access to optimal diagnosis and treatments when they need them.

To achieve the goals in the countries where I work, initiatives are taken in close collaboration with national programs to develop targeted solutions. For example, some of the work involved developing a case to demonstrate the value of shifting procurement toward one formulation that would benefit the global market, thereby reducing fragmentation. Some other examples involved developing drug inventory tools with decision-making support in order to avoid commodity stock-outs, and developing pilots of sample transport systems in order to ensure that patients can get appropriate testing and diagnosis and be put on optimal treatments. Understanding where these inefficiencies are and developing innovative ways to change systems are needed in a disease area that continues to persist and grow more challenging. New research, tools, and products can now help countries in changing their approach to TB in a more dynamic and responsive manner.

In this age when technological advances progress in leaps and bounds, it is unconscionable that people still die of diseases that have plagued the world for centuries.

Countries now have access to new products improving TB services and outcomes in high-burden settings and, thanks to increased data availability, a clearer understanding of the gaps and challenges in programs. This progress is heartening, and there is new hope in reducing the burden of TB and eventually living in a TB-free world.

Recommended Reading

Banerjee, A. W., & Duflo, E. (2011). *Poor economics.* New York, NY: Random House.

Bynum, H. (2012). *Spitting blood: The history of tuberculosis.* Oxford, United Kingdom: Oxford University Press.

Frost, L. J., & Reich, M. R. (2008). *Access: How do good health technologies get to poor people in poor countries?* Retrieved from http://apps.who.int/medicinedocs/documents/s18776en/s18776en.pdf

References

Cohen, J. M., Smith, D. L., Cotter, C. Ward, A., Yamey, G. Sabot, O. J., & Moonen, B. (2012). Malaria resurgence: A systematic review and assessment of its causes. *Malaria Journal, 11*(122). doi:10.1186/1475-2875-11-122

Unitaid. (2014). *Tuberculosis medicines technology and market landscape.* Retrieved from https://www.unitaid.eu/assets/UNITAID-TB_Medicines_Landscape-2nd_edition.pdf

World Health Organization. (2013). Tuberculosis financing and funding gaps. Retrieved from http://www.who.int/tb/WHO_GF_TB_financing_factsheet.pdf

World Health Organization. (2014). *Antimicrobial resistance: Global report on surveillance.* Retrieved from http://apps.who.int/iris/bitstream/10665/112642/1/9789241564748_eng.pdf

World Health Organization. (2015). *Global TB report.* Retrieved from http://apps.who.int/iris/bitstream/10665/191102/1/9789241565059_eng.pdf

CHAPTER 29

LINKING RESEARCH TO APPLIED FIELD WORK
EBOLA AND THE PUBLIC HEALTH LABORATORY

Devy Emperador, MPH

Disclaimer: The findings and conclusions in this chapter are those of the author and do not necessarily represent the official position of the Centers for Disease Control and Prevention.

If you had asked any infectious disease expert in 2014 what the next big epidemic would be, the Ebola virus would have been in the bottom of the list. Influenza virus, drug-resistant bacteria, or MERS-CoV were more likely contenders due to such factors as ease of transmission, lack of appropriate tools to diagnose and treat these pathogens, and the challenge of alleviating systemic barriers such as poor sanitation and access to health care. But in August 2015, I found myself on a plane to Sierra Leone to assist with laboratory coordination in the largest Ebola epidemic since 2001. And although my first love and training were in the biology research laboratory, this was a chance to apply my research and laboratory skills to assist in a larger global public health response.

From Basic to Applied Research: The Public Health Laboratory Scientist

When one hears or sees the word *laboratory* in terms of health, what may come to mind are images of a researcher looking under a microscope in a university research laboratory or of a medical technologist running diagnostic tests on a patient at a hospital

Foundations for Global Health Practice, First Edition. Lori DiPrete Brown.
© 2018 John Wiley & Sons, Inc. Published 2018 by John Wiley & Sons, Inc.

laboratory. Laboratories are an integral part of the health care system. However, most people are unaware of a type of laboratory that serves the wider purpose of protecting health: the public health laboratory.

Public health laboratories are specialized government laboratories that serve to protect the public's health. These laboratories, located at local, state, and federal levels, work to monitor, detect, and research health threats ranging from infectious disease outbreaks to environmental disasters (Association for Public Health Laboratories, n.d.). Similar to research and clinical labs, the public health lab is staffed with highly trained scientists and outfitted with sophisticated equipment. However, on any given day, a public health laboratory can respond to calls of an oil spill off the coast in the morning, conduct research on vaccine-resistant strains of pertussis in the afternoon, and run confirmatory tests on a clinical lab sample of a patient linked to an ongoing measles outbreak.

Along with medical professionals, the first line of defense when it comes to a health threat or outbreak is a team comprising epidemiologists, specialized scientists who conduct data and surveillance activities; public health educators and information specialists; local community members; and laboratory scientists. Because of this interdisciplinary approach to public health, the type of training and experience needed to be a public health laboratory scientist is broad, requiring not only expertise in laboratory techniques but also knowledge in logistics, management, and communication. These latter few skill sets are not normally taught in traditional research programs, so the knowledge really comes from experience. It was this, the desire to apply my lab knowledge, that ignited my interest in field-based global public health.

Public Health Laboratory in a Resource-Limited Setting

At the time that I worked on the 2014–2015 Ebola response, my exposure to the global public health space was just starting. Prior to joining the response, I was an eager research fellow at the Centers for Disease Control and Prevention (CDC) in Atlanta, conducting laboratory research on rotavirus vaccine effectiveness in resource-limited settings. Previously, I was a Global Health Corps fellow based at the Infectious Diseases Institute in Uganda, coordinating training programs for frontline health care workers, including laboratory workers. And before going into public health, I worked in research and biotechnology laboratories, learning microbiology and molecular biology techniques. The laboratories and systems I worked in were well equipped, had reliable logistical support, and possessed working sample transport and management systems, among other requirements for a functioning public health laboratory. So, although I was not wholly unprepared for a six-week deployment into West Africa, I understood that working in the context of an outbreak was going to be a challenge different from those I had previously experienced.

The "Countdown to Zero" in Sierra Leone was just starting when I arrived in Freetown. By that time, there were over 28,000 cases in the three most affected countries (Guinea, Liberia, and Sierra Leone), and an average mortality rate of 40% (Centers for Disease Control and Prevention [CDC], 2016). Sierra Leone had the highest burden of disease, with almost 14,000 cases and over 8,000 deaths (CDC, 2016). The rate of infection increased exponentially in late 2014 to early 2015 as transmission overwhelmed the already stretched public health infrastructure in the region. However, aggressive case finding and contact tracing, community engagement, proper infection and prevention controls, and laboratory testing increases resulted in the continued decline of cases by mid-2015.

The focus of my deployment was twofold: to support the Ebola response and assist with post-Ebola recovery activities. The first task was to support the CDC field laboratory in southern Sierra Leone. At the height of the epidemic, there were more than 20 testing laboratories set up to handle the thousands of samples needing results daily. The scientists who worked in the field laboratories, almost all volunteers, tested and reported on hundreds of suspected Ebola-positive samples each day. It was especially important to practice proper infection control as the majority of deaths that occurred early in the response were among health care workers (World Health Organization, 2015).

Interestingly, my most pressing responsibilities as the lab coordinator did not involve hands-on lab work. When there was a fuel shortage in the country, I worked with the logistics team to send gasoline from Freetown to ensure that the laboratory had enough to maintain the generator that powered all the testing equipment. When an unknown sample arrived at the entrance to the field lab, I liaised with other partners to track where the sample had come from and where the results should go. And when a confirmed Ebola-positive case was found after weeks of zero cases, we all realized the importance of continuing to test and report results as quickly and accurately as possible.

The few cases that continued to occur brought to light the importance of my second, more challenging task: that of supporting post-Ebola recovery activities. As I assisted the field laboratory, I sat with other international partners and contributed as plans to put a national public health laboratory system in place began to take shape. I had little experience in policy development, but I quickly learned the importance of advocacy and partnership building, working with different individuals, teams, and organizations to include laboratory representation in decisions related to both response and post-Ebola recovery activities.

Conclusion

As I reflect on the Ebola response, I have come to appreciate the importance of the laboratory in public health, as well as to realize that the activities of public health laboratory scientists go far beyond their bench skills. I entered the global public health space because I wanted to apply my laboratory background to effect larger change. There is a lot to learn from the Ebola response that applies to other diseases of importance to public health (Barash, 2016; Kanji, 2016; Mayhew, 2016). For me, working on the response was both exhilarating and humbling, and truly highlighted the amazing work of the public health laboratories, and the scientists who work in them, as a part of the larger system that responds to health threats as well as protects the public's health.

Recommended Reading

Ned-Sykes, R., Johnson, C., Ridderhof, J. C., Perlman, E., Pollock, A., & DeBoy, J. M. (2015, May 15). Competency guidelines for public health laboratory professionals: CDC and the Association of Public Health Laboratories. *MMWR Supplements, 64*(1), 1–81. Retrieved from http://www.cdc.gov/mmwr/preview/mmwrhtml/su6401a1.htm

Nkengsasong, J. N., & Skaggs, B. A. (2015, November). Are post-Ebola reconstruction efforts neglecting public health laboratory systems? *The Lancet: Global Health, 3.* doi:10.1016/S2214-109X(15)00159-X

World Health Organization. (2015, May 1). *Health worker Ebola infections in Guinea, Liberia and Sierra Leone: Preliminary report.* Retrieved from http://www.who.int/csr/resources/publications/ebola/health-worker-infections/en/

References

Association for Public Health Laboratories. (n.d.). About public health laboratories. Retrieved from https://www.aphl.org/aboutAPHL/pages/aboutphls.aspx

Barash, D. (2016, June 6). The time is now: How we can work together to address the Global Health Security Agenda. *Huffington Post*, p. 1. Retrieved from http://www.huffingtonpost.com/david-barash/the-time-is-now-how-we-ca_b_10319716.html

Centers for Disease Control and Prevention. (2016, June 22). 2014–2016 Ebola outbreak in West Africa. Retrieved from https://www.cdc.gov/vhf/ebola/outbreaks/2014-west-africa/

Kanji, L. (2016, April 15). Hidden dangers: The implications of the Global Health Security Agenda. *Harvard International Review, 37*(2), 1.

Mayhew, M. (2016, May 17). As Ebola wanes, Guinea, Liberia, Sierra Leone, and world look to curb next pandemic. World Bank. Retrieved from http://www.worldbank.org/en/news/feature/2016/05/13/as-ebola-outbreak-wanes-guinea-liberia-sierra-leone-show-what-could-have-been-done-to-prevent-ebolas-spread-and-what-can-be-done-now-to-stop-the-next-pandemic

World Health Organization. (2015, May 1). *Health worker Ebola infections in Guinea, Liberia and Sierra Leone: Preliminary report.* Retrieved from http://www.who.int/csr/resources/publications/ebola/health-worker-infections/en/

CHAPTER 30

A CALL TO SURGEONS TO ADVANCE GLOBAL HEALTH

Girma Tefera, MD, FACS

Surgery is an indivisible and indispensable part of health care.
—Dr. Jim Yong Kim, president of the World Bank, 2012–present

"The vast majority of the world population has no access whatsoever to skilled surgical care and little is being done about it." These remarks by Dr. Halfdan Mahler, director general of the World Health Organization, at the 1980 International Surgical Congress remain true today. Globally, five billion people lack access to safe, timely surgery with anesthesia and protection from financial catastrophe. This burden is borne disproportionately by lower- and middle-income countries, where 94% of the population lack access, compared to 14.9% in high-income countries. It is estimated that health systems around the world fail to provide 143 million needed surgeries annually.

In spite of this need, infectious diseases and, more recently, non-communicable diseases have been funding priorities in global health, whereas surgical interventions continue to be a lower priority. Misconceptions fuel this lack of investment (Bae, Groen, & Kushner, 2011), and these same misconceptions are the source of fundamental challenges related to the global workforce. In this chapter, I will discuss these misconceptions and challenges, and suggest a path forward for global surgeons.

■ ■ ■

Misconceptions about the global disease burden related to surgery. One misconception is that failure to access needed surgical care accounts for only a small fraction of the global burden of disease. In fact, 11% of global disease burden can be associated with the need for surgical care (Meara et al., 2015). For 2010, mortality from conditions needing surgery was estimated at 16.7 million, representing 32.9% of all deaths. In 2013 alone, injury-related mortality was 4.8 million (Haagsma et al., 2015). This mortality figure is higher than for HIV/AIDS (1.46 million), tuberculosis (1.20 million), and malaria (1.17 million) combined.

Foundations for Global Health Practice, First Edition. Lori DiPrete Brown.
© 2018 John Wiley & Sons, Inc. Published 2018 by John Wiley & Sons, Inc.

Misconceptions about the complexity and scalability of surgery. Another misconception is that surgery is too complicated to be made universally available, and requires the presence of highly trained surgeons wherever surgery is practiced. In reality, some surgical procedures, such as circumcision to protect against HIV, can, with proper preparation, be shifted to health care providers without surgical expertise (Bae et al., 2011). Although this is feasible, it requires investment. In addition to training for health care workers, basic equipment and infrastructure must be in place to sustain a surgery program. A 2011 report of hospitals in six sub-Saharan countries stated that none of the surveyed hospitals had adequate infrastructure to meet the World Health Organization's minimum standards for the provision of emergency and surgical care, and less than 50% had 24-hour services (Hsia, Mbembati, Macfarlane, & Kruk, 2011). Thus we must be prepared to advocate for infrastructure and training investments if global surgery is to be a reality.

Misconceptions about cost. Finally, many perceive that surgery is prohibitively expensive. In fact, the cost-effectiveness, as measured by cost per disability-adjusted life year (DALY) averted, for basic surgical interventions is comparable to that of nonsurgical services. Trauma care, cataract surgery, cleft lip surgery, safe abortion, reproductive surgery, and acute emergency abdominal surgery have all been shown to be cost-effective. In Bangladesh, surgical obstetric care costs US$10.93 per DALY averted, and in Sierra Leone, general surgery costs US$32 per DALY averted. This compares with US$9 for Vitamin A supplementation, US$20 for treatment for acute respiratory infection, and US$30 for measles vaccination (Bae et al., 2011).

Conditions that require surgery, especially when left untreated, result in substantial losses in terms of economic productivity (Meara et al., 2015). If this deficit is not addressed, up to 2% of the gross domestic product—US$12.3 trillion—can be expected to be lost in low- and middle-income countries (LMICs) between 2015 and 2030. Globally, an estimated 33 million people per year will face catastrophic health expenditure for surgical care, unless financial protection plans are put in place through universal health coverage policies (Meara et al., 2015).

Addressing the Surgical Workforce Shortage

In recognition of the need to expand access to surgery globally, the World Health Assembly put forth a resolution to strengthen basic emergency and essential surgery as an integral component of universal health coverage. This resolution was adopted by all participating nations. This very important first step will lead to more health care, and more health care will require a larger health workforce.

According to a World Health Organization (2014) report, the Americas have 14% of the world's population, 10% of the disease burden, and 42% of the health care workers. In contrast, sub-Saharan Africa has 11% of the population, 25% of the disease burden, and only 3% of the world's health care workers. The report estimates a global shortage of 7.2 million health care workers, most severe in sub-Saharan Africa. In the eastern, central, and southern parts of Africa, there are a total of 1,609 surgical specialists (including anesthesiologists and gynecologists) for a population of over 300 million people. The ratio is 0.5 surgeon per 100,000 people in this region, whereas high-income countries have about 57 surgical specialists for every 100,000 people.

The health workforce shortage is not limited to low-income countries. The Association of American Medical Colleges (2016) reported that there is a projected shortage, in the range of 37,400 to 60,300, of non-primary-care physicians in the United States by 2025. Shortages in high-income countries are not new. For decades, the United States, the United Kingdom, and others have recruited foreign medical graduates into their health care systems. In the United States, over 25% of the physician workforce were born and trained in LMICs. This is a complex ethical dilemma that we should no longer ignore. A comprehensive evaluation needs to be undertaken to find solutions that honor the investments that lower-income countries have made in training professionals, that respect individual preferences and choices, and that distribute heath care equitably in our interconnected world. One activity that will be an essential part of this solution is collaboration to train more health care workers through global surgery education.

Ethics and Professionalism in Global Surgery Education

The rules for surgical engagement in global partnerships, collaboration, medical missions, and service are not well defined. There are more questions than answers: Which rules apply and what kind of ethical boundaries and safeguards apply when we work in LMICs? What licensing and malpractice arrangements are needed? Do international collaborators, whether paid or volunteers, show awareness of ethical issues, and are they prepared to navigate ethical challenges? How is informed consent obtained when we don't speak the language? How are patients' rights defined? Do we have cultural competency trainings? Does the local culture support physicians as decision makers? What kind of code of professional conduct do we adhere to while working or teaching in LMICs? Do different subspecialties have unique needs and standards?

I believe there is a great opportunity to join hands across US surgical subspecialties and societies that are engaged in global health to develop a unique program that can clearly define the rules of engagement, learning objectives, and expectations. We need predeployment training programs to better prepare our fellow surgeons, residents, and students before they engage in global health. We should recognize that teaching, learning, assisting, encouraging, and collaborating in research with LMICs are very important in global health, and that these activities can and must be accomplished with the highest ethical standards and cultural sensitivity.

Another Task for Surgeons: Advocacy

Surgeons and the public at large in the United States cannot imagine our health care system without a strong surgical component. Yet the surgical community has not, to date, been vocal enough about the importance of access to surgery globally. It is my hope that in the era of the Sustainable Development Goals, with their call for universal health care, surgeons alongside other health care providers will work to advocate for global health. This advocacy has already begun thanks to organizations such as the Global Initiative for Essential and Emergency Surgical Care (GIEESC), the World Health Organization, the American College of Surgeons, the American Society of Anesthesiologists, the International College of Surgeons, the Association for Academic Surgery, the International Surgical Society, and others. Their support for implementation of the resolution to strengthen emergency and essential surgical and anesthesia care is encouraging.

The Way Forward: Partnerships

Although peer-to-peer relationships are the building blocks of partnerships, institutionalizing relationships among health care institutions, medical schools, and departments of surgery is key to success and long-term sustainability. We can and should work with a framework of mutual benefit and two-way learning. In the past, institutions have been forced to compete for limited funding, resources, staff and leadership, or prestige. We need to develop a common platform and functional networks among universities, research institutions, funders, and other groups to develop collaborative partnerships that achieve impactful results. Such organizations as GIEESC, the American College of Surgeons, and the Consortium of Universities for Global Health are ideally positioned to develop the platform and infrastructure needed.

The potential advantages of developing a collaborative framework for capacity building include providing a well-supervised, curriculum-based educational opportunity for our residents and students; career development opportunities for junior faculty; and safety and continuity for patients.

In addition to working together on educational efforts, we should collectively advocate for the inclusion of surgery as a critical component of universal health coverage. This moment provides us with an opportunity to define the moral and ethical principles that will ensure equal partnership, so that we can share knowledge and skills, and treat all underserved patients with respect and dignity, be it here in our backyard or in the developing world.

We live in a globalized society where economies have become interdependent, and mobility of populations has clearly shown the vulnerability of these economies to rapidly spreading pandemics. It is well known to all that diseases have no boundaries in our global society. Now it is time to make it equally well known that despite our societal advances, five billion people do not have access to basic surgical care. As clinicians, teachers, and students of surgery, we must recognize that there is a global need. We need to be global surgeons and reach out to the world.

Recommended Reading

Disease Control Priorities. *Essential surgery* (3rd ed., Vol. 1). Retrieved from http://dcp-3.org/surgery

Meara, J. G., Leather, A.J.M., Hagander, L., Alkire, B. C., Alonso, N., Ameh, E., … Yip, W. (2015). Global surgery 2030: Evidence and solutions for achieving health, welfare, and economic development. *Lancet, 386,* 569–624. doi:10.1016/S0140-6736(15)60160-X

World Health Organization. (2017). Emergency and essential surgical care. Retrieved from http://www.who.int/surgery/en/

References

Association of American Medical Colleges. (2016). New research confirms looming physician shortage. Retrieved from https://www.aamc.org/newsroom/newsreleases/458074/2016_workforce_projections_04052016.html

Bae, J. Y., Groen, R. S., & Kushner, A. L. (2011). Surgery as a public health intervention: Common misconceptions versus the truth. *Bulletin of the World Health Organization, 89,* 395. doi:10.2471/BLT.11.088229

Haagsma, J. A., Graetz, N., Bolliger, I. Naghavi, M., Higashi, H., Mullany, E. C., … Vos, T. (2015, December 3). The global burden of injury: Incidence, mortality, disability-adjusted life years and time trends from the Global Burden of Disease study 2013. *Injury Prevention.* doi:10.1136/injuryprev-2015-041616

Hsia, R. Y., Mbembati, N. A., Macfarlane, S., & Kruk, M. E. (2011). Access to emergency and surgical care in sub-Saharan Africa: The infrastructure gap. *Health Policy and Planning, 27,* 234–244. doi:10.1093/heapol/czr023

Meara, J. G., Leather, A.J.M., Hagander, L., Alkire, B. C., Alonso, N., Ameh, E., … Yip, W. (2015). Global surgery 2030: Evidence and solutions for achieving health, welfare, and economic development. *Lancet, 386,* 569–624. doi:10.1016/S0140-6736(15)60160-X

World Health Organization. (2014). *A universal truth: No health without a workforce.* Retrieved from http://www.who.int/workforcealliance/knowledge/resources/GHWA-a_universal_truth_report.pdf?ua=1

CHAPTER 31

STORIES AND BALANCE
LOCAL TO GLOBAL PERSPECTIVES ON PAIN POLICY AND PALLIATIVE CARE

James F. Cleary, MD, FAChPM

Statistics are just people with the tears wiped away.
—Victor Sidel

To bring about change in global health, we need to tell stories about what we see, what we do, and the changes being made, especially in poorly understood fields, such as palliative care. Mortality is often seen as just a global health statistic, but the reality is that 100% of us will die, and we will need appropriate care as we approach the end of our lives. In my work as a practicing medical oncologist and palliative care physician, the stories of patients for whom I care enable me to be a more effective global health advocate throughout the United Nations (UN) and its agencies. As the leader of the Pain and Policy Studies Group—a WHO Collaborating Center for Pain Policy and Palliative Care at the University of Wisconsin Carbone Cancer Center (UWCCC)—I find that my clinical practice greatly assists my interactions with government and clinical leaders in health care.

The stories of significance that I share are of interactions I have had with people with cancer around the world: A middle-aged man in Calcutta with head and neck cancer that had eroded through his cheek and who has no access to pain relief. The mother of a young man who had died from a brain tumor and who during the course of his illness had attempted to throw himself out of a 12th-story window because of the lack of pain control. A woman in rural India whose left breast is replaced with a large cancer causing severe pain for which there is no pain relief. A US pharmacist with metastatic

Foundations for Global Health Practice, First Edition. Lori DiPrete Brown.
© 2018 John Wiley & Sons, Inc. Published 2018 by John Wiley & Sons, Inc.

pancreatic cancer who felt like a "drug addict" every time he went to collect the medicines that were the only ones that reduced his pain. The young child in Kenya who cried as she had her burn dressings changed without analgesia. The retired colonel from the Soviet army who had severe pain from metastatic prostate cancer; because of inadequate pain control, he sleeps with his service revolver under his pillow for when the pain becomes intolerable.

Devastating Impacts

The story of Artur, the retired KGB colonel, was one of the more startling. I was accompanying some University of British Columbia journalism students to the Ukraine as part of their masters project (thepainproject.org) on the global lack of access to opioids. Artur had prostate cancer that had spread to the bone, and he had severe back pain even after receiving radiotherapy to his spine. Ukrainian laws mandated that injectable morphine was the only opioid available for his pain control (Cherny, Baselga, de Conno, & Radbruch, 2010) and regulations required that the morphine could be given only by a visiting nurse no more than four times a day. The nurse had to collect the used ampoules before getting any new ones. Artur suffered greatly, drinking a bottle of brandy daily to take the edge off the pain. But even that was not enough. While showing us a military commendation, received for his service in Afghanistan and signed by President Gorbachev, he reached under his pillow and produced his military pistol. He told us he would use this when his pain became too severe, no longer controlled by the limited morphine made available to him. Artur died some three months after our visit, fortunately not as a result of a bullet from his own gun.

Artur's situation is not an isolated one when it comes to the treatment of cancer pain. Eighty percent of the world's population lack access to opioids, essential medicines as defined by WHO since 1977. Their role in the treatment of pain is enshrined in the 1961 United Nations (UN) Single Convention on Narcotic Drugs (1977). This convention establishes a framework to

1. Prevent abuse and diversion
2. Ensure the availability of drugs for medical purposes

The preamble of the Convention, agreed to by the nations of the world, states that "the medical use of narcotic drugs continues to be indispensable for the relief of pain and suffering. . . .[A]dequate provision must be made to ensure the availability of narcotic drugs for such purposes."

However, the primary focus of the UN Commission on Narcotic Drugs (CND) has largely been on abuse and diversion as part of the global war on drugs. The UN bodies that play leading roles in opioid control—the UN Office on Drugs and Crime

(UNODC) and the International Narcotic Control Board—are both based in Vienna; the UN health body, the World Health Organization (WHO), is based in Geneva. Even though both are in Europe, they could be thousands of miles apart given the little interaction between them over the first decades of the Convention.

The last 30 years has seen increased attention to cancer pain relief, first in Geneva. The WHO Cancer Control Program focused on palliative care and cancer pain relief in guidelines released in the 1980s (WHO, 1986). In 2000, a WHO working group met in Madison, Wisconsin, to write a report titled *Achieving Balance in Access to Opioids.* Balance became the key to implementing the Single Convention (World Health Organization [WHO], 2000): "National policy should establish a drug control system that prevents diversion and ensures adequate availability for medical use. Drug control measures should not interfere with medical access to opioids." These guidelines were updated in 2011 (WHO, 2011).

Still, the focus in Vienna and many of the world's capitals was on reducing the risk and harm that can be associated with opioids, rather than ensuring pain relief for those with unmet medical needs. Fear of addiction, cost, and overregulation were among the main reasons identified as major barriers to accessing opioids for pain relief (Berterame et al., 2016). How could anyone change the combined culture of those involved with CND, as well as the individual mind-set of those representing their countries, many of whom had their administrative home in police and justice departments?

The combination of advocacy by a number of nongovernmental organizations (NGOs) and a few sympathetic governments together with committed officials from within the UNODC ensured that the issue of balance was raised, discussed, and eventually adopted by members of the working group. Education was critical, and educational events outside of the main meeting schedule (side events) focused on the issues. These events often consisted of government and civil society representatives telling stories from their own countries about the need for pain control and the impetus for change. The director of India's Narcotics Control Bureau, for example, told of his country's restrictive policies, whereby major penalties were imposed for simple administrative errors. He spoke of his own realization that as a result of the actions of the government of India, 17% of the world's population was denied access to pain relief. India consumes approximately 0.1 mg of morphine per capita per year, whereas the United States and Canada consume over 700 mg of morphine equivalence per capita when including morphine and four other opioids. This gap in opioid availability measured by this (Hastie, Gilson, Maurer, & Cleary, 2014) and other similar metrics (Gilson, Maurer, Ryan, Rathouz, & Cleary, 2012) is one of the most dramatic discrepancies in global health (Knaul, Gralow, Atun, & Bhadelia, 2012) and has been used to compare countries with their regional neighbors and across the world.

My relationship with the director of the Narcotics Control Bureau in India came about through the International Pain Policy Fellowship that has been held at the UWCCC since 2006 (Bosnjak et al., 2016). In this program, we recruit clinical champions in cancer pain relief and palliative care together with senior government officials committed to bringing about change in the medical access to opioids. In Kenya, they worked out that a tax on morphine was making the cost prohibitively high. In Jamaica, regulations precluded the delivery of morphine to rural pharmacies; changes to those regulations improved access around the island. Nepal had difficulty importing opioids from its southern neighbor, India, due to the requirement for multiple export licenses; by the time all were collected, the original approval had expired and had to be applied for again. As a result of this impediment, Nepal started to produce its own morphine tablets. Consumption has increased in all of these countries, with little evidence of increase in misuse or diversion. The federal government of India amended the Narcotic Drug and Psychotropic Substances Act in 2014, and new regulations are being applied on a state-by-state basis (Vallath et al., 2016).

Balance

These stories reflect global realities that have to be "balanced" with the situation in the United States (Centers for Disease Control and Prevention, 2012). Much of the early work on balance took place in the United States in an effort to ensure that patients with advanced cancer had access to opioids for pain relief. Soon other groups of patients living with chronic pain began to request opioids for severe pain. Pharmaceutical companies heavily marketed newly developed opioid products such as sustained-release tablets and transdermal patches. Many states made changes to allow the appropriate use of opioids for medical purposes. However, Florida continued to allow physicians not only to prescribe opioids but also to dispense them. Florida had over 600 pill mills where physicians were illegally dispensing tablets when this "loophole" was closed, resulting in 500 of them closing and a reduction in opioids prescribed and opioid-associated deaths.

These deaths are more likely to occur when opioids are used with sedatives such as benzodiazepines and alcohol. The influx of very cheap heroin from Mexico and illegally manufactured fentanyl from China has led to a public health care crisis in which more deaths are associated with opioids than with car accidents. Despite these stories, the reality is that most people who are prescribed opioids for medical purposes do not become "addicted" to them. This crisis is being addressed at many levels of government, and it is imperative that we fully understand the nature of the problem, minimizing the risk of misuse and diversion while ensuring that people who need these essential medicines continue to have access. The crises of untreated pain in most of the world and of opioid abuse in a small percentage of people in high-income countries need a public health approach to ensure that we bring about a global solution (Cleary, Husain, & Maurer, 2016).

We need not only to understand the statistics we use but also to listen to the stories of those whose lives and deaths are impacted by untreated pain.

Recommended Reading

Berterame, S., Erthal, J., Thomas, J., Fellner, S., Vosse, B., Clare, P., . . . Mattick, R. P. (2016). Use of and barriers to access to opioid analgesics: A worldwide, regional, and national study. *The Lancet, 387,* 1644–1656. doi:10.1016/S0140-6736(16)00161-6

Cleary, J. F., Husain, A., & Maurer, M. (2016). Increasing worldwide access to medical opioids. *The Lancet, 387,* 1597–1599. doi:10.1016/S0140-6736(16)00234-8

References

Berterame, S., Erthal, J., Thomas, J., Fellner, S., Vosse, B., Clare, P., . . . Mattick, R. P. (2016). Use of and barriers to access to opioid analgesics: A worldwide, regional, and national study. *The Lancet, 387,* 1644–1656. doi:10.1016/S0140-6736(16)00161-6

Bosnjak, S. M., Maurer, M. A., Ryan, K. M., Popovic, I., Husain, S. A., Cleary, J. F., & Scholten, W. (2016). A multifaceted approach to improve the availability and accessibility of opioids for the treatment of cancer pain in Serbia: Results from the International Pain Policy Fellowship (2006-2012) and recommendations for action. *Journal of Pain and Symptom Management, 52,* 272–283. doi:10.1016/j.jpainsymman.2016.01.005

Centers for Disease Control and Prevention. (2012, July 3). Prescription painkiller overdoses: Use and abuse of methadone as a painkiller. Retrieved from http://www.cdc.gov/vitalsigns/MethadoneOverdoses/index.htm

Cherny, N. I., Baselga, J., de Conno, F., & Radbruch, L. (2010). Formulary availability and regulatory barriers to accessibility of opioids for cancer pain in Europe: A report from the ESMO/EAPC Opioid Policy Initiative. *Annals of Oncology, 21,* 615–626. doi:10.1093/annonc/mdp581

Cleary, J. F., Husain, A., & Maurer, M. (2016). Increasing worldwide access to medical opioids. *The Lancet, 387,* 1597–1599. doi:10.1016/S0140-6736(16)00234-8

Gilson, A. M., Maurer, M. A., Ryan, K. M., Rathouz, P. J., & Cleary, J. (2012). Using a morphine equivalence metric to quantify opioid consumption: Examining the capacity to provide effective treatment of debilitating pain at the global, regional, and country levels. *Journal of Pain and Symptom Management, 45*(4), 681-700. doi:10.1016/j.jpainsymman.2012.03.011

Hastie, B. A., Gilson, A. M., Maurer, M. A., & Cleary, J. F. (2014). An examination of global and regional opioid consumption trends 1980–2011. *Journal of Pain & Palliative Care Pharmacotherapy, 28,* 259–275. doi:10.3109/15360288.2014.941132

Knaul, F. M., Gralow, J. R., Atun, R., & Bhadelia, A. (2012). *Closing the cancer divide.* Cambridge, MA: Harvard University Press.

United Nations. (1977). *Single convention on narcotic drugs, 1961.* New York, NY: Author.

Vallath, N., Tandon, T., Pastrana, T., Lohman, D., Husain, S. A., Cleary, J., . . . Rajagopal, M. R. (2016). Civil-society driven drug policy reform for health and human welfare - India. *Journal of Pain and Symptom Management, 53,* 518–532. doi:10.1016/j.jpainsymman.2016.10.362

World Health Organization. (1986). *Cancer pain relief.* Retrieved from http://apps.who.int/iris/handle/10665/43944

World Health Organization. (2000). *Achieving balance in national opioids control policy.* Retrieved from http://apps.who.int/medicinedocs/pdf/whozip39e/whozip39e.pdf

World Health Organization. (2011). Ensuring balance in national policies on controlled substances: Guidance for availability and accessibility of controlled medicines. Retrieved from http://apps.who.int/iris/bitstream/10665/44519/1/9789241564175_eng.pdf

CHAPTER 32

THE GLOBAL BURDEN OF AVOIDABLE CHILDHOOD BLINDNESS

AN ISSUE THAT CAN EXTEND BEYOND JUST SIGHT

Luxme Hariharan, MD, MPH

There can be no keener revelation of a society's soul than the way in which it treats its children.

—Nelson Mandela

Last week, my adorable, freckle-faced, five-year-old patient surprised me. Dismayed that she did not need eyeglasses like her brother, she looked at her mother, who stated, "The grass is always greener on the other side." My patient smiled, then curiously responded, "Dr. Lux, isn't the grass greener where you water it most?" Magic moments while helping children like her are the icing on the cake in my work as a pediatric ophthalmologist. Each day, I strive to make the "grass greener" for my patients as a surgeon, a clinician, and a public health leader by advocating tirelessly for high-quality, accessible eye care for all children, no matter what zip code or country they may be born in, so that they can maximize their full and true potential.

According to the World Health Organization (WHO, 2002), every five seconds a child somewhere in the world goes blind. Over a third of these children never graduate high school, and half will grow up to become permanently unemployed. In low- and middle-income countries (LMICs), only 5%–10% of blind children even attend school, let alone go to high school and graduate. The burden that childhood blindness places

Foundations for Global Health Practice, First Edition. Lori DiPrete Brown.
© 2018 John Wiley & Sons, Inc. Published 2018 by John Wiley & Sons, Inc.

on society extends far beyond vision impairment alone and has significant social and economic impacts on families, communities, and countries worldwide. Even though up to 80% of blindness in childhood is avoidable, many areas have limited resources to specifically address eye conditions in children. In addition, there is often suboptimal coordination and collaboration among existing organizations that work to implement effective vision screening programs and timely treatment (WHO, 2013).

The economic impact of childhood blindness is significant and is therefore a priority that ministries and departments of health and finance should address jointly. We know that when a person's sight is restored, greater than 10 times the cost of the surgery is returned to the economy within the first year (Thylefors, 1998). In addition, 80% of learning is through vision; therefore, children who are visually impaired from early in life are often unable to develop normally or fully realize their ambitions, especially if they lack access to high-quality and timely visual rehabilitation or disability services. Furthermore, the impact of blindness in children is often greater than that in adults, as one study highlights that the number of "blind years" due to all causes of blindness in children is almost equal to the number of blind years due to cataracts in adults (Gilbert & Foster, 2001).

The main causes of decreased vision and blindness in children vary widely by the geographic region and socioeconomic status of the country. For example, in wealthier nations, blindness from uncorrected refractive error, amblyopia ("lazy eye"), central nervous system disorders, genetic retinal dystrophies, strabismus (eye muscle misalignment), and diseases of the optic nerve predominate. In poorer countries, corneal scarring secondary to largely preventable conditions such as measles, trachoma, and vitamin A deficiency; the use of harmful traditional eye remedies; and ophthalmia neonatorum are the main causes of blindness. In middle-income countries, with the rise in premature births and the varying development of neonatal care infrastructure, there is a higher incidence of childhood blindness from retinopathy of prematurity. Other significant causes worldwide include cataracts, glaucoma, congenital abnormalities, and hereditary retinal dystrophies (WHO, 2007). One study estimates that in almost half the children who are blind today, the underlying cause could have been prevented, or the eye condition could have been treated to preserve vision or restore sight (Gilbert, Foster, Negrel, & Thylefors, 1993). These differing causes of childhood blindness are also highly dependent on the availability of primary health care and eye care services, accessible instruments, and effective vision screening programs. The major causes of blindness in children have changed rapidly over the past 20 years as a result of improving socioeconomic conditions, improved public health interventions such as measles vaccines and Vitamin A supplementation, as well as improved eye care services for children.

Effective vision screening is particularly important, as pediatric vision problems often have no symptoms and may largely go undetected, especially in younger children. Fortunately, vision screening using evidence-based screening methods can help detect vision problems. In the developed world, 1 in every 20 children has a vision problem, including 5%–10 % of preschoolers and up to 25% of school-age children (WHO, 2000; Gilbert et al., 2003). In the developing world, these numbers are often unknown because of limited measuring tools, published studies, and standardized programs.

Ample evidence supports vision screening as the best way to detect potential visual problems early in children. A child's visual system is different from an adult's, as their visual pathways are continually developing and are malleable to interventions until the age of 10 years. Timely interventions in a child, such as glasses, can thus mitigate permanent vision loss from common treatable conditions such as refractive error and amblyopia (Rahi, Gilbert, Foster, & Minassian, 1999). Unfortunately, in developing countries particularly, only a minority of children receive effective vision screening that could detect their refractive error or amblyopia risk at an age when treatment can have the best outcome. Early detection and timely treatment are critical for preventing permanent vision loss. Timeliness of screening is crucial, as the effectiveness of amblyopia therapy declines starting at age five years. In addition to identifying children who may benefit from early interventions to improve or correct vision, screening and evaluation of the visual system can also help identify vision-threatening conditions such as retinal anomalies, retinopathy of prematurity, cataracts, glaucoma, life-threatening retinoblastoma, strabismus, and neurological disorders. It is often difficult in LMICs to set up preschool screening; therefore, services for prevention and detection of blinding eye diseases should become an integral component of services for mothers and preschool-age children, such as the WHO Integrated Management of Neonatal and Childhood Illness. Reports from the American Academy of Pediatrics recommend vision screening for all children starting at the age of one to three years. New screening tests using mobile phones and digital photos make it possible to detect vision problems more efficiently and in resource-poor settings. Innovative breakthroughs in technology continue not only to help us treat eye diseases more effectively but also to detect them earlier. Such screening would ensure that conditions such as amblyopia could no longer silently steal the vision of our children.

The control of childhood blindness is a priority of WHO and the International Association for the Prevention of Blindness's VISION 2020 global initiative (WHO, 2007). The strategies in this initiative are largely region specific, based on activities to prevent blindness at different levels of service delivery. For example, in the community, measles immunization, health education, and control of vitamin A deficiency are required. The strategies also include tertiary-level eye-care facilities for conditions that require treatment by specialists—for example, cataracts or glaucoma—or for interdisciplinary care.

The following VISION 2020 priorities have been agreed on for blindness prevention:

1. To reduce the global prevalence of childhood blindness from 0.75 per 1,000 children to 0.4 per 1,000 children.
2. To eliminate corneal scarring caused by vitamin A deficiency, measles, or ophthalmia neonatorum.
3. To eliminate new cases of congenital rubella syndrome.
4. All children with congenital cataracts to receive appropriate surgery, with immediate and effective optical correction, in suitably equipped specialist centers.
5. All babies at risk of retinopathy of prematurity to have fundus examination, by a trained observer, six to seven weeks after birth. Laser treatment to be provided for all those with treatable disease.
6. All schoolchildren to receive a simple vision screening examination, with glasses provided for all those with significant refractive error. This should be effectively integrated into school programs.

In addition to the VISION 2020 initiative, many nongovernmental organizations such as Orbis, Peek Vision, and Combat Blindness International have as a priority in their organizational missions the elimination of avoidable childhood blindness through effective screening methods and programs, innovative technology, telemedicine outreach, and development of well-equipped tertiary eye centers.

Other strategies to eliminate avoidable causes of blindness in children include implementing effective public health policies, advocacy initiatives, and legislation specifically addressing the causes. These additional tools may augment traditional medical and surgical methods to eliminate avoidable causes of blindness in children. For example, effective legislation and policies passed at the local and country levels can enforce proper vision screenings in schools, screenings for retinopathy of prematurity, and access to timely treatment effectively embedded into health care systems. This multipronged approach to preventing avoidable causes will have a greater impact than focusing purely on developing clinical and surgical services.

Global programs that appropriately prioritize childhood blindness prevention by utilizing multiple, varied, and interdisciplinary strategies are key to ensuring that the future of our children's eyesight is protected. This will extend beyond saving sight alone for those at risk of limited opportunities. Through effective vision screening, medical and surgical treatment, polices, legislation, advocacy, and sustainable programs, no child will go silently blind from conditions we now know how to timely identify and effectively treat.

Discussion Questions

1. Did you or someone you know wear glasses as a child, and if so, do you know or remember whether the vision problem was identified through a failed vision screening in the schools? Or was the vision problem first detected by the child, a teacher, a parent, or a pediatrician?
2. What are some ways to educate communities about the importance of childhood blindness prevention and early detection and treatment?
3. How can advocacy and legislation play an effective role in childhood blindness prevention?

Recommended Reading

Gogate, P., Gilbert, C., & Zin, A. (2011). Severe visual impairment and blindness in infants: Causes and opportunities for control. *Middle East African Journal of Ophthalmology, 18,* 109–114. doi:10.4103/0974-9233.80698

Kong, L., Fry, M., Al-Samarraie, M., Gilbert, C., & Steinkuller, P. G. (2012). An update on progress and the changing epidemiology of causes of childhood blindness worldwide. *Journal of the American Academy of Pediatric Ophthalmology and Strabismus, 16,* 501–507. doi:10.1016/j.jaapos.2012.09.004.

References

Gilbert, C., & Foster, A. (2001). Childhood blindness in the context of VISION 2020—The right to sight. *Bulletin of the World Health Organization, 79,* 227–232.

Gilbert, C., Foster, A., Negrel, D., & Thylefors, B. (1993). Childhood blindness: A new form for recording causes of visual loss in children. *Bulletin of the World Health Organization, 71,* 485–489.

Gilbert, C., Rahi, J., West Jr., K., Sommer, A., Klauss, V., Schaller, U... Quinn, G. (2003). Visual impairment and blindness in children. In G. J. Johnson, R. A. Weale, D. C. Minassian, & S. K. West (Eds.), *The epidemiology of eye disease* (2nd ed., pp. 260–286). London, United Kingdom: Arnold.

Rahi, J. S., Gilbert, C. E., Foster, A., & Minassian, D. (1999). Measuring the burden of childhood blindness. *British Journal of Ophthalmology, 83,* 387–388.

Thylefors, B. (1998). A global initiative for the elimination of avoidable blindness. *Indian Journal of Ophthalmology, 46,* 129–130.

World Health Organization. (2000). *Preventing blindness in children: Report of a WHO/IAPB scientific meeting.* Retrieved from: http://apps.who.int/iris/handle/10665/66663

World Health Organization. (2002, October 10). World sight day: 10 October. Retrieved from http://www.who.int/mediacentre/news/releases/pr79/en/

World Health Organization. (2007). *Vision 2020: The right to sight: Global initiative for the elimination of avoidable blindness.* Retrieved from http://www.who.int/blindness/Vision2020_report.pdf

World Health Organization. (2013). *Universal eye health: A global action plan, 2014–2019.* Retrieved from http://www.who.int/blindness/actionplan/en/

CHAPTER 33

GLOBAL HEALTH NURSING
CONTRIBUTIONS AND CHALLENGES

Linda C. Baumann, PhD, RN, FAAN
Karen D. Solheim, PhD, RN

Constant attention by a good nurse may be just as important as an operation by a surgeon.

—Dag Hammarskjöld, secretary general of the United Nations, 1953–1961

As members of the largest health profession in the world, nurses are uniquely positioned to effectively impact health worldwide. The nursing profession is based on the principles of caring for the whole person (physical, emotional, spiritual, interpersonal) within the context of that person's family and community, with the goals of enhancing a person's ability to care for themselves at whatever level of function is possible and realistic. Nurses bring a broad range of skills—technical, communication, leadership, and education and counseling about health and illness—to any setting. In fact, whether providing care to individuals in hospitals, providing reproductive health care in rural clinics, or assessing community health in a refugee camp, nurses work directly with individuals, families, and communities as they strive for better health. Whether a nurse is working in their home setting or in a remote location, it is increasingly critical to address health challenges with a global perspective (Baumann & Hartjes, 2013; Hunter & Fineberg, 2014).

Global Perspective of Nursing

A global perspective involves recognizing the global context of health determinants, risks, and opportunities and that care to individuals and populations takes place in a complex global context (Hunter & Fineberg, 2014). *Globalization* refers to the increased interconnection and interdependence of people and countries due to the flow of ideas,

Foundations for Global Health Practice, First Edition. Lori DiPrete Brown.
© 2018 John Wiley & Sons, Inc. Published 2018 by John Wiley & Sons, Inc.

people, other life forms, knowledge, capital, and goods and services across national boundaries (World Health Organization [WHO], 2016a). For example, countries are interdependent in ensuring an adequate nursing workforce through recruitment and migration, generally from less developed to more developed countries. Forces of globalization are reflected in health determinants from economic, political, cultural, technological, and environmental realms of life (Lee, Yach, & Kamradt-Scott, 2011; Upvall, Leffers, & Mitchell, 2014). Although the dynamics of globalization are not new, the intensity and scope are increasingly prominent. Realizing how global themes impact health and nursing and how nurses in turn impact global issues has the potential to make our endeavors and outcomes more effective, powerful, and meaningful. Baumann and Hartjes (2013) describe global health nursing as the adoption of a global perspective by nurses seeking collaborative and sustainable solutions to health problems, irrespective of national boundaries. Global health nurses respect differences in language, culture, customs, and health beliefs. They approach health issues in partnership with communities to mutually identify expectations, resources, and strategies best suited to the local context.

Nursing's long history of social responsibility and working toward social justice so that people everywhere can live healthy, productive lives underlies nurses' interest in bettering the health of the global population. Nurses bring these values when they contribute to global challenges and develop and implement solutions to such issues as poverty, health equity, access to care in politically unstable climates, and environmental conditions that affect global health (Mill, Astle, Ogilvie, & Gastaldo, 2010; Tyer-Viola et al., 2009).

Contributions

Nurses contribute to global health through leadership, research, education, and practice, and as entrepreneurs. Nurses can lead at the broadest levels of global health. For example, Dr. Judith Shamian, president of the International Council of Nurses, is a commissioner on the United Nations secretary-general's High-Level Commission on Health Employment and Economic Growth (World Health Organization [WHO], 2016b), and Dr. Naeema Al-Gasser is the WHO representative in Sudan (WHO, 2015). Leadership groups, such as the expert panels of the American Academy of Nursing, develop and disseminate policy papers on global health topics, such as emerging infectious diseases and human trafficking.

Working in collaboration with colleagues from other countries, nurses also make an impact through research. Examples include research on a peer intervention for HIV/AIDs prevention in Malawi (Crittenden, Kaponda, Jere, McCreary, & Norr, 2015); diabetes self-care using peer support in Uganda (Baumann, Nakwagala, Nankwanga, Ejang, & Nambuya, 2014); and the development of an international school nurse asthma care coordination model with nurse collaborators in Iceland and the United States (Garwick, Svavarsdottir, Seppelt, Looman, Anderson, & Orlygsdottir, 2015). Nurses are working together to strengthen nursing education worldwide by joining the faculty of schools of nursing for short-term assignments and through school-to-school partnerships. Many nurse faculty have received Fulbright Awards to address nursing curricular needs in other countries, and these have often evolved into ongoing faculty exchanges and collaborative research projects. A bachelor's-prepared pediatric nurse developed a program to teach youth with HIV/AIDs about reproductive health in Kenya through a Fulbright scholarship (International Division, University of Wisconsin–Madison, 2014). The University of Illinois at Chicago College of Nursing (2016) has partnered with Bel-Air College of Nursing since 2004 to educate nurses in India.

Examples of global health nursing practice include faculty from West Africa College of Nursing taking on the task of creating awareness and sensitizing nurses to Ebola in four regions of Sierra Leone ("West Africa College of Nursing . . . ," 2014); a US nurse helping coordinate a response to the cholera outbreak in Haiti through Samaritan's Purse (Wisconsin Alumni Association, 2012); and nurses working in humanitarian crises as field leaders, community health nurses, or educators with refugees and displaced people. Finally, nurses with a global perspective are creative and entrepreneurial, using their expertise as innovators to improve health for others. An example is the Health by Motorbike program (http://healthbymotorbike.wix.com/healthbymotorbike), which delivers women's health care to remote regions of Kenya by using motorbikes to visit villages and increase women's access to care.

Challenges

There are a number of nursing-related challenges in global health, having to do with leadership, practice, education, and research. Too few nurses hold leadership roles—for example, serving on governing boards or editorial boards, and being members of policy-making bodies—in the delivery of health care. The roles of nurses in advanced practice roles and as interprofessional colleagues will continue to expand in managing chronic conditions such as HIV and diabetes. However, in most countries there is no statutory change in the scope of nursing practice to recognize these changing roles. Nurses globally have had a significant role in providing education to patients and other nurses, to improve their knowledge and increase access to higher education. The challenge is that although nurses from another country, such as the United States, can help develop and deliver a curriculum, they have more difficulty sustaining this support over time. Many nursing faculty in developing countries are working on master's and doctoral degrees to be able to continue their faculty employment in a university program. Faculty members' leaving their positions to obtain more education creates frequent disruptions in leadership.

Nurses lead and are part of many research initiatives globally that focus on collaborative efforts to address global health topics relevant to the country in which they are conducted. However, there is a need to enable more nurses to engage in research by providing time, funding, and recognition for their contributions. The global arena provides opportunities for entrepreneurship and testing new ideas for health care delivery. There are growing needs for caring for an aging population and improving the delivery of preventive services and health education. These opportunities occur in a global context of a severe shortage of qualified health care workers in many regions of the world.

Resources

Resources for nurses preparing for a role in global health are varied. The International Council of Nurses (2012) has developed international guidelines and standards for practice, education, and research. Sigma Theta Tau International (2017) is launching the Institute for Global Healthcare Leadership to prepare leaders for a global context and to enhance the success of projects. In many schools of nursing, students can gain global health experience through clinical rotations in communities of need, both in the United States and abroad. These programs emphasize mutual respect, understanding other cultures and health care systems, interprofessional practice, and the role of nurses in diverse settings. Working nurses often donate their time as volunteers in nongovernmental organizations, such as Health Volunteers Overseas (HVO; www .hvousa.org), that aim to build capacity to strengthen the global workforce. HVO's success in sustaining global programs stems from matching the clinical and personal skills of a volunteer with the needs of a host partner (Leffers & Plotnick, 2011).

Insights

The personal insights of author Linda Baumann complement the ideas presented thus far. First, never make promises you cannot keep. Although this sounds like a rather simple idea, it has been the most challenging promise to keep. Upon an initial visit to a site, one is often overwhelmed with the needs, the challenging environmental conditions, and the cultural gaps. It is a reflex reaction to nod and agree that you will try to meet requests. However, often the requests are too costly or impractical, and don't really address the root cause of a problem. Also, keeping promises requires that one returns. Medical tourism is criticized because it often provides only a "visit" to a project or country with no plans to return.

Start where your partners are, or even better, be invited to consult or work on an issue relevant to your partners. I was an adult nurse practitioner and public health nurse when I first visited Vietnam in 1989. The community was seeking to improve hospital nursing;

public health nursing didn't exist, and the expanded role of a nurse in primary care was unimaginable in a rigid hierarchy of doctors and nurses. However, after my experience working on projects to enhance teaching, research, and clinical skills, the need for nurses to take a more active role in patient education and chronic disease management became apparent. My patience and commitment proved valuable. I still consult in these areas as nurses expand their roles worldwide. And finally, sustainability can be achieved not just with more funding but through a relationship over time with international partners to develop systems and materials that support engagement in practice, education, and research.

Reflective Questions

1. How would you plan to learn more about the health care system and the role of nurses in another country?
2. What are critical elements in the sustainability of global health efforts?
3. You are considering volunteering to work as a nurse abroad. What do you want to know about an organization before making a commitment to volunteer?

Suggested Reading

Baumann, L. C., & Hartjes, L. (2013). Perspectives on nursing in a global context. In L. Purnell (Ed.), *Transcultural health care: A culturally competent approach* (pp. 74–87). Philadelphia, PA: F. A. Davis.

Davis, S. (2012, November 20). Why nurses are the unsung heroes of global health. *Huffington Post*. Retrieved from http://www.huffingtonpost.com/sheila-davis-dnp-anpbc-faan/international-nurses-week_b_1499802.html

Global Health Nursing & Midwifery (http://www.ghdonline.org/nursing/)
From the website: "Nurses and midwives provide the backbone of health care delivery systems worldwide. Members of this community share experiences and exchange information in efforts to raise the standard of nursing care and training."

Nightingale, F. (1860). *Notes on nursing*. Retrieved from http://digital.library.upenn.edu/women/nightingale/nursing/nursing.html
This is an online version of Florence Nightingale's writing, which has become the basis of modern nursing. It contains timeless elements that are relevant in any contemporary setting.

References

Baumann, L. C., & Hartjes, L. (2013). Perspectives on nursing in a global context. In L. Purnell (Ed.), *Transcultural health care: A culturally competent approach* (pp. 74–87). Philadelphia, PA: F. A. Davis.

Baumann, L. C., Nakwagala, F., Nankwanga, B., Ejang, J., & Nambuya, A. (2014). A demonstration of peer support in Ugandan adults with type 2 diabetes. *International Journal of Behavioral Medicine, 22*, 374–383. doi:10.1007/s12529-014-9412-8

Crittenden, K. S., Kaponda, C. P., Jere, D. L., McCreary, L. L., & Norr, K. F. (2015). Participation and diffusion effects of a peer-intervention for HIV prevention among adults in rural Malawi. *Social Science & Medicine, 133*, 136–144. doi:10.1016/j.socscimed.2015.03.055

Garwick, A. W., Svavarsdottir, E. K., Seppelt, A. M., Looman, W. S., Anderson, L. S., & Orlygsdottir, B. (2015). Development of an international school nurse asthma care coordination model. *Journal of Advanced Nursing, 3*, 535–546. doi:10.1111/jan.12522

Hunter, D., & Fineberg, H. (2014). Convergence to common purpose in global health. *New England Journal of Medicine, 370*, 1753–1755. doi:10.1056/NEJMe1404077

International Council of Nurses. (2012). *Code of ethics for nurses*. Retrieved from http://www.icn .ch/who-we-are/code-of-ethics-for-nurses/

International Division, University of Wisconsin–Madison. (2014). Gold's Fulbright experience comes back to benefit UW–Madison students. Retrieved from http://international.wisc.edu/ golds-fulbright-experience-comes-back-to-benefit-uw-madison-students/

Lee, K., Yach, D., & Kamradt-Scott, A. (2011). Globalization and health. In M. Merson, R. Black, & A. Mills (Eds.), *Global public health: Diseases, programs, systems and policies* (3rd ed., pp. 885–913). New York, NY: Jones & Bartlett.

Leffers, J. M., & Plotnick, J. (2011). *Volunteering at home and abroad: The essential guide for nurses*. Indianapolis, IN: Sigma Theta Tau International.

Mill, J., Astle, B., Ogilvie, L., & Gastaldo, D. (2010). Linking global citizenship, undergraduate nursing education, and professional nursing: Curricular innovation in the 21st century. *Advances in Nursing Science, 33*(3), E1–E11. doi:10.1097/ANS.0b013e3181eb416f.

Sigma Theta Tau International. (2017). Institute for Global Healthcare Leadership. Retrieved from / http://www.nursingsociety.org/connect-engage/our-global-impact/institute-for-global -healthcare-leadership

Tyer-Viola, L., Nicholas, P. K., Corless, I. B., Barry, D. M., Hoyt, P., Fitzpatrick, J. J., & Davis, S. M. (2009). Social responsibility of nursing: A global perspective. *Policy, Politics & Nursing Practice, 10*(2), 110–118. doi:10.1177/1527154409339528

University of Illinois at Chicago College of Nursing. (2016). Partnerships & global efforts: Current memoranda of understanding. Retrieved from http://www.nursing.uic.edu/about-us/ global-health#partnerships-amp-global-efforts

Upvall, M. J., & Leffers, J. M. (Eds.). (2014). *Global health nursing: Building and sustaining partnerships*. New York, NY: Springer.

Upvall, M., Leffers, J., & Mitchell, E. (2014). Introduction and perspectives of global health. In M. Upvall & J. Leffers (Eds.), *Global health nursing* (pp. 1–18). New York, NY: Springer.

West Africa College of Nursing takes on Ebola. (2014, July 10). *Global Times*. Retrieved from http://www.globaltimes-sl.com/west-africa-college-of-nursing-takes-on-ebola/

Wisconsin Alumni Association. (2012). Maggie Rodgers '09. Retrieved from https://www .uwalumni.com/awards/forward_rodgers/

World Health Organization. (2015). Sudan – WHO Country Office. Retrieved from http://www .who.int/hac/network/who/co_sudan/en/

World Health Organization. (2016a). Globalization. Retrieved from http://www.who.int/topics/ globalization/en/

World Health Organization. (2016b). High-level commission on health employment and economic growth. Retrieved from http://www.who.int/hrh/com-heeg/en/

CHAPTER 34

CONTRIBUTIONS OF PHARMACISTS IN GLOBAL PUBLIC HEALTH

Trisha Seys Ranola, PharmD, CDE, BCGP
Connie Kraus, PharmD, BCACP

Of all the forms of inequality, injustice in health care is the most shocking and inhumane.

–Dr. Martin Luther King Jr.

What role does a pharmacist play in the health care system? Given the vast array of roles for pharmacists, this question is complex. You may not always know whether a pharmacist is on the clinical team, but you will definitely be able to tell when they are not. A pharmacist's role is to ensure the smooth distribution of medications, provide clinical decision making on complicated therapies, and educate patients and providers on correct and safe use of medications.

Globally and domestically, pharmacists seek to address complex pharmacy-related issues impacting the care of millions. Some of these include the need to standardize pharmacy practice worldwide, the global burden of counterfeit and falsified medications, low rates of health literacy affecting safe use of pharmaceuticals, and ensuring high-quality pharmacy education. International pharmacy organizations, pharmacy educators and researchers, and pharmacy students have made progress in addressing these issues by working toward universal professional standards, educational change, and population-based public health outreach.

The professional roles that pharmacists play in the health care system continue to evolve. At the foundation of pharmacy practice is the tenet that the right drug at the right dose should get to the right patient at the right time. Although this seems straightforward, a well-designed health system is required in order to ensure that this uniformly occurs. Second, pharmacists ensure the safe and effective use of medications

Foundations for Global Health Practice, First Edition. Lori DiPrete Brown.
© 2018 John Wiley & Sons, Inc. Published 2018 by John Wiley & Sons, Inc.

by all patients. The International Pharmaceutical Federation has defined the roles of the profession of pharmacy as follows (International Pharmaceutical Federation [FIP], 2012c, pp. 10–14):

> Role 1: Prepare, obtain, store, secure, distribute, administer, dispense, and dispose of medical products
> Role 2: Provide effective medication therapy management
> Role 3: Maintain and improve professional performance
> Role 4: Contribute to improve effectiveness of the health care system and public health

Regarding the provision of safe and effective medications, the World Health Organization (WHO, 2016) estimates that 25% of medications in low-resource countries are counterfeit—and as high as 50% in some areas. By contrast, approximately 1% of medications in high-resource countries, including the European Union, Canada, and the United States, are counterfeit. A January 2016 WHO statement reveals that this issue, once thought to be confined to low-resource countries, is now a global problem in part due to the wide availability of medications through Internet purchases. This issue is complex due to the lack of a global consensus on clear definitions regarding *counterfeit,* a legal term referring to patented medications made without permission, versus *falsified medications,* referring to medications made without regard to quality or safety by illegal organizations for financial gain (Attaran et al., 2012).

Lack of access to medications may fuel demand met by falsified medications obtained through illegitimate supply chains. Globally, an estimated 20%–40% of the population in low-resource countries has access to safe and effective medications at affordable prices (WHO, 2015). Up to 24% of patients in the United States cannot afford their medications (Cox, Kamal, Jankiewicz, & Rousseau, 2016).

In addition to providing medications, pharmacists also ensure the ongoing efficacy and safety of medications received by patients. Internationally and domestically, there are barriers to provision of ongoing pharmaceutical care, but also strong efforts toward improvement.

Even though the United Nations estimates that 84% of the adult population globally is literate, health literacy may be much lower, with one in three literate adults misinterpreting medication directions on their prescription bottles (FIP, 2012a). Many patients (e.g., those with HIV or heart failure) take eight or more medications daily; incorrect administration is possible due to the sheer number of medications. Many adverse events may be traced back to a lack of health literacy resulting in incorrect medication use. FIP has developed internationally recognized pictograms, or pictures, that providers can use to create "storyboard-like" visual images for patients on how, when, and how often to take medications.

To provide effective medication therapy management, pharmacists need to be readily available to patients. In the United States, community pharmacists provide comprehensive medication reviews (Wisconsin Pharmacy Quality Collaborative, 2016). Some pharmacists may also practice in clinics, including federally qualified health centers (FQHCs) using a medical home model, that provide services to patients who many not regularly receive care due to lack of adequate health insurance. Working as part of the health care team in these settings, pharmacists perform comprehensive medication therapy reviews to highlight issues of concern to the providers and patients, optimize complex therapy, and offer alternatives to high-cost medications. Inclusion of pharmacists in the medical home is important, as only 33%–50% of patients on chronic medications are completely adherent to medications, and only 32% of patients with adverse reactions seek emergency care. One of the current barriers to expansion of pharmacist services in medical homes is lack of uniform reimbursement strategies to support provision of their services (Smith, Bates, Bodenheimer, & Cleary, 2010).

In the international arena, an inadequate workforce may limit access to ongoing care by pharmacists. According to the World Bank (FIP, 2012b), the number of pharmacies in lower-middle, upper-middle, and high-income economies varies little, but the number of pharmacists working at these sites varies dramatically, with higher density in high-income economies. Furthermore, many African countries have neither pharmacies nor pharmacists. This unequal connection to dispensing and ongoing services presents a challenge, not only to equal access and distribution of medications but also to the crucial patient education component necessary for safe and effective medication use.

Pharmacists' contributions to global health depend on the advancement of pharmaceutical education worldwide. FIP has taken a lead in promoting development of educational standards to advance the pharmacy profession, stating that the profession must have "a professionally educated health-care workforce, an appropriate academic and institutional infrastructure and high quality competency-based education" (FIP, n.d.). FIP has worked to prepare global educational leaders to effect change, using train-the-trainer methods whereby faculty members in schools of pharmacy that have well-developed competency-based education and quality assurance programs collaborate with educators in schools of pharmacy globally to exchange educational best practices. One such example is the US-Thai Consortium for Pharmacy Education, which was established over 20 years ago (US-Thai Consortium, 2016). Efforts toward a Global Competency Framework are also under way, which will provide a framework for schools of pharmacy to facilitate the improvement and standardization of professional requirements for clinically trained pharmacists, including requirements for work in public health (FIP, n.d.).

The US-based Accreditation Council for Pharmacy Education shares an educational advancement vision similar to FIP's. In addition to educational standards designed to ensure that pharmacy students learn to provide high-quality individual patient care, current standards also highlight the need for development of skills to provide population-based care and to function as part of health care teams, the cornerstone of public and global health (Accreditation Council for Pharmacy Education, 2015). In addition, standards call for students to gain skills in evaluating the health needs of the community, understanding medication-use systems, and optimizing medication procurement and distribution.

Students learn best by doing. One such example can be found on the streets of New York: Project Renewal (www.projectrenewal.org/home), where a pharmacy professor holds his clinic in a mobile van, caring for homeless patients with acute care issues related to the diagnosis of HIV/AIDS (St. John's College, n.d.). In collaboration with other health care providers, the professor and his students (closely supervised by the professor) provide care to patients who would otherwise not receive it, and also provide information on medication optimization and strategies to overcome adherence barriers that accompany the challenges of homelessness.

There are other ways pharmacy students can learn about global health through local engagement. Pharmacy students at University of Wisconsin–Madison regularly engage with the local community to address unmet needs. Several years ago, a few pharmacy students interested in global health, in collaboration with community leaders, identified an opportunity to teach elementary school-age children healthy habits as the foundation for healthy living. Together, they identified elementary schools located in lower-resource areas that were interested in hosting a health fair for their students, as well as for the broader community. Pharmacy students partnered with school nurses, public health providers, community clinics, charitable pharmacies, a dental office, and nutrition experts, as well as medical and nursing students, to orchestrate this unique health outreach program. Elementary students participated in a daylong multilingual program with topics including nutrition, exercise, poison control, and dental hygiene. Activities were presented at an age-appropriate level with many hands-on experiences. After school, parents and community members were also invited to come to the health fair to learn about a variety of health topics. Adults were offered free blood pressure, cholesterol, and diabetes screenings with licensed health professionals on site to help navigate next steps should further follow-up be required. This community-based health outreach model, now in its fourth year, has been sustainable and scalable, now reaching multiple elementary schools throughout the city.

Pharmacy-based research also contributes to improvement in the health care system and public health (Vivian, Colbert, & Remington, 2013). One example is that of a pharmacist educator at UW–Madison whose community-based, participatory research program engages and trains adolescents with type 2 diabetes to mentor their peers who also have type 2 diabetes in making healthier choices. An unexpected, but welcome, by-product of the intervention was that the parents and guardians of both groups learned from their children what it means to eat healthily and the importance of regular, routine exercise. These community health and wellness programs, including peer-to-peer mentoring, have been shown to improve the health of individuals and communities, but also require considerable time to create the deep relationships necessary to develop and keep the trust of the community.

Pharmacists are making a global impact through a comparative health systems approach to quality improvement and implementation of best practices (Seys Ranola, Kraus, & DiPrete Brown, 2014). This is accomplished through pharmacists' involvement not only in direct patient care, education, and access to medicine but also in the monitoring and evaluation of programs to ensure quality outcomes and promote sustainability.

A global comparative approach to population-based health systems improvement was recently developed at UW–Madison (Seys Ranola et al., 2014). Pharmacist researchers from UW–Madison and colleagues from an international partner institution met to discuss needs-based quality improvement ideas of mutual interest. Together, they chose a quality improvement theme of antimicrobial stewardship, a prominent topic around the globe considering the rise of "superbugs" that no longer respond to gold-standard antimicrobial therapies. The systems in which these pharmacists work, and the types of antibiotic resistance they work with, may look different. However, the goals of decreasing the improper use of antibiotics and implementing system-wide protocols to influence prescribing are the same. Initially, pharmacist researchers were trained in the principles of continuous quality improvement (CQI). This framework bridges the gap between research and practice and provides a foundation to assess the effects of the intervention. To deepen the knowledge base of CQI, these same pharmacists were also trained in the tenets of implementation science to conduct and publish their research, thereby contributing to the body of literature related to best practices.

■ ■ ■

Pharmacists work to ensure access to high-quality medications worldwide, and also work with patients to ensure safe and effective use of medications. International collaborations between pharmacist practitioners, educators, and researchers are crucial for strengthening pharmacy practice standards, preparing student pharmacists for providing high-quality pharmaceutical care to individual patients, evaluating the health needs of the community, and improving use of medications in the health care system through research and scholarship.

Suggested Reading

Gogo, A. (2012). Combatting the counterfeit drug trade. TedxBoston. Retrieved from https://www.youtube.com/watch?v=4ZIwOoaCPxI

Smith, M. (2014). Pharmacists' role in public and population health. *Annals of Public Health and Research, 1*(2), 1006.

Ulbrich, T. (2013). Medication therapy management: Utilizing the pharmacist to control our health care costs. TedxUniversity at Buffalo. Retrieved from https://www.youtube.com/watch?v=QnCGD05u58k

References

Accreditation Council for Pharmacy Education. (2015). Accreditation standards and key elements for the professional program in pharmacy leading to the doctor of pharmacy degree. Retrieved from https://www.acpe-accredit.org/pdf/Standards2016FINAL.pdf

Attaran, A., Barry, D., Basheer, S., Bate, R., Benton, D., Chauvin, J., . . . McKee, M. (2012). How to achieve international action on falsified and substandard medicines. *BMJ, 345*, e7381. doi:10.1136/bmj.e7381

Cox, C., Kamal, R., Jankiewicz, A., & Rousseau, D. (2016). Recent trends in prescription drug costs. *Journal of the American Medical Association, 315*, 1326. doi:10.1001/jama.2016.2646

International Pharmaceutical Federation. (n.d.). FIP Foundation and pharmacy education. Retrieved from http://fip.org/www/index.php?page=awardsandthefipfoundation_fipfoundation_education

International Pharmaceutical Federation. (2012a). About health literacy. Retrieved from http://fip.org/www/index.php?page=about_health_literacy

International Pharmaceutical Federation. (2012b). *Global pharmacy workforce report 2012.* Retrieved from http://apps.who.int/medicinedocs/documents/s20206en/s20206en.pdf

International Pharmaceutical Federation. (2012c). *Good pharmacy practice: Joint FIP/WHO guidelines on GPP: Standards for quality of pharmacy services.* Retrieved from http://fip.org/www/uploads/database_file.php?id=331&table_id=

Seys Ranola, T., Kraus, C., & DiPrete Brown, L. (2014). *Comparative health systems global pharmacy fellowship.* Unpublished proposal, University of Wisconsin–Madison School of Pharmacy.

Smith, M., Bates, D. W., Bodenheimer, T., & Cleary, P. D. (2010). Why pharmacists belong in the medical home. *Health Affairs, 29*, 906–913. doi:10.1377/hlthaff.2010.0209

St. John's College. (n.d.). Pharmacy professor John Conry takes his expertise to the streets of Manhattan. Retrieved from http://www.stjohns.edu/sites/default/files/documents/FaithService/pharmacy_professor_john_conry_takes_his_expertise_to_the_streets_of_manhattan.pdf

US-Thai Consortium. (2016). About US THAI Consortium. Retrieved from http://www.usthaiconsortium.org/site/about_conference

Vivian, E. M., Colbert, L. H., & Remington, P. L. (2013, September). Lessons learned from a community based lifestyle intervention for youth at risk for type 2 diabetes. *Journal of Obesity & Weight Loss Therapy, 13*(1). doi:10.4172/2165-7904.1000191

Wisconsin Pharmacy Quality Collaborative. (2016). What is the Wisconsin Pharmacy Quality Collaborative? Retrieved from http://www.pswi.org/WPQC/About-WPQC/About-WPQC

World Health Organization. (2015). *Median availability of selected generic medicines: Data by country.* Global Health Observatory Data Repository. Retrieved from http://apps.who.int/gho/data/view.main.660

World Health Organization. (2016). Substandard, spurious, falsely labelled, falsified and counterfeit (SSFFC) medical products. Retrieved from http://www.who.int/mediacentre/factsheets/fs275/en/

CHAPTER 35

REFLECTIONS AND STEPPING-STONES TO A CAREER IN GLOBAL HEALTH

Cindy Haq, MD

Don't ask yourself what the world needs. Ask yourself what makes you come alive, and go do that, because what the world needs is people who have come alive.

—Howard Thurman

What follows in this chapter are reflections on the life of a woman, mother, and family physician engaged in local and global health over three decades. These reflections reveal an intertwining of personal and professional aspirations. Love and commitment to family drove my career choices and, in turn, career influenced my family and life circumstances. I share steps that enabled me to address personal, family, and professional goals through local and global efforts. This is an invitation for health professionals, young and old, to reflect on their own lives, professional priorities, and critical decisions.

Family and Values

Born to an American mother and (Asian) Indian father, I was raised in and between two cultures. I witnessed profound poverty, prejudice, and oppression, and I developed appreciation for beauty, dignity, kindness, and basic human rights. Drawn to medicine by the opportunity to integrate science with humanitarian work, I was determined to develop skills to help others who were less fortunate. Early marriage and child rearing required me to address personal and professional needs throughout my career.

Foundations for Global Health Practice, First Edition. Lori DiPrete Brown.
© 2018 John Wiley & Sons, Inc. Published 2018 by John Wiley & Sons, Inc.

Medical School and Residency

As I nervously prepared for my first interview for medical school, a college counselor coached me through common questions. "What will you tell them you do in your spare time?" I replied, "I enjoy cooking, gardening, and time with my husband and one-year-old son." My advisor said, "No! Never tell them you have a child or you'll never get into medical school."

Early on, I was told that it was not be possible to be a mother and a physician. "You must be married to medicine and willing to give up the rest of your life to be worthy of the honor of being a physician." "Women [medical students] waste spots that could be used more effectively by men." These messages resulted in a fearful suppression of my identity. I felt that I had to pretend to be someone other than who I was in order to be a good physician.

However, my love of life, a supportive husband, and beautiful children kept me going and drew me out of the sucking vortex of medicine. During residency, I was plagued with exhaustion, self-doubt, and guilt. There was not enough time to be a good parent and physician, let alone pursue work abroad. I had to find time to cook, play, and garden, for these were activities that sustained me and my family. Only after I negotiated to extend three years of training into four did I find space to breathe.

Early International Experience

I wanted to work abroad because that is where I felt the needs were greatest. However, it was challenging to find such work with a husband and, by then, three children. The *Journal of the American Medical Association* published a list of physician volunteer opportunities abroad each year. I poured through the lists and wrote—this was before the Internet—to every organization that might accept a new doctor with her family. We were excited when I was accepted by the Minnesota International Health Volunteers to train village health workers in rural Uganda. This was in 1986 at the end of a brutal civil war that had devastated the health system. One in three children died before the age of five; malaria, tuberculosis, and HIV were rampant. I was to be the only physician serving a population of about 500,000, many of whom were internally displaced refugees.

We were too naïve to know what we were getting ourselves into. We could not begin to fathom the devastation that had occurred in Uganda, the strength and resilience of the local people, the cohesion and power of the community to heal, and the ways that this experience would influence our lives. Fortunately, our family survived and thrived. This experience strengthened my resolve to build a career that would enable me to promote high-quality primary health care for disadvantaged populations.

Negotiating Professional Responsibilities

As I gained experience, I recognized that my values and skills could enhance my abilities as a healer. Given my love of patient care, teaching, international work, and my family, I negotiated for an 80% job that would include at least one month off per year to work in low-resource settings. "Part-time" work, limited to three to four days per week until my children were in elementary school, allowed me to savor mothering as I developed my academic skills. International work was not considered as part of my formal duties, as the university was focused on local needs. My colleagues supported my practice through my periodic leaves of absence from local duties.

I loved patient care. Yet I learned that I needed to look beyond caring for individual patients to design and lead educational programs; to cultivate my skills to influence medical education; to recruit, train, and retain motivated health professionals where they are needed most; and to raise my voice as an advocate for justice in health care. I needed to find others with similar goals, build teams to strengthen medical education and health systems, and target efforts where they had a chance to have long-lasting impact. I carefully sought opportunities to pursue my passion for international work in Pakistan, China, Afghanistan, and elsewhere.

Reflecting back, I could not have predicted how my seminal experience in Uganda more than 30 years ago would influence my career as a medical educator and in global health. This experience heightened my awareness of the social determinants of health, the power of community, and the resilience of the human spirit. It galvanized my commitment to work with medically underserved people, to promote health equity and humanism in medicine, and to hone my skills as a health advocate for individuals and communities at home and around the world. It strengthened my resolve to work for health system improvement and the expansion of access to high-quality primary health care for all.

Stepping-Stones

These stepping-stones outline some of the principles that can help guide you as you reflect on your aspirations and take action to make them a reality.

■　■　■

Honor your history and relationships. Each of our lives is shaped by a complex web of historical circumstances, experiences, and relationships. Each of us has a unique background and motivations. Our values, behavior, and choices emerge from these conditions. Your decisions will be strongly influenced by your stage in life, whom you love, and how you can make a living. These conditions will determine whether you can work abroad, when, for how long, and in which locations.

Follow your passions and pursue your core values. Whatever gives you energy and gets you excited will fuel your drive, determination, and creativity. Pursue your dreams! When you're excited about a goal, you're more likely to remain committed and to overcome what may be numerous challenges. Given the current and projected global shortages of human resources for health, there is an endless supply of global health needs and opportunities where you can make a contribution. When you match your passion with an area of need, you will be able to sustain your motivation to find the resources and time to pursue these interests.

Create your own opportunities. Building a career in global health is like choosing your own adventure. Each choice you make opens doors that will lead to others. Each experience can lead to a dead end or to additional opportunities. Initially, you may feel like an overwhelmed observer and unsure of your abilities. If you don't yet have all the skills needed to pursue your dreams, seek additional training and/or experienced mentors who have those skills so that you can learn from them and contribute to their efforts. You will be able to do more as you gain experience and confidence. Don't give up. Keep moving!

If you are negotiating between a domestic and global health career, be sure to honor your local colleagues and obligations. Work hard so that you become a valued colleague and member of your group. Support your colleagues when they need time away from practice. Carefully communicate and plan your leaves of absence and help your colleagues make backup plans. As you add value to your domestic work group, you will gain credibility, negotiating power, and the ability to attract additional resources.

Strive for balance between personal and professional obligations. This may be the greatest challenge, as there is always more work to be done in global health. Yet you are the only person who can care for yourself and honor your relationships with loved ones. Each of us needs to find and maintain a healthy equilibrium. Your energy and commitment may change due to personal and family circumstances and life's seasons.

Finally, take time to have fun, cultivate new friendships, savor pleasures, catch the sunset, and smell the flowers. These experiences add depth, value, and rewards that will fuel your fires. Remember, given the world's vast unmet health needs, your career is a marathon and not a sprint. The world needs you to remain energized and engaged for the long term!

Consider the prompts in Box 35.1 as you reflect on your own personal and professional goals.

BOX 35.1
STEPPING-STONES

Honor your history and relationships

- Whom do you love? Who loves you?
- Sustain loving relationships.

Discover your passion and core values

- What do you enjoy?
- What gets you excited and energized?
- What areas of need match your passions?
- What are you good at?

Create your own opportunities

- Work hard! Aim high!
- Add value near and far.
- Negotiate for your career interests.
- Look for a good fit; support your colleagues, and they will support you.
- Seek supportive mentors.

Strive for balance between personal and professional responsibilities

- Hone yourself, your most important tool.
- Take time for self-care and renewal.
- Don't try to do it alone; reach out to family, friends, mentors, and colleagues.
- Honor your life seasons; don't try to do it all at once.
- Discover, explore, and enjoy!

CHAPTER 36

GLOBAL HEALTH AND EDUCATION

Nancy Kendall, PhD

An educated, enlightened, and informed population is one of the surest ways of promoting the health of a democracy.

—Nelson Mandela

The Sustainable Development Goals (SDGs) call on the global community to end poverty, protect the planet, and ensure prosperity for all. In order to achieve the SDGs, I believe we will need a new approach to synchronizing the global education, health, and equity efforts that underlie our capacity to achieve all other SDGs. Without good health and general well-being (SDG 3), without education and lifelong learning for all (SDG 4), and without gender equity and women's empowerment (SDG 5) occurring in tandem, most other SDGs simply cannot be attained. There are large and well-established relationships between education and health (Cutler & Lleras-Mooney, 2006) and between gender equity and equitable health and education outcomes. Yet the current organization of the SDGs may make it harder for sustainable development efforts, ideas, and resources to respond holistically (and, therefore, effectively) to people's daily lives and the complex realities that impact their well-being. A vignette from research conducted in Malawi in 2009 (Box 36.1) illustrates this point.

Teresa's story illustrates clearly how education, health, and gender equity work together in complex ways to shape young people's outcomes, and in turn our capacity as an international community to achieve the SDGs.

We did not, as a global community, meet the 2015 Millennium Development Goals (MDGs). Although we made the most progress on meeting the education MDGs (MDGs 3 and 4), education efforts focused largely on getting all children to attend existing schools. This single-sector, "add new children to existing interventions and stir" approach worked for some children, but it did not work for the most marginalized, who, like Teresa, face

Foundations for Global Health Practice, First Edition. Lori DiPrete Brown.
© 2018 John Wiley & Sons, Inc. Published 2018 by John Wiley & Sons, Inc.

BOX 36.1

THE INTERRELATIONS AMONG GENDER, EDUCATION, HEALTH, AND CHILD WELL-BEING IN A TIME OF AIDS

Teresa is 19 years old. Her father left when she was six; her mother died, likely of AIDS, when she was nine. She remembers her mother with great love and fondness. When her mother died, Teresa and her two brothers were sent to live with their uncle in Blantyre, Malawi's largest city. The children attended a good school, and Teresa describes this period as "very happy." Her uncle was wealthy, and treated them as his own. When Teresa was 12, however, her uncle became ill and died. It appears from her description that he likely suffered a heart attack that left him partially paralyzed, then suffered a second, fatal attack soon after.

Teresa and her brothers were then sent to their home village to live with their maternal grandmother. Their grandmother lived in a tiny house with one small farm plot. Although it was a major transition to move to a rural area and to suffer much higher levels of material poverty than before, Teresa says that her grandmother was very loving and did her best to ensure that the children were fed and clothed and that they went to school each day. The children worked hard, including hours of farm labor each day, but they saw a path toward a brighter future through schooling. It was hard to keep up their studies at the local school, though; the children were sometimes teased for being orphans, and the school had very few teaching and learning resources. Nonetheless, their grandmother encouraged them, just as their mother had.

The children suffered a third shock when their grandmother died about two years later. Teresa will not speak about that time. But in the weeks after their grandmother's death, it became increasingly clear to the children that they were stranded in the village. With no access to capital, irregular rains, and no access to irrigation, their tiny "child-headed home" soon faced increasing food insecurity. Teresa and her older brother left school to try to fend for the family. Then, miraculously, another uncle said that he would support Teresa's older brother's education, so that he could finish secondary school, get a job, and take full responsibility for the family. The uncle sent Teresa's older brother to town, where he would stay for the next four years. In the meantime, Teresa was responsible for her younger brother, and the uncle provided no support for their family. After a few months of trying desperately to farm on her own, 15-year-old Teresa decided that her only option was to find a husband. She married a relatively wealthy man in the village, sent her younger brother to school with money she received from her husband, and soon became pregnant.

Four years later, as we interview her, she tells us that her elder brother finished school, could not find a job, and returned home to the village. But friends from secondary school pooled funds to start a business with him, growing and transporting tomatoes. The business is going well, and her brother has even been able to build a good home. Teresa's younger brother moved in with her older brother, and is himself planning to start secondary school soon. Teresa, by contrast, has two children, no primary school degree, and no way to escape a husband whom other community members described as "cruel." Her husband travels a great deal, and Teresa tells us in a soft whisper that her greatest fear was that she, like her mother, would "become ill."

multiple, complex constraints on their capacity to survive and thrive in and out of school. These constraints include deep poverty, the multigenerational effects and traumas of the AIDS syndemic, environmental degradation, limited access to sexual and reproductive health services, fraying community safety nets, no access to psychosocial support services, inequitable gender relations, and climate change, among others.

For young women like Teresa to complete their education, schools themselves will need to change. They will need to provide wraparound health, nutrition, and psychosocial services. They will need to be gender responsive in their curricula and pedagogies. They will need to reassess their goals and focus on supporting each child's well-being within a healthy community (Wallerstein & Bernstein, 1994), instead of primarily preparing each child for a test. Likewise, to achieve the SDGs pertaining to education, health, gender equity, climate change, peace building, and water and sanitation, among others, our efforts will need to be coordinated, multisectoral, multigenerational, and directly responsive to the lived experiences of the world's most disenfranchised children and communities. This is particularly true in sub-Saharan Africa and South Asia—the regions with the greatest numbers of girls and children out of school.

Achieving the SDGs will require a multisectoral and coordinated effort, and education will need to play a key role in these efforts. In Malawi, as in many of the countries furthest from reaching the SDGs, the average age of the population is 16.5 years, the average age of first childbirth is 18, and the fastest-growing HIV infection rates are occurring in girls ages 15–24. Schools are central to reaching these children and youth. Most children are not directly served by institutions other than schools—for example, health efforts (e.g., SDG 4) often do not prioritize the needs of children between age five and reproductive age; wealth-creation efforts (e.g., SDGs 8 and 9) will not usually target people under age 18; and other SDGs may be tied to legal practices (such as land ownership or legal adulthood) that also constrain their focus on children. Schools are widely distributed throughout much of the world, and can therefore serve as effective distribution centers for resources and care provision for the world's most vulnerable children (Kendall & O'Gara, 2007).

Beyond schools' potential role as service provision centers for children and youth, education itself underlies the processes of empowerment and citizenship building that will fuel progress on the SDGs. Where will the next generation learn about climate change or sex education or solar power or the system of government in which they live? Where will girls experience being as smart as boys, and as deserving of adult support? Although there are many potential answers to these questions, we as a global community have agreed that schools should play a key role in preparing children to live in a sustainable 21st century, and the infrastructure to educate, enlighten, and empower through schools now exists throughout much of the world, thanks to the Education for All movement and the MDGs.

In summary, there are many ways in which schools can play a role in achieving the SDGs. First, schools are the only state institutions in most countries that are distributed widely enough to serve as delivery points for food, medicine, ideas, practices, and many more of the resources essential to reaching the SDGs. Second, schools can serve as key sites of collaboration and learning among the various actors involved in improving well-being (e.g., teachers, health workers, agricultural extension workers, veterinary workers, and so forth), so that our efforts to improve well-being can be coordinated and synergized. Third, schools can provide marginalized children with safe spaces, regular routines, and adult care that may no longer be available in their homes or communities. Fourth, schools also offer the promise of transforming the mind-set of a generation of world citizens by aligning their beliefs, attitudes, knowledge, skills, and practices (e.g., SDGs 12, 13, 14, 15, and 16) with those that will support attainment of the SDGs.

For schools to play this robust role in supporting the education, health, and other SDGs, school systems will need to be strengthened and realigned around a holistic model of child, family, and community well-being. Schools will need additional resources to fulfill these new roles, as well as new collaborations across governmental and nongovernmental bodies. Schooling continues to be a cost-effective investment in children's—particularly girls'—well-being (Patrinos, 2008; Sperling & Winthrop, 2015). Many of the world's poorest families, communities, and countries are already investing heavily in schooling, but their resources are strained, and thus their impact is limited. The international community will therefore need to invest heavily in a new, intersectoral model of schooling, health, and equity to achieve the SDGs.

New forms of partnership and collaboration grounded in and responsive to the daily realities of people's lives offer the best chance of leveraging current resources into future fulfillment of the SDGs. Professionals in education and health are best positioned to lead this charge. Although there are important differences between the two sectors, health and education systems and providers can play similar roles in nurturing the root stability from which individual and social well-being can grow. An important first step in achieving this goal is for education and health practitioners and policymakers to learn from each other about children's and youth's lives and to begin to talk to each other about how education and health systems might collaborate to more holistically address young people's—particularly marginalized young people's—needs. Points of initial collaboration are multifarious: from HIV/AIDS education and prevention, to deworming, to school feeding, to empowering girls and boys to transform harmful economic, political, or cultural practices, and many more. There are examples of scaled and sustained health–education collaboration successes around the world, including Tostan and the Bangladesh Rural Advancement Committee, from which we can draw inspiration. There are also developing problem areas—such as how to support the health and well-being of grandmothers caring for orphans in southern Africa in order to ensure that vulnerable children remain protected and supported in their home and in their schooling, or how to understand the links among and long-term repercussions of environmental degradation, malnutrition, and early pregnancy on individual and community well-being—around which collaborations can and should be organized. With political will, economic resources, respect for marginalized communities, and international support for the notion that every person has an inalienable right to basic education and health, we can significantly improve educational and health outcomes—and thus all SDG outcomes.

Suggested Reading and Resources

Education Rights

Bourdillon, M., & Musvosvi, E. (2014). What can children's rights mean when they are struggling to survive? In A.T.D. Imoh & N. Ansell (Eds.), *Children's lives in an era of children's rights: The progress of the Convention on the Rights of the Child in Africa* (pp. 105–122). London, United Kingdom: Routledge.

International Labor Organization. (2008). *Combating child labour through education.* Retrieved from www.ilo.org/ipecinfo/product/download.do?type=document&id=7850

UNESCO. (n.d.). Education for All movement. http://www.unesco.org/new/en/education/themes/leading-the-international-agenda/education-for-all/

Education and Health

Cutler, D. M., & Lleras-Muney, A. (2006). *Education and health: Evaluating theories and evidence* (No. w12352). Cambridge, MA: National Bureau of Economic Research.

Global Campaign for Education. (2014). Global education as a vaccine against HIV/AIDS. Retrieved from http://campaignforeducationusa.org/global-action-week/impact-detail/global-education-as-a-vaccine-against-hiv-aids

Vandemoortele, J., & Delamonica, E. (2000). The "education vaccine" against HIV. *Current Issues in Comparative Education, 3*(1), 6–13.

Education, Health, and Vulnerable Children

Kendall, N., & O'Gara, C. (2007). Vulnerable children, communities and schools: Lessons from three HIV/AIDS affected areas. *Compare: A Journal of Comparative and International Education, 37*(1), 5–21.

Nyambedha, E. O., & Aagaard-Hansen, J. (2010). Educational consequences of orphanhood and poverty in Western Kenya. *Educational Studies, 36,* 555–567.

Skovdal, M. (2010). Children caring for their "caregivers": Exploring the caring arrangements in households affected by AIDS in Western Kenya. *AIDS Care, 22*(1), 96–103.

Education and Gender

Patrinos, H. (2008). Returns to education: The gender perspective. In M. Tembon & L. Fort (Eds.), *Girls' education in the 21st century: Gender equality, empowerment and economic growth* (pp. 53–64). Washington, DC: World Bank.

Tomasevski, K. (2005). *Girls' education through a human rights lens: What can be done differently, what can be made better?* London, United Kingdom: Overseas Development Institute and Rights in Action.

Winthrop, R., & McGivney, E. (2014). *Raising the global ambition for girls' education.* Policy Paper 5. Retrieved from https://www.brookings.edu/wp-content/uploads/2016/06/Winthrop-NextGenGirls-v3.pdf

Community Empowerment and the SDGs

Kendall, N., Kaunda, Z., & Friedson-Rideneur, S. (2015). Community participation in international development education quality improvement efforts: Current paradoxes and opportunities. *Educational Assessment, Evaluation and Accountability, 27*(1), 65–83.

Wallerstein, N., & Bernstein, E. (1994). Introduction to community empowerment, participatory education, and health. *Health Education Quarterly, 21,* 141–148.

Video Resources

Choudry, N. (Producer, director, writer), & Fredericks, A. (Writer). *Time for school: 2003–2016.* Retrieved from http://www.pbs.org/wnet/time-for-school/

Creative Media. (2015, October 16). BRAC education program. YouTube. Retrieved from https://www.youtube.com/watch?v=keogXpIePXY

Kendall, N. (2014). The granny corps. TEDxUWMadison. Retrieved from https://www.youtube.com/watch?v=AUHJh8BUm2w

Media for Development Trust (Producer) & Dangarembga, T. (Director). (1996). *Everyone's child* [Motion picture]. Media Development Trust.

Tostan International. (2010). Tostan: Empowering communities to abandon female genital cutting (FGC). YouTube. Retrieved from https://www.youtube.com/watch?v=JcX32btTU48

References

Cutler, D. M., & Lleras-Muney, A. (2006). *Education and health: Evaluating theories and evidence* (No. w12352). Cambridge, MA: National Bureau of Economic Research.

Kendall, N., & O'Gara, C. (2007). Vulnerable children, communities and schools: Lessons from three HIV/AIDS affected areas. *Compare: A Journal of Comparative and International Education, 37*(1), 5–21.

Patrinos, H. (2008). Returns to education: The gender perspective. In M. Tembon, & L. Fort (Eds.), *Girls' education in the 21st century: Gender equality, empowerment and economic growth* (pp. 53–64). Washington, DC: World Bank.

Sperling, G. B., & Winthrop, R. (2015). *What works in girls' education: Evidence for the world's best investment.* Washington, DC: Brookings Institution Press.

Wallerstein, N., & Bernstein, E. (1994). Introduction to community empowerment, participatory education, and health. *Health Education Quarterly, 21,* 141–148.

CHAPTER 37

THE IMPORTANCE OF NARRATIVE TO GLOBAL HEALTH RESEARCH AND PRACTICE

Louise Penner, PhD

Addressing global health problems requires accurate and robust collection of data about the diverse populations and locations from which global health issues emerge and spread. Although we cannot "see" percentages of people or know much about their lives by interpreting graphs or charts, we can imagine what kinds of benefits, suffering, or harms might be represented in these abstract representations of facts. That this data suggests stories about the people whose lives it represents is important: we interpret the plot details, who the players are, and the significance of the narratives that lie behind that data by combining our imaginative powers with our knowledge of history and context. Consciously or not, we interpret data in part through the stories, fiction and nonfiction, that we have previously encountered.

This chapter suggests that, especially at a time when scientific data is coming under increased scrutiny from those who doubt the arguments of natural and social scientists on key issues such as climate change, we might benefit from focusing on the issue of how narratives emerge from data. Learning to interpret narratives about particular settings and communities—whether those narratives are offered in fiction, memoir, poetry, drama, film, graphic novel, creative nonfiction, or some other form—actually helps us do a better job of contextualizing the public health data we encounter about those settings and communities. In turn, the skills of apt narrative interpretation help us become more affective presenters of public health data to others. Critical reading of literature reminds us that all stories emerge from patterns of information, in the numbers, words,

Foundations for Global Health Practice, First Edition. Lori DiPrete Brown.
© 2018 John Wiley & Sons, Inc. Published 2018 by John Wiley & Sons, Inc.

objects, or behaviors that a storyteller notices in the world and represents for readers or listeners. Reading literature with an eye attuned to storytelling methods, particularly the strategies narrators employ to help us, as readers, see the significance in the patterns of information they represent, can make us better interpreters of what we observe in our lives. It can, as well, help us become better and more effective narrators and interpreters of the stories that lie behind global health data.

Practicing the skills of interpreting and writing imaginative literature gives us the power to shape, analyze, and critique our methods of interpreting stories and data. And literary stories can offer crucial insight that data alone may not. In 1722, Daniel Defoe published his *Journal of the Plague Year,* in which he drew from London parish records of the great plague to tell the story of a shopkeeper recording the stress and despair of the untenable decisions he and his neighbors faced in living through the wave of deaths occurring in his and surrounding neighborhoods in London. The narrative's power lies in part in the vivid portrait of societal collapse that follows the disease outbreak. The parish records are real, verifiable data; Defoe's story is invented. He himself was seven at the time of the plague; his family, other than his grandfather, was not in London at the time. Readers learning these biographical details are tempted to call Defoe's work fraudulent or entirely fictional, and therefore not useful in understanding the plague's effect on real people's lived experience. But, of course, his story is neither fraudulent nor entirely fictional.

As Defoe's example shows, we create narratives to explain our world: as J. Hillis Miller (1990) has written, those narratives can be a reinforcement or confirmation of what we think we already know, or they can shake us up. They can offer us "repetition with a difference," in which case a narrative offers us a familiar and thus predictable setup and then ruptures our expectations, and we are forced to question why we were so secure in our expectations in the first place. The importance of how the repetition of particular kinds of narratives can shape the way we discuss health, illness, and disease was made manifest in Susan Sontag's *Illness as Metaphor* (1978), which served as a call to the Western biomedical community to recognize the ways that language, figurative and otherwise, can shape patients' experiences of health and health care providers. Her work made evident patterns in the creative arts that established and reinforced the unscientific notions that tuberculosis sufferers were more artistic and fragile than other people, whereas cancer patients were victims of their own emotional repression, patterns that, if anything, made patients' struggling with illness vulnerable to the cultural perception that their illness was derived from flaws in their temperament.

The interdisciplinary work of medical humanities scholars, such as Rita Charon (2008), has prompted biomedical professionals to consider how their practices might be improved to take "whole person" and "life course" approaches to their interactions with patients, thus helping them recognize the key role that risk factors such as stress play in chronic health problems. One example of this is the attention Charon brought to the limitations in how patient histories had conventionally been taken and recorded in charts generally focused on vital statistics data. She began training medical students in the taking of "parallel charts" to capture details of patients' narratives that would otherwise have no place in patient records. Medical education has adjusted to the insights of Charon and others: students are now trained to ask open-ended questions about patients' experience of their health, rather than questions focused specifically on physical pain or discomfort, including such previously overlooked matters as patients' work environments and their feelings of personal safety.

But health, illness, and disease are dynamic and permanent features of landscapes that can exist in places far removed from biomedical settings, and our understanding of each requires that we attend to the lives of those who may never make it to a health professional's office. Contemporary public health surveillance has allowed for the production of data about the health of many people around the globe who make up such populations. But interpreting what that data means and how best it can be used requires that we establish complex, nuanced perceptions of the individual and communal lives that the data represents. Only then can we begin to gauge the ways that international and national government policies shape these individual lives and the health of their communities, and thus their lived experience, thereby ensuring that their priorities are attended to, despite the other measures of success we so often prioritize.

As Rajini Srikanth (2016) says in an essay about how literature can encourage empathy, literary texts enable authors "to practice 'what if' scenarios about our own capacity for understanding the 'pain of others' and for recognizing how our power and privilege can contribute to others' injury, whether that be material, political or emotional." This observation is vital if we are to recognize how important it is that we read the stories of others whose experiences of the world and relative positions of privilege—whether economic, racial, gendered, or other—differ from ours. Making the effort to read those stories critically, attempting to remain cognizant of how our own social positioning in relation to the lives depicted within these stories influences how we read, helps us develop skills for interpreting our world and conveying our understanding to others. Consider the importance of reading the stories of and by people living in the areas most vulnerable to environmental devastation that is the result of policies and pollution over which they have had little, if any, say. Leslie Marmon Silko's (1991) *Almanac of the Dead* tells just such a story of indigenous peoples of the United States and Mexico who had generations ago been removed as stewards of land now subject to human-made drought. The multiple narratives of Silko's novel clearly seek to inspire indigenous alliances to serve as land protectors. These stories, like all stories, may show us the personal biases of the writers and a focus on priorities that may or may not be our own. But they can and should focus us, for a time, on the effects of the choices made by people who, like me, live in areas where resources, as well as power over the distribution of resources, tend to be concentrated. They help us recognize where our priorities and our seemingly mundane choices may intersect profoundly with those of others.

The dangers of disregarding the stories of those whose lives are studied largely through data are made evident in literary works focused not just elsewhere but also in US communities. In *My Own Country,* for example, Abraham Verghese (1994) details the period when HIV/AIDS began to spread to rural areas of the southern United States, but was still assumed to be an urban epidemic. He describes how HIV-positive individuals in the Johnson City, Tennessee, area were repulsed by their local physicians. As the area's only infectious disease specialist, Verghese recognized that for him to intervene in a way that would prevent an even larger outbreak would require him to move outside the biomedical setting, to enter the outcast queer community's "safe spaces," including gay bars and trailer park homes, to provide disease and treatment literacy to the community and initiate the spread of that literacy. In *Waist-High in the World: A Life among the Nondisabled,* Nancy Mairs (1997) reorients readers' perspectives to see communities of the nondisabled as foreign environments, thus prompting nondisabled readers' recognition of their own privilege and the potential damage that can be caused to others by perceiving one's own privileged position as "normal." Similarly, Tony Kushner's (1993) play *Angels in America: A Gay Fantasia on National Themes* shows us how power and privilege allow the character Roy Cohn to gain access to antiretrovirals then unavailable to far more sympathetic figures in the play; but Kushner also shows us how the struggles of HIV-positive gay men in America of the 1990s share features with those of other immigrants and isolated individuals who seek a place and a community in which their beliefs, stories, and burdens will be shared or at the very least recognized and understood.

Without such stories, in fact, the lives of those most disadvantaged, the illiterate and disenfranchised, would almost certainly not be known, and the interpretation of public health data about them would be far less meaningful. For example, Rohinton Mistry's (1997) novel *A Fine Balance* offers an unrelentingly harrowing portrait of the severe health and psychological challenges of the "untouchable" class in India and the government's utter neglect of their health challenges (including sources of employment, food, safe housing, sanitation) and its enactment of a mass sterilization campaign during the time of "Emergency" rule (1975–1977). This history informs many of the public health challenges that contemporary India faces, a context that contemporary morbidity and mortality data cannot provide.

The United States has its own examples of such political and societal neglect leading to the erasure of stories from which public health policy would benefit. Sapphire's (1996) novel *Push* offers a more hopeful, if equally disturbing, account of a black pre-teenage girl's journey from illiteracy and familial abuse to literacy and self-sufficiency aided by a teacher and social worker. In an early scene, the child, Precious, recognizes how her future is circumscribed by the school file bearing her name, sitting on top of her principal's desk. Later in the novel, she steals her social worker's file and uses her nascent reading ability to try to decipher the words contained on the pages in front of her. A powerful scene ensues, in which Precious realizes that the information the folder contains—her data, the listing of events from her life as interpreted by the school and her social worker—doesn't represent the dedicated mother, student, and aspiring poet she now knows herself to be. Precious's moment of recognition here helps begin her (and, one hopes, the reader's) outright rejection of the narrative of failure being attached to her. This is a fictional moment from which any public health professional might learn. Sapphire's narrative offers a powerful argument for the need for community engagement in setting the priorities necessary to bring about positive health outcomes, particularly in financially and socially disadvantaged communities. Those who study populations with poor public health outcomes need to recognize that the lives of those they study—their lived experiences of struggle—matter in the setting and implementation of public health and policy agendas.

Public health data is vital to our understanding of our world and the challenges we face in making it a healthier place for all; but the stories produced from that data have the potential either to reveal or obscure details that matter to those who often don't narrate their own stories. The privilege of narrating the stories our data produce requires that all narrators, whatever their mode of producing stories, strive to engage with and understand the lived experience of people whose data they try to contextualize. Reading stories by and about those people may be the best way we have to ensure that our efforts to be objective about data are recognized as themselves limited and situated by our knowledge of history and context and our desire to empathize; we show our recognition that our attempts to be objective in representing others are always necessarily incomplete, and thus we sustain our openness to and invitation for input from those people, lives, and narratives the data represents. We thus enable ourselves to offer not only better analytical accuracy but also more nuanced and accurate presentations of information for all.

References

Charon, R. (2008). *Narrative medicine: Honoring the stories of illness.* New York, NY: Oxford University Press.

Defoe, D. (2003). *A journal of the plague year.* New York, NY: Penguin Classics. (Original work published 1772)

Kushner, T. (1993). *Angels in America: A gay fantasia on national themes.* New York, NY: Theatre Communications Group.

Mairs, N. (1997). *Waist high in the world: A life among the nondisabled.* Boston, MA: Beacon Press.

Miller, J. H. (1990). Narrative. In F. Lentricchia & T. McLaughlin (Eds.), *Critical terms for literary study* (pp. 66–79). Chicago, IL: University of Chicago Press.

Mistry, R. (1997). *A fine balance.* New York, NY: Vintage.

Sapphire. (1996). *Push*. New York, NY: Knopf.

Silko, L. M. (1991). *Almanac of the dead*. New York, NY: Simon & Schuster.

Sontag, S. (1978). *Illness as metaphor*. New York, NY: Farrar, Straus, and Giroux.

Srikanth, R. (2016). Why literature matters in debate about race and immigrants. *AP*. (Original work published on *The Conversation* website) Retrieved from http://bigstory.ap.org/article/2c1a49caaa804bcb8f3375247ad1600e/why-literature-matters-debate-about-race-and-immigrants

Verghese, A. (1994). *My own country*. New York: NY: Simon & Schuster.

CHAPTER 38

THE URBAN OPPORTUNITY FOR GLOBAL HEALTH

Jason Vargo, PhD, MPH, MCRP

Cities have the capability of providing something for everybody, only because, and only when, they are created by everybody.

—Jane Jacobs

Global health and urban health are more closely linked today than at any point in human history. With more than half of the world's population now living in urban areas—and that number expected to rise to nearly three quarters by the end of the century—there's no question that this century is the urban century. Cities have become the dominant human habitat on the planet, and as it is a habitat that we directly and purposefully create, shape, and destroy, there is a huge opportunity to influence the lives of billions with the urban decisions we make. The urban growth that will take place between now and 2100 will be equivalent to everything constructed between Mesopotamian times and the present (United Nations, 2014), and there's little chance that it will, or should, resemble urban growth up to this point. The scale, pace, and reach of this physical, social, and cultural change happening across the globe offer unprecedented opportunities to rethink resource use, distribution, and sharing to benefit global health in profound ways.

The organizational advantages of moving closer to one another and staying in one place have contributed to some of our greatest innovations as a species—agriculture, government, rights, writing, trade—and today cities remain the hubs of creativity, science, and economic activity. These benefits come from agglomeration or, more specifically, from the proximity of people to one another, which results in idea exchange, specialization, and benefits for firms, including decreased transport costs and access to labor (Dawkins, 2003).

This phenomenon, of course, has impacts for health, and stark inequality in cities means that they include both the best and worst conditions for health and health outcomes (World Health Organization & UN Habitat, 2010). The proximity of people to one another presents problems, as density and overcrowding can increase transmission of communicable diseases. The colocation of populations and industry also means that people sometimes have little choice but to live in close proximity to hazardous levels of pollution. But cities also house amenities that protect and preserve health, such as water treatment plants or the largest hospitals with the most expertise. The density of cities offers economies of scale that make such investments possible. It's a part of what can make removing a single pump handle so effective in halting a cholera epidemic.

A question central to making cities as healthy as possible is how to best capitalize on urban advantages and to secure accessibility for all. The fundamental thread tying together urban planning and public health is a principal interest in preempting problems and addressing them by focusing on underlying, root, or upstream conditions. For the physical environment, this begins with infrastructure.

Shared infrastructure can be crucial to long-term public health in cities and thus, on a larger scale, to global health. It is an investment that is used by many or all of a city's residents on a regular basis. Basic infrastructure can determine access to health care, exposures to risk, and economic opportunities for individuals. Investments in infrastructure are important to get right because they are long lasting, expensive, and difficult to retrofit, and they determine many other future decisions.

Some of the most common infrastructures to be associated with urban development are networks, such as electric grids, roads and sewers, pipes, and treatment facilities, to facilitate energy delivery, transport, water provision, and waste removal. These "hard infrastructure" elements provide essential services and have enabled tremendous decreases in communicable diseases as populations have developed. The overall increase in a nation's or population's wealth has been seen in parallel with urban and epidemiological transitions, where childhood mortality, family size, and communicable disease incidence decrease, and chronic diseases and lifespan increase as a group urbanizes and becomes more wealthy. The disparity between nations along these trajectories also exists within nations along urban-rural lines. In today's global economy, cities are often the drivers of national economic growth and thus experience earlier a larger share of the development. The benefits of outsized investment for urban infrastructures contribute to greater health improvements for urban dwellers compared to rural counterparts.

As new cities are constructed around the world, infrastructure will be some of the first things to be put in place. The physical infrastructures noted earlier are often thought to be a necessary first step to development—providing basic services like clean water, energy, and mobility. Indeed, little else can be developed in a place without a road first connecting it to outside people and resources. However, the presence of such transportation infrastructure is not enough to guarantee health. Access is often limited due to inequalities and inequities, be they economic, cultural, or spatial. For example, the utility of a new road depends on the availability of a vehicle and one's ability to purchase a vehicle. Even if a person has access to capital for a vehicle, the use of a car or motorcycle may be restricted, formally and informally, on the basis of age or gender.

Urban health, and thus major public health efforts around the globe, can be aided by more dedicated and focused consideration of infrastructure. In the most obvious way, this may accomplished by paying greater attention to the factors related to disparity in accessing existing infrastructures. This involves, for example, providing subsidies directly to individuals to cover the costs of utility hookups and energy, or implementing other city-wide programs to increase usage—for example, in the form of transit that makes certain routes and roads more useful to those without a car. Still, these fixes are compensating for flaws in the infrastructure networks themselves. In new and emerging cities, where there is an opportunity to design and build such systems initially, these issues may be resolved more effectively.

Bogotá, Colombia—a city infamous as one of the most dangerous in the world—was transformed, largely under the leadership of mayors Antanas Mockus and Enrique Peñalosa, into a model of citizen-focused planning. The period of change covered a decade and involved financial and civic efforts in addition to large construction projects. The investments and construction done around the city, particularly around projects that sought to equalize per capita metrics of transportation and public spaces, received specific attention and encapsulated what Peñalosa calls "democratic equality." For example, a bus with 80 people on it has the right to 80 times the space of an individual driver in their car alone. This principle was embodied in large projects to build a bus rapid transit system with dedicated lanes, and networks of bicycle and pedestrian paths (*ciclorutas*). The improvements in the transportation network for nonmotorized modes improved the options available to many of Bogotá's residents and increased the amount of travel by these modes in the city (Verma, Lopez, & Pardo, 2014). The benefits of these shifts include increased physical activity, decreased air and noise pollution, fewer injuries, and reductions in emissions that cause climate change (De Nazelle et al., 2011).

Bogotá's approach was additionally innovative in that it expanded the scope of necessary public infrastructures for supporting the well-being of the city's residents. In addition to transportation, there was an emphasis placed on public spaces, including libraries and parks. The quality and number of parks were improved. Such spaces are important for giving people places to exercise, socialize, and mentally recover. Libraries have long been seen as an informational resource, but are increasingly being rethought as places for creative exploration, skill building, and community organization; thus libraries are fundamental to facilitating the best aspects of idea exchange that we associate with cities and urban living.

A couple of themes run through the investments in Bogotá. The first is that they are widely accessible and usable for residents, regardless of age and ability. The universal utility of the infrastructures focused on by Bogotá is captured in the name "8 80 Cities" (http://www.880cities.org/), a nonprofit that is working to improve cities and well-being globally (led by Enrique Peñalosa's brother, Gil, who formerly directed Bogotá's Parks Department). Unlike a traditional road, which requires a trained and capable driver and vehicle, ciclorutas are open to and utilized by children (age 8) and grandparents (age 80) on foot, bike, or skates, or in a wheelchair. Central to this idea is the involvement of citizens in the city's decision making itself.

An important factor in the success of the program was the emphasis placed on the quality of these new investments. There was a conscious effort to ensure that these new paths, buildings, and spaces were not seen as second-class projects. Such attention is important for ensuring that the desired outcome of the investment is accomplished— namely, that people will use the new building, plaza, or park. Low-quality public spaces will be used, but only by those who have little other choice. High-quality public spaces become destinations, the kinds of places people go out of their way to enjoy and that continue to stimulate development in adjacent properties (Gehl, 2013).

Design alone, however, is not enough to ensure that infrastructure will maximally contribute to well-being in cities. Infrastructures interact with policy—in particular, land use—and thinking about how to combine these facets can ensure efficiency and success for public investments. The emergence of relatively new ideas such as transit-oriented development (TOD) aim to unite physical infrastructures (a rail or bus station) with policy (mixed-use zoning) and affordable housing so that transportation investments reach as many people as possible and ensure that those with the greatest need have secure access.

The sharing of ideas and innovations globally among cities is important for making the most of our urban opportunity for global health. The pace of urbanization requires that cities adopt and adapt the best practices of city planning, infrastructure design, public finance, and civic engagement. There is a tremendous opportunity for cities to "leapfrog" urban development practices and avoid the pitfalls of previously pursued paths. The consequences of infrastructure decisions are far reaching, difficult to foresee, and sometimes unintended. It is important that governments, engineers, and planners facing these decisions today are aware of the context and long-term impacts of their decisions.

Consider, for example, the legacy in the United States of pursuing investments in high-speed, high-volume, auto-focused road projects that have expanded America's metropolitan areas. Although those policies opened access to cheap land on the fringe of urban areas for many Americans, they've also promoted sprawling growth that is linked to unsustainable dependencies on automobiles and fossil fuels and to the consumption of valuable productive farmland, and that has left some communities isolated both physically and socially.

■ ■ ■

The story of global urbanization is one that keeps me optimistic. The raw numbers of human population growth and movement make cities a focal point for improving global health. Beyond shaping the physical environment that billions of people inhabit, cities also play an important role in developing, supporting, and rolling out larger public health initiatives and interventions. They are the seats of economic, cultural, and political power and thus have major influence over the laws, regulations, and conditions for healthy and just development well beyond their borders. Moreover, they are places of constant dynamism, eager to learn and try new things. Individually, they are places that can improve the lives of their residents; collectively, cities can improve the health of us all.

Recommended Reading

Cities: An interactive data visual. International Institute for Environment and Development. Retrieved from http://www.iied.org/cities-interactive-data-visual

Harvey, D. (2008, September-October). The right to the city. *New Left Review, 53,* 23–40. Retrieved from https://newleftreview.org/II/53/david-harvey-the-right-to-the-city

McGranahan, G., & Satterthwaite, D. (2014, August). *Urbanisation: Concepts and trends.* International Institute for Environment and Development. Retrieved from http://pubs.iied.org/10709IIED/

Rydin, Y., Bleahu, A., Davies, M., Dávila, J. D., Friel, S., De Grandis, G., . . . Lai, K. M. (2012). Shaping cities for health: Complexity and the planning of urban environments in the 21st century. *The Lancet, 379,* 2079–2108. Retrieved from http://www.ucl.ac.uk/healthy-cities/outputs/lancet

World Health Organization. (2016). *Global report on urban health: Equitable healthier cities for sustainable development.* Retrieved from http://who.int/kobe_centre/measuring/urban-global-report/en/

References

Dawkins, C. J. (2003). Regional development theory: Conceptual foundations, classic works, and recent developments. *Journal of Planning Literature, 18,* 131–172.

De Nazelle, A., Nieuwenhuijsen, M. J., Antó, J. M., Brauer, M., Briggs, D., Braun-Fahrlander, C., . . . Hoek, G. (2011). Improving health through policies that promote active travel: A review of evidence to support integrated health impact assessment. *Environment International, 37,* 766–777.

Gehl, J. (2013). *Cities for people.* Washington, DC: Island Press.

United Nations, Department of Economic and Social Affairs. (2014). *World urbanization prospects: The 2014 revision: Highlights* (ST/ESA/SER.A/352). Retrieved from https://esa.un.org/unpd/wup/publications/files/wup2014-highlights.Pdf

Verma, P., Lopez, J. S., & Pardo, C. (2014). *Bicycle account: Bogotá 2014.* Bogotá, Colombia: Despacio. Retrieved from http://www.despacio.org/wp-content/uploads/2015/01/Bicycle-Account-BOG-2014-20150109-LR.pdf

World Health Organization & UN Habitat. (2010). *Hidden cities: Unmasking and overcoming health inequities in urban settings.* Retrieved from http://www.who.int/kobe_centre/publications/hidden_cities2010/en/

CHAPTER 39

BUILDING EFFECTIVE HEALTH SYSTEMS IN TRANSITIONAL SOCIETIES

LESSONS FROM POSTWAR ETHIOPIA, RWANDA, AND SOUTH SUDAN

Augustino Ting Mayai, PhD

Political violence has deleterious long-term effects on health care and other social systems. Transition to stability takes tremendous amounts of resources, time, and wisdom. In eastern Africa, Ethiopia, Rwanda, and South Sudan have experienced devastating civil wars. Restoring health services delivery became a top objective of these countries' governments, which subsequently invested millions or billions of dollars in the sector. In this chapter, I analyze the importance of decentralization, financial investment, and good governance in the development of health care systems in transitional states, focusing on Ethiopia, Rwanda, and South Sudan.

Investments and Impacts in Health

Rebuilding health systems in transitional states has dominated the international development agenda for decades. This is partly so because health systems recovery implies restoration of peace and stability (Kruk, Freedman, Anglin, & Waldman, 2010; OECD, 2012). These incentives not only engender good health but also encourage economic growth, for quality health translates into productive economic outcomes (Deaton, 2003; World Bank, 2013). More specifically, Bloom, Canning, and Sevilla (2004, p. 1) find

Foundations for Global Health Practice, First Edition. Lori DiPrete Brown.

that "good health has a positive, sizable, and statistically significant effect on aggregate economic output." In sub-Saharan Africa, publicly funded service programs are largely aimed at alleviating economic hardships among the rural poor and raising living standards in these communities (Basinga et al., 2011; Gertler & Vermeersch, 2013). This relationship between health and economic opportunity is readily invoked because economic vulnerabilities are associated with poor health outcomes (Deaton, 2003).

There is ample evidence of success in health care investments. For instance, in Ethiopia, infant and child health improved significantly following a substantial investment in public health programs (Central Statistical Agency/Ethiopia and ICF International, 2012). Between 2005 and 2011, Ethiopia saw a reduction of nearly 30% in childhood mortality, a substantial increase in the proportion of rural residents with access to safe drinking water, and a reasonably declining poverty incidence across historically disadvantaged districts (Central Statistical Agency/Ethiopia and ICF International, 2012; Human Development Africa [HDA], 2013). Further research suggests that these significant health transitions in Ethiopia align sufficiently with the introduction of the Promoting Basic Service (PBS) program, which now supports the Health Extension Program (HEP), Ethiopia's premier health system designed mainly to improve basic health for the country's rural poor (Asefa, Drewett, & Tessema, 2000).

The Rwandan public health system has also achieved remarkable results in the last 20 years (Logie, Rowson, & Ndagije, 2008; Basinga et al., 2011; Morgan, 2009; Gertler & Vermeersch, 2013; Ministry of Health Rwanda [MoH] et al., 2014). Rwanda's health improvements are primarily owed to a host of governance factors, most significantly the health care system, which distributes health services to municipalities or districts, with each district supplying all necessary health services to roughly 20,000 people (Logie et al., 2008). The system is also supported through workers' and health centers' performance incentives, as well as a number of inexpensive nationwide health insurance premiums. Since 2000, Rwanda has enjoyed drastic declines in early-age and maternal mortality (MoH et al., 2014; Bucagu, 2016).

South Sudan's health care system, in contrast, has not been as effective as the Ethiopian and Rwandan systems have been. After more than 10 years since the new health system was introduced, when self-rule as a region of Sudan was acquired, South Sudan's health conditions remain the worst in the entire region (Mayai, 2015). These differential health outcomes across similar health care systems are expected, as arrays of contributing factors, including application of governance tools, are likely to differ, sometimes radically. The government of South Sudan makes marginal budgetary contributions toward health service delivery. This situation is compounded by pervasive corruption due to lack of robust oversight and accountability measures. Consequently, the country's health outcomes do not correlate with its public spending level (Mayai, 2015, 2016).

Successful Practices: Health Extension Workers in Ethiopia

Ethiopia emerged from violent conflicts around the turn of the 20th century, and committed to various development programs, both locally and internationally, including the Millennium Development Goals (MDGs). Service delivery became one of the country's main development priorities, and its government designed programs aimed at investing in service sector institutions such as health, education, and infrastructure (HDA, 2013; Central Statistical Agency/Ethiopia and ICF International, 2012; Susuman, 2012; El-Saharty, Kebede, Dubusho, & Siadat, 2009). To promote better health, Ethiopia instituted the HEP in 2003 (World Bank, 2013). The HEP was birthed by the Ethiopian government to address problems of universal coverage of primary health care in the country (World Bank, 2013). The HEP was first introduced in 2003 in agrarian communities before it was subsequently scaled up and expanded to pastoral and urban areas. The program currently delivers a host of health packages falling under three broad service branches: preventive, promotive, and curative (World Bank, 2013). All of these services are available for free to all Ethiopians in need.

There have been significant improvements in the health of Ethiopians after the installation of the HEP (Central Statistical Agency/Ethiopia and ICF International, 2012). More specifically, morbidity has decreased, access to family medicine has increased, and hygiene and environmental conditions have improved. The HEP is now credited with a decrease in under-five mortality from 123 per 1,000 live births to 88 per 1,000 live births between 2005 and 2011; access to contraceptives rose from 15% to 29%; under-five stunting declined by 8%; there has been 10% reduction in anemia incidence among women; and access to and use of insecticide-treated nets increased by nearly 40% (Central Statistical Agency/Ethiopia and ICF International, 2012). In addition, access to safe drinking water in the rural areas has improved—rising from 35% to 71% (Central Statistical Agency/Ethiopia and ICF International, 2012; HDA, 2013). Overall, the HEP has been highly effective in improving early-age health in Ethiopia. It has reduced infant mortality by 30% and under-five mortality by 28% (Mayai, 2015).

Successful Practices: Decentralization, Access, and Coordination in Rwanda

Following the 1994 genocide, many social and economic institutions in Rwanda collapsed, and its real income plummeted to a record low, subsequently exacerbating poor socioeconomic circumstances in the country (Akresh & de Walque, 2008). Rwanda's under-five mortality went from 151 in 1992 to 196 in 2000, and maternal mortality went from 611 to 1,071 during the same period (MoH et al., 2014). After stabilization,

Rwanda instituted a substantial reform agenda, both social and political, to confront these enormous recovery tasks brought about by destructive political violence. Between 1996 and 2013, Rwanda adopted a range of health policy and poverty reduction programs, beginning with mutual health insurance meant to enhance maternal health surveillance (MoH et al., 2014).

A postconflict Rwanda has become popular among development partners and in the region for its reputed three-track health care system that combines aid coordination with nationwide health insurance schemes and a performance-based reward program for health facilities and service providers (Logie et al., 2008; Morgan, 2009). With decentralized health care governance shared between national and subnational governments, these peace-dividend programs were primarily designed to respond to dismal child and maternal health conditions.

Rwanda understood that its reconstruction commitments would face the impediments of weak institutions and governance, conditions that are often pervasive in a postconflict environment, so it instituted a range of measures that guaranteed the government's political support and promoted transparency and accountability. First, to meet the health system reform objectives, especially the MDGs, as the country transitioned out of war, the Rwandan government demonstrated a regionally unparalleled political will by mobilizing closely monitored foreign aid, as well as setting up decently coordinated structures across health services providers, private or otherwise (MoH et al., 2014). Early-age, maternal, and reproductive health and improvement in nutrition took center stage in the new system. Thus, integrating private and public health systems under the supervision of the National Ministry of Health of Rwanda ultimately eased the system's monitoring and evaluation, empowered the providers, and enabled the effective delivery of essential health services nationwide. Second, the government established monitoring and evaluation policies and frameworks (i.e., a health management information system) to continuously appraise returns on investments for improvements, aid in priorities realignment, and keep the stakeholders informed of the progress (MoH et al., 2014). Lastly, Rwanda made significant investments in producing skilled health professionals. This enabled a per capita increase in the number of qualified human resources offering basic services across the country. These trained health workers have been reinforced with performance incentives, essentially nudging them toward greater productivity.

Ongoing Efforts in South Sudan

South Sudan, which recently gained independence, is struggling to reap meaningful outcomes from its prevailing health development programs. Instead, ineffective governance, corruption, and institutional weakness seem to thwart the country's health initiatives, hence limiting returns on strategic health investments there.

South Sudanese health care governance is shared between the central government and state governments. After the country attained peace in 2005, restoring the health system to provide direly needed services became a priority in the region, with substantial health financing required (Carrin, Evans, & Xu, 2007; Mayai, 2008). At independence in 2011, the country had fewer than 500 professionally trained medical doctors and fewer than 10 public hospitals nationwide (MoH & National Bureau of Statistics, 2013; Mayai, 2015, 2016).

Between 2006 and 2011, the South Sudanese central government funded health services at the state level with little regard to differences in needs. The country's health care administration has been operating under two forms of decentralization—devolution and delegation—to help restore primary health care standards. However, only 4% of the government's total annual spending has been going toward health, less than recommended in the 2000 Abuja Declaration (African Union, 2001; Gubbins & de Walque, 2012). In particular, South Sudan spent on average US\$3.19 (\$0.41–\$17.05) per person on health between 2006 and 2010 (Mayai, 2015). The per capita transfers at the national level varied annually between a low of \$0.78 in 2008 to a relatively high \$7.97 in 2006. Although the national government's average transfers to states differ modestly across states, there have been significant per capita spending variations due to differences in population size. For instance, the state of Western Bahr el Ghazal, whose population size is much smaller than that of the rest of the states, averaged \$7.79 per person over five years, whereas Jonglei, the most populous state of all, averaged \$1.77 per person during the same period. There are also within-state differences in per capita spending. More specifically, the state of Upper Nile spent \$0.57 per person in 2008, down from \$5.47 in 2006. By far, Western Bahr el Ghazal spent more (\$17.05) on health than any other state in 2006. Overall, in the 2006 fiscal year, there seems to have been relatively higher health spending compared to the periods that followed. In contrast, the 2008 fiscal year saw funding for salaries only.

Lessons for South Sudan and Other Transitional Societies

Why are the health systems designs delivering in Ethiopia and Rwanda but not in South Sudan, and how can transitional societies provide health care effectively? Review of the earlier case studies suggests three strategies to consider.

First, it is important to note that all of the three nations, upon emerging from violence, adopted a decentralization mechanism for their health care administration (Bossert & Beauvais, 2002; Bossert, Chitah, & Bowser, 2003; Bossert & Mitchell, 2011). Decentralization, as many studies suggest, engenders positive health returns because it promotes good governance (Faguet, 2004; Crook & Sverrisson, 1999). This is imperative in societies whose fundamental systems of governance have been ruined by war.

Second, Ethiopia and Rwanda partly owe their outstanding performance to adequate financial commitments to primary health care. Both countries allocate significant portions of their annual national gross economic production toward health. Ethiopia spends over a billion US dollars on health annually. Rwanda provides performance incentives on top of basic budgetary distributions to boost health production.

Third, and perhaps the most important lesson, is that good governance plays a fundamental role in the effectiveness of basic services programming more generally and particularly in health. This finding complements insights from prior research, especially in the Sudan, Philippines, and China (World Bank, 2013; Uchimura & Jütting, 2009; Azfar & Gurgur, 2008). In particular, a number of critical measures, which have not yet been pursued in South Sudan, enabled positive health returns in Ethiopia and Rwanda. Chiefly, the two countries prioritized a joint supervisory role of health care delivery programming among central, state or provincial, and subnational governments. This minimizes corruption and maximizes the likelihood of achieving positive results. Ethiopia took extra strides by encouraging civil society institutions to participate in and enhance health services planning, transparency, and accountability decisions. This participatory governance allowed local players to identify their most pressing priorities and strengthened relevant bureaucratic processes, hence increasing accountability and potent health results.

In summary, effective health care in transitional states demands more than just the financial resources international aid institutions offer soon after the state emerges from civil violence. Although these resources are essential in accelerating transition, participatory governance, increased transparency and accountability, and demonstrated political will by national and subnational authorities appear to be more imperative in ensuring effective health care recovery in those states (Cometto, Fritsche, & Sondorp, 2010). The efficacy of decentralized administration is also associated with the nature of political arrangements and institutional guarantees (Litvack, Ahmad, & Bird, 1998). Appropriate arrangements and sufficient political support boost investment in various aspects of integrated decentralization measures, including enhanced human resources, public participation, and sufficient financial allocations in health care decision making (Faguet, 2004).

Therefore, local governance measures, factors that tend to be ignored in postviolence health care recovery arrangements, should be given high priority when rebuilding health systems in transitional states.

References

African Union. (2001). Abuja declaration on HIV/AIDS, tuberculosis and other related infectious diseases. Retrieved from http://www.un.org/ga/aids/pdf/abuja_declaration.pdf

Akresh, R., & de Walque, D. (2008). *Armed conflict and schooling: Evidence from the 1994 Rwandan genocide.* Policy Research Working Papers. World Bank. doi:10.1596/1813-9450-4606

Asefa, M., Drewett, R., & Tessema, F. (2000). A birth cohort study in South-West Ethiopia to identify factors associated with infant mortality that are amenable for intervention. *Ethiopian Journal of Health Development, 14*, 161–168.

Azfar, O., & Gurgur, T. (2008). Does corruption affect health outcomes in the Philippines? *Economics of Governance, 9*, 197–244.

Basinga, P., Gertler, P. J., Binagwaho, A., Soucat, A. L., Sturdy, J., & Vermeersch, C. M. (2011). Effect on maternal and child health services in Rwanda of payment to primary health-care providers for performance: An impact evaluation. *The Lancet, 377*, 1421–1428.

Bloom, D. E., Canning, D., & Sevilla, J. (2004). The effect of health on economic growth: A production function approach. *World Development, 32*(1), 1–13.

Bossert, T. J., & Beauvais, J. C. (2002). Decentralization of health systems in Ghana, Zambia, Uganda and the Philippines: A comparative analysis of decision space. *Health Policy and Planning, 17*(1), 14–31.

Bossert, T. J., Chitah, M. B., & Bowser, D. (2003). Decentralization in Zambia: Resource allocation and district performance. *Health Policy and Planning, 18*, 357–369.

Bossert, T. J., & Mitchell, A. D. (2011). Health sector decentralization and local decision-making: Decision space, institutional capacities and accountability in Pakistan. *Social Science & Medicine, 72*(1), 39–48.

Bucagu, M. (2016). Improving maternal health in Rwanda: The role of community-based interventions: A systematic review (2005–2015). *Journal of Community Medicine & Health Education, 6*, 434. doi:10.4172/2161-0711.1000434

Carrin, G., Evans, D., & Xu, K. (2007). Designing health financing policy towards universal coverage. *Bulletin of the World Health Organization, 85*, 652–652.

Central Statistical Agency/Ethiopia and ICF International. (2012). Ethiopia demographic and health survey 2011. Addis Ababa, Ethiopia: Authors. Retrieved from http://dhsprogram.com/publications/publication-FR255-DHS-Final-Reports.cfm

Cometto, G., Fritsche, G., & Sondorp, E. (2010). Health sector recovery in early post-conflict environments: Experience from southern Sudan. *Disasters, 34*, 885–909.

Crook, R. C., & Sverrisson, A. S. (1999). To what extent can decentralized forms of government enhance the development of pro-poor policies and improve poverty-alleviation outcomes? World Bank. Retrieved from http://siteresources.worldbank.org/INTPOVERTY/Resources/WDR/DfiD-Project-Papers/crook.pdf

Deaton, A. (2003). Health, inequality, and economic development. *Journal of Economic Literature, 16*, 113–158.

El-Saharty, S., Kebede, S., Dubusho, P. O., & Siadat, B. (2009). Ethiopia: Improving health service delivery. Washington, DC: World Bank.

Faguet, J. P. (2004). Does decentralization increase government responsiveness to local needs? Evidence from Bolivia. *Journal of Public Economics, 88*, 867–893.

Gertler, P., & Vermeersch, C. (2013). *Using performance incentives to improve medical care productivity and health outcomes.* Cambridge, MA: National Bureau of Economic Research.

Gubbins, P., & de Walque, D. (2012). *Progress and challenges for improving child & maternal health in a post-conflict setting: The case of South Sudan.* Washington, DC: World Bank Group.

Human Development Africa. (2013). Q&A: Ethiopia's Promoting Basic Services (PBS) III Program. Retrieved from http://siteresources.worldbank.org/INTAFRICA/Resources/257994-1337109990438/et-q-a-ethiopia-s-promoting-basic-services-pbs-iii-program.pdf

Kruk, M. E., Freedman, L. P., Anglin, G. A., & Waldman, R. J. (2010). Rebuilding health systems to improve health and promote statebuilding in post-conflict countries: A theoretical framework and research agenda. *Social Science & Medicine, 70*(1), 89–97.

Litvack, J. I., Ahmad, J., & Bird, R. M. (1998). *Rethinking decentralization in developing countries.* Washington, DC: World Bank.

Logie, D. E., Rowson, M., & Ndagije, F. (2008). Innovations in Rwanda's health system: Looking to the future. *The Lancet, 372,* 256–261.

Mayai, A. T. (2008). Child mortality differentials in the Sudan: The case of the southern region (Unpublished paper). University of Wisconsin–Madison.

Mayai, A. T. (2015). *Essays in child health and health systems in Eastern Africa: Evidence from South Sudan and Ethiopia.* (Doctoral dissertation). ProQuest Dissertations. (3703563)

Mayai, A. T. (2016). The impact of public spending on infant and under-five health in South Sudan. *American Journal of Medical Research, 3*(1), 207–243.

Ministry of Health and National Bureau of Statistics. (2013). *South Sudan Household Survey 2010, Final Report.* Juba, South Sudan.

Ministry of Health Rwanda, PMNCH, WHO, World Bank, AHPSR, & Participants in the Rwanda Multistakeholder Policy Review. (2014). *Success factors for women's and children's health: Rwanda.* Retrieved from http://www.who.int/pmnch/knowledge/publications/rwanda_country_report.pdf

Morgan, L. (2009). Signed, sealed, delivered? Evidence from Rwanda on the impact of results-based financing for health. World Bank. Retrieved from http://documents.worldbank.org/curated/en/824231468147299185/pdf/541030BRI0RBF110Box345636B01PUBLIC1.pdf

OECD. (2012). International support to post-conflict transition: Rethinking policy, changing practice. DAC Guidelines and Reference Series. OECD Publishing. doi:10.1787/9789264168336-en

Susuman, A. S. (2012). Child mortality rate in Ethiopia. *Iranian Journal of Public Health, 41*(3), 9–19.

Uchimura, H., & Jütting, J. P. (2009). Fiscal decentralization, Chinese style: Good for health outcomes? *World Development, 37,* 1926–1934.

World Bank. (2013). Rwanda: Can bonus payments improve the quality of health care? From evidence to policy. Retrieved from https://openknowledge.worldbank.org/handle/10986/22606

CHAPTER 40

GRAND CHALLENGES IN GLOBAL HEALTH AND THE ROLE OF UNIVERSITIES

Keith Martin, MD, PC

There can be no greater gift than that of giving one's time and energy to help others without expecting anything in return.

—Nelson Mandela

Over the last 30 years, remarkable improvements to human well-being have been achieved. Life spans have increased, maternal and child mortality has declined, the number of people living in absolute poverty has decreased dramatically. But these advances have not been evenly distributed. Billions of people are still excluded from enjoying the advances that have improved the lives of many in high- and middle-income communities. These are the communities that suffer from the highest burden of disease. It is where the global health and development community should focus the bulk of its efforts.

Universities as Partners in Global Health

The good news is that we know how to address most of these problems. Our challenge is to overcome the persistent knowledge–needs gap and scale up known solutions for those communities in greatest need. Universities have a unique and remarkable opportunity to do this. Academia's role has been to engage in research and education and to provide service to society. Many university-ranking services assess a university's performance across research, teaching, employability, and internationalization. Institutions are judged according to their reputation as measured through the eyes of academics

Foundations for Global Health Practice, First Edition. Lori DiPrete Brown.
© 2018 John Wiley & Sons, Inc. Published 2018 by John Wiley & Sons, Inc.

and employers around the world; the student-to-faculty ratio; the number of citations the institutions' research receives; and the proportion of foreign students and faculty at the university. These metrics are useful, but they omit a vital, underutilized role that is within academia's mandate: service.

Research is a vital underpinning of society's ability to advance effective policies for the public good. However, most research and many outstanding solutions lie dormant in academic journals, never to be translated. We need a much better connection between research produced and policies made and implemented. It is in this area that academia has an extraordinary opportunity.

Academic institutions, particularly those in high-income areas, should convene representatives from NGOs, civil society, the private sector, and all levels of government to address specific challenges in their communities. Academic institutions, particularly the large ones in high-income nations, have abundant relationships with institutions in low-income countries. These usually involve faculty engaging in research and students having experiential learning opportunities. There is little in these relationships for the low-income institution. This must change. These relationships should be used as a platform to provide trainers and access to online libraries and curricula to improve the training and research capabilities of the resource-constrained institution. Benefits from these relationships must accrue to all partners, but particularly to those in low-income settings. It is unethical to utilize a low-income institution for research and training opportunities without ensuring that the institution receives long-term, sustainable benefits that strengthen its training, research, and service capabilities.

Universities should also have a formal program that continuously brings children from low-income areas on campus so that they can be exposed to the academic possibilities they may not be aware of.

Politics moves policy, and the public moves the political. Academia must be far more fearless in educating the public and policymakers about evidence-based solutions that can address the challenges society faces. Keeping the dialogue within the ivory tower does a disservice to the remarkable work that academia produces.

By strengthening its service role, academia would actually open up a range of new research and training opportunities for faculty and students. It is remarkable to see well-known institutions that produce vast quantities of superb research sitting within or close to communities suffering from numerous challenges.

The Consortium of Universities for Global Health

At the Consortium of Universities for Global Health (CUGH), we are using our committees and platforms to integrate medical and nonmedical disciplines through education, research, advocacy, and service initiatives. The website (www.cugh.org) has been modernized, and interest groups have been created on the site that parallel many of the global health challenges we face. It is an open-access platform for knowledge sharing, collaboration, implementation, and advocacy. CUGH's committees have compiled a wide selection of training modules and other education products, identified competencies in global health, created a capacity-building mechanism to connect trainers and curricula with needs, and has advocated for a range of global health initiatives. CUGH also runs webinars, workshops, and an annual conference. Further, we use our convening power to bring academia, governments, NGOs, the private sector, and our overseas colleagues together to identify ways they can collaborate.

We will also collaborate with University of Washington and Johns Hopkins University, which are engaging their local communities to address the social determinants of health for those who are most vulnerable. We have been working with the Global Health Fellows Program (GHFP) II to reach out to minority-serving institutions in the United States and work with them to strengthen their global health programs. Our goal with GHFP-II is to increase opportunities for minority students in this field so that ultimately, the US overseas development workforce will more accurately reflect American demographics.

Against this backdrop, there is much to do. Old threats remain, and new ones are rapidly careening toward us. The following are some of the neglected challenges we face and what we can do about them.

A Triple Challenge

Although HIV, tuberculosis, and malaria mortality has steadily declined, millions still perish from these and other infectious diseases. As we saw with the Ebola virus and now with the yellow fever and Zika virus epidemics, communicable disease outbreaks remain a persistent threat. Antimicrobial resistance and pandemics are of increasing concern. This prompted the international community to convene and create the Global Health Security Agenda (GHSA; www.ghsagenda.org), which will help prevent, detect, and respond to infectious disease outbreaks. Although this agenda is well thought out, most nations have yet to fulfill their commitments to it.

Our second challenge is the global increase in non-communicable diseases (NCDs): cardiovascular disease, diabetes, pulmonary diseases, cancer, mental health disorders, substance abuse, and injury. They account for 70% of the world's deaths, or 40 million deaths per year ("Global Burden of Disease," 2016). Although they are increasing in incidence in high-income countries (HICs), they are even more devastating in low- and middle-income countries (LMICs) where NCDs are the leading cause of death and disability (Council on Foreign Relations, 2016). Furthermore, as our life spans increase, we are living for longer periods with disabilities associated with NCDs. This is producing an enormous, increasing strain on economies and health systems ill-prepared to deal with this problem. We need to create healthier life spans with fewer years of disability.

Our third challenge is to heal the planet. Human activity is destroying Earth's life-support systems. This threatens the very existence of our species and that of most others on the planet (Whitmee et al., 2015). Climate change is contributing to extreme weather events, food insecurity, drought, rising sea temperatures, ocean acidification, migration, changing disease patterns, and biodiversity losses. Human activity in the Anthropocene is causing a massive loss of species: the sixth great extinction (Convention on Biological Diversity, 2015).

Addressing the Neglected Foundation of Development

One of the most important reasons why we have not seen even greater gains in human well-being, particularly in the world's poorest nations, is our neglect of two crucial preconditions for development: a stable, responsible government accountable to its citizens, and a competent public service. Both are vital to implementation of effective public policies. If these conditions do not exist, the durability of development initiatives and the stability of a nation are compromised.

Decisions about whether a vaccine is used, a hospital is built, sanitation is provided, health workers are trained, health care is funded, or conflict incited are political decisions. They are choices. They are not based on whether policymakers have the best data and research at their disposal. Information is important, but it is a mercurial mix of interests, benefits, costs, and relationships across sectors that determines what is actually done. The matrix of each decision-making situation is unique to the environment in which it occurs. The failure to understand the political environment in which a problem exists and how to navigate it hampers significantly the ability to have effective public policies adopted. If you are involved in global health and you want a problem addressed, you must become politically active. It is insufficient to solely develop solutions and expect them to produce an impact. Research published does not equal research used.

A political environment where elected leaders are accountable to the people is not enough to create a stable environment for investment, commerce, innovation, and sustainable development. Stable nations need a competent, noncorrupt public service and functional ministries, not only of health but, also important, of finance, justice, public works, agriculture, the environment, education, housing, and more. They are pillars of a stable national infrastructure.

Conditions for stability also include the presence of an effective, independent judicial system, open media, and a vibrant civil society. These are essential to maintain strong accountability mechanisms between the elected and their citizens. Where these bonds are weakened or severed, governments cease being accountable to the people, and social conditions can deteriorate. These sectors all have a profound impact on the social determinants of health.

If you examine those countries with the worst health outcomes, they all suffer from some combination of bad governance, weak political systems, and ineffective institutions. This breeds corruption, poverty, poor access to public services, terrible health outcomes, and often conflict (e.g., Syria, Zimbabwe, Venezuela, Angola, the Democratic Republic of the Congo, the Central African Republic, South Sudan, Iraq, and Afghanistan) (Transparency International, 2016).

In this the international community is partially responsible. We have turned a blind eye to the financial loopholes that allow a small number of people in countries that are rich in natural resources yet impoverished to use their positions to loot their nations and stash these monies in opaque, overseas tax havens or through the purchase of real estate and other assets in some of the richest countries in the world. It is estimated that in Africa alone, approximately $333 billion is stolen from the continent every year through corruption, a number that is eight times larger than the official development assistance the continent receives. The international financial architecture must be reformed, loopholes closed, and the perpetrators of these massive acts of corruption prosecuted.

Priorities for Action

The following section highlights several of the critical areas toward which different actors in the global health and development community should direct their efforts.

Action for Government and Society

Focus on the world's poorest nations and the communities with the worst health outcomes. This is where we will achieve the biggest impact on human well-being. For this to work, though, there must be a commitment in will and resources from the governments in those nations to address the challenges they face. If they do not want to do this, then there is little hope of external actors and resources having a long-term impact.

Strengthen governance and public service capabilities. Public service strengthening should be undertaken by partnering with other public services, academia, and NGOs to establish domestic, context-relevant training capabilities. The timeline must be decades in length.

Invest in public health systems. This is the common platform not only to address NCDs but also to prevent, detect, and respond to communicable disease outbreaks. Despite its proven effectiveness in addressing the biggest causes of mortality and morbidity, public health system investment receives a fraction of the funding allocated to health. We need to do a much better job of allocating funds to where they will have the biggest impact. Advocacy by all sectors is needed to make this shift to support greater investments in public health.

Train and retain primary care physicians with surgical capabilities, nurses, community care workers, and administrative support staff. Africa alone currently has a deficit of one million health workers. This number will only grow with time. Training and retaining people where they are needed with these skill sets will enable a health system, with the appropriate infrastructure, to address most acute and chronic health challenges.

Strengthen infrastructure, procurement processes, and access to material. Access to electricity, clean water, the Internet, drugs, medical devices, sanitation, roads, and so on must be supported by a reliable procurement mechanism, which is often missing in low-resource settings.

Adopt universal health coverage (UHC). Quality health care without universal access only benefits the few. The poor will not have access to care unless they can afford it. Without UHC, the poor and often the middle class will be deprived of the care they need or may be driven into penury by being compelled to pay for it.

Address climate change and incorporate conservation and the protection of ecosystem services into development policies. Climate change is *the* existential threat to our survival. Mitigation is useful, but it will not aggressively reduce the rise in atmospheric carbon. An integrated approach whereby individuals, communities, and businesses can reduce their carbon footprint is needed now. The massive environmental degradation we are enduring, with its concomitant loss of biodiversity and destruction of ecosystems that provide vital resources essential to human health (fresh water, food, bulwarks against climate change), has, until recently, been neglected. To address this massive challenge, we need, among other things, to aggregate and share sustainable development practices; advocate for the protection of identified critical ecosystems; and implement the range of policies that will create sustainable cities, given that the next two billion people will live in urban areas, primarily in LMICs.

Action for Trainees in Global Health

Acquire the skills of implementation. In addition to honing your discipline, learn about project management, finance, monitoring and evaluation, grant writing, and communications, and pick up another language if you can.

Become politically active; be an advocate. Get involved in the political process. If you do, you will greatly enhance your ability to translate knowledge into public policies that affect people's lives. Effective advocacy is the lifeblood of change.

Action for Academic Institutions

Take a hard look at the partnerships you have in low- and middle-income countries. Although our students may have exciting opportunities abroad and our researchers are able to carry out trials and investigations overseas, we must ask: How does this partnership benefit the LMIC institution? Existing partnerships can be leveraged to strengthen the training capabilities in the overseas institution; curricula should be shared; opportunities should be created for publication and coauthorship with LMIC colleagues; and free online access to HIC libraries should be provided. These actions, relatively easy to implement, will assist in strengthening research and training capabilities in LMICs.

Conclusion

Improving the health of people and our planet is the existential challenge of our time. It will require the collaboration of all sectors to sustainably implement what we know will address the problems that our planet and we as a species face and to identify solutions where none exist. Inaction or insufficient actions will have grave consequences for us and the other species that inhabit our planet. In this global effort, academia has an extraordinary opportunity to use its research, training, advocacy, and service capabilities in ways that have yet to be realized. Opportunities beckon.

References

Convention on Biological Diversity. (2015). *Health and biodiversity.* Retrieved from https://www .cbd.int/health/

Council on Foreign Relations. (2016). The emerging global health crisis: Non-communicable diseases in low- and middle-income countries. Retrieved from http://www.cfr.org/diseases -noncommunicable/emerging-global-health-crisis/p33883

Global burden of disease. (2016). *The Lancet.* Retrieved from http://www.thelancet.com/gbd

Transparency International. (2016). *Corruption perceptions index: Overview.* Retrieved from http:// www.transparency.org/research/cpi/overview

Whitmee, S., Haines, A., Beyrer, C., Boltz, F., Capon, A. G., Ferreira, B., . . . Yach, D. (2015, November 15). Safeguarding human health in the Anthropocene epoch: Report of the Rockefeller Foundation–*Lancet* Commission on planetary health. *Lancet, 386,* 1973–2028. http://www .thelancet.com/journals/lancet/article/PIIS0140-6736(15)60901-1/fulltext

GLOSSARY

Accountability: The obligation of an individual or organization to account for its activities, accept responsibility for them, and disclose the results in a transparent manner

Active listening: The practice of listening to a speaker while providing feedback indicating that the listener both hears and understands what the speaker is saying

Adaptation: In the context of climate change, a strategy that corresponds with secondary prevention or preparedness, and aims to reduce the public health impacts of climate change

Agriculture: A spectrum of practices that produce food, fiber, and fuel

Amino acids: Building blocks of carbon, oxygen, hydrogen, and nitrogen that joint together to make up proteins

Basic mental health treatment packages: In the context of mental health, treatment packages for mental disorders comprising evidence-based treatments that can include psychosocial, psychotherapeutic, and psychopharmacologic treatments that, taken together, can greatly increase the chances of a person benefiting from safe, effective care for a mental disorder

Behavioral medicine: An interdisciplinary field that aims to integrate biological and psychosocial perspectives on human behavior and to apply them to the practice of medicine

Beveridge model: A health care system in which health care is provided by the government and financed through tax payments

"Big data": Data sets that are large enough that sophisticated analytics can produce new insight from these data

Biofuels: Fuels derived from renewable sources of organic matter, such as plant material

Bismarck model: A health care system in which providers and payers are private; plans cover everyone, employed or not; and insurance companies do not make a profit

Building Resources Across Communities (BRAC): A development organization based in Bangladesh

Capacity building: The development and strengthening of human and institutional resources

Cap-and-trade: A system in which the government sets a cap on total emissions and distributes permits to companies as a strategy to manage emissions and create incentives for reduction of emissions

Carbon tax: A government tax on emissions

Case fatality ratio: The proportion of deaths within a designated population of cases

Climate change: Changes in climate beyond natural variability that stem directly or indirectly from human activities and their impact on the global atmosphere

Climate justice: Efforts that consider inequitable vulnerabilities, hold those who produce harm accountable, and emphasize the importance of community voice and participation in addressing the consequences of climate change

Foundations for Global Health Practice, First Edition. Lori DiPrete Brown.
© 2018 John Wiley & Sons, Inc. Published 2018 by John Wiley & Sons, Inc.

Collaborative, team-based care: A method of care delivery whereby there is effective communication, and task-sharing of care delivery functions across disciplines in contexts where there are few specialists

Commercial farm: As used in this text, farming activities with the primary objective of selling goods for income rather than of growing food for personal consumption

Communicable disease: Infectious disease that is contagious and that can be transmitted from one source to another by infectious bacteria or viral organisms

Community-based participatory research (CBPR): In the context of public health, a mixed-methods collaborative approach to research that equitably involves, for example, community members, organizational representatives, and researchers in all aspects of the research process

Community engagement: Collaboration among institutions of higher education and their larger communities (local, regional/state, national, global) for the mutually beneficial exchange of knowledge and resources in a context of partnership and reciprocity

Community mapping: A technique whereby a selected group of people from the community are asked to draw their community, label its features, and then talk about community assets and risks.

Community survey: A tool used to collect information on a population in a community

Competency: The ability to do something successfully

Composite measures: Summaries or combined information needed to make comparisons or allocation decisions

Convenience sample: An informal sample chosen from a population of interest without reference to a complete sampling frame and without randomization; generally, subjects that are easier to study because of geographic or other factors are more likely to be chosen

Convention on the Rights of Persons with Disabilities (CRPD): A 2006 treaty that took effect in 2008 and recognizes that disability is an evolving concept

Coverage: The extent to which health systems enable people to access and benefit from an intervention, service, or program

Cultural competency: The ability to understand, appreciate, and interact with people from cultures or belief systems different from one's own

Declaration of Alma-Ata: A 1978 declaration endorsed by 134 countries that stated, "The main goal of governments and the World Health Organization in the coming decades should be the attainment by all people of the world by the year 2000, a level of health that would permit them to lead a socially and economically productive life"

Deep listening: To be fully present to what is happening in any given moment so that you may hear with clarity the fullness of what is unfolding

Demographic transition: The change in birth and death rates that has historically accompanied economic growth and the shift to modern society

Depression: A state of sustained feeling of low mood, sadness, and hopelessness that causes a significant decrease in functioning

Digital health or connected health: The current paradigm of information communication technology in health, in which, in addition to developing new innovations that take advantage of mobile and cloud-based solutions, we now recognize the importance of bridging earlier generations of fixed-site technologies, such as hospital computer systems and servers, with compatible and complementary mobile platforms

Directly Observed Treatment Short Course (DOTS): Name given to the tuberculosis control strategy recommended by the World Health Organization

Disability: A physical or mental condition that limits a person's movements, senses, or activities

Disability-adjusted life years (DALYs): Years of healthy life lost to premature death and disability

Discernment: A reflective practice that pursues understanding and/or decision making through assumption analysis, contextual exploration, imaginative speculation, and reflective skepticism

Diversification: A form of scale-up in which interventions are tested and added into an existing package of services already being delivered by an organization or institution

Double burden of disease: The persistent burden of infectious disease typically associated with lower-income countries, combined with an increasing non-communicable disease burden that occurs as life expectancy increases

Electronic health record (EHR): An electronic version of a person's medical record

Endangerment finding: A government determination that greenhouse gas emissions could be expected to pose a threat to public health

Extensive agriculture: A production system that uses low-to-no synthetic inputs of labor, fertilizers, and capital, relative to the land area being farmed

Fiber: Inedible agricultural commodities that become items such as cotton clothing or the paper used to print a book

Field course: Type of course that "brings the classroom to the community" and is often characterized by visiting the locations where the learning topics take place

Food: The agricultural products that people and animals eat

Food security: Reliable access to a sufficient quantity of affordable, nutritious food

Food system: A collection of interconnected resources that produce food and bring food to people

Framework Convention on Global Health (FCGH): A framework to bring the benefits of medical and broader public health advances to all people, including the poorest and most marginalized

Fuel: The products that we burn for energy outside of our bodies

Gender: Term that refers to the roles, behaviors, activities, and attributes that a given society at a given time considers appropriate for men and women; gender is part of the broader sociocultural context, as are other important criteria for sociocultural analysis, including class, race, poverty level, ethnic group, sexual orientation, and age

Gender and feminist analysis: The critical examination of how differences in gender roles, activities, needs, opportunities, and rights and entitlements affect men, women, girls, and boys in certain situations or contexts

Gender equality: Term that refers to the equal rights, responsibilities, and opportunities of women and men and girls and boys; gender equality implies that the interests, needs, and priorities of both women and men are taken into consideration, recognizing the diversity of different groups of women and men

Gender equity: Term that refers to fairness and—rather than requiring equality, or the same treatment for all—recognizes that specific measures must be designed to eliminate inequalities between women and men, end discrimination, and ensure equal opportunities

Genetically modified organisms (GMOs): Seeds that have been developed for specific purposes, including but not limited to drought tolerance and herbicide resistance

Germ theory of disease: Theory which states that disease can be caused by specific microorganisms

Global burden of disease: The gap between optimal versus actual health, caused by all disease and disability in the world

Global health: The endeavor to achieve solutions to health problems that cross geographic and socioeconomic boundaries

Global mental health: A field of study that focuses on mental health in a global context, considering varying resource constraints, different community assets, and cultural differences, while at the same time invoking the protection of the human rights of all those living with mental illness around the world

Global South: Term that refers to lower-income countries, which are located primarily in the Southern Hemisphere

Governance: The way in which a system is managed

Gray literature: Document types produced at all levels of government, academics, business, and industry in print and electronic formats that are protected by intellectual property rights, of sufficient quality to be collected and preserved by libraries and institutional repositories, but not controlled by commercial publishers

Greenhouse gases: Gases such as carbon dioxide (CO_2), methane (CH_4), and nitrous oxide (N_2O), which absorb outgoing radiation and redirect it back toward the earth's surface

The Green Revolution: A period of scientific advances in agriculture that took place in the 19th century, which led to a better understanding of how plants grow and increased agricultural production

Group interviews: A dialogue with community members to explore topics of interest, with key questions to guide discussion

Harmful algal blooms: Blooms of algae that release toxins

Health care system: A set of relationships in which structural components, or means, and their interactions are associated and connected to the goals that the system desires to achieve, or the ends; the key means in a health care system are financing, payment, macro-organization of the health care delivery, regulations, and persuasion

Health cobenefits: Advantages of climate change or other environmental strategies that not only benefit the environment in the ways intended but also have a beneficial impact on human health

Health disparity: A preventable difference in the burden of disease, injury, violence, or opportunities to achieve optimal health that are experienced by socially disadvantaged populations

Health equity: The extent to which a society minimizes differential access to health care and other services that lead to a healthy life, usually assessed by comparisons in morbidity and mortality across groups

Health in All Policies: A term used to express that many of the factors that create health are not under the jurisdiction of the health sector, so that we need to be able to engage sectors other than health to contribute to the health and well-being of the population

Health statistics: Both empirical data and estimates related to health

Health system: People, institutions, and resources arranged together in accordance with established policies to improve the health of the population they serve

Health/technical expertise: Technical knowledge and skills that have become relevant to global health over the years

Heat island: Urban areas that generate and retain heat as a result of human and industrial activities, buildings, and other factors, such as the lack of trees

Horizontal scale-up: Expansion of an intervention to new geographic areas and new populations

Hygiene: Conditions and practices that help maintain health and prevent the spread of disease

Implementation science: The scientific study of methods to promote the systematic uptake and/or adaptation of proven clinical treatments, practices, and organizational and management interventions into routine practice, and hence to improve health

Improved sanitation facility: A facility that hygienically separates human excreta from human contact

Improved water source: A collection point that adequately protects the source from outside contamination, particularly fecal matter

Incidence: The rate of new cases for a given disease during a defined time interval

Informant interview: An interview conducted with an identified leader to whom you can talk about a specific subject matter, such as descriptive information, historical information, and social or cultural information

Information communication technology (ICT): An umbrella term that includes any communication device or application, such as radio, television, cellular phones, or computer

Intensive agriculture: A production system that involves increased levels of input and output per unit of agricultural land area

Intercept survey: A survey of individuals at a central location, such as a clinic, school, marketplace, or town square

International Covenant on Economic, Social and Cultural Rights (ICESCR): A multilateral treaty adopted by the United Nations General Assembly that commits its parties to work toward the granting of economic, social, and cultural rights

International Health Regulations (IHR): A WHO treaty protecting against the international spread of disease

Interoperable data: Data that are organized such that disparate data sets can be aggregated and integrated for larger more meaningful analysis

Interpersonal effectiveness: Desired outcomes achieved through interpersonal strategies such as communication, compassion, trust building, and good communication

Interprofessional collaboration: Development and maintenance of effective working relationships with learners, health care providers, patients, families, and communities to maximize health

Knowledge management: Systematic and effective handling of information so that data can be interpreted and used effectively

Knowledge transfer: Teaching the technical and operational elements of an intervention to other implementers

Kyoto Protocol: International agreement (1992) that committed developed countries and emerging market economies to reduce their overall emissions of six greenhouse gases by at least 5% below 1990 levels over the period between 2008 and 2012, with specific targets varying from country to country

Leadership competencies: Skills and behaviors that contribute to impactful performance

Macronutrients: The fats, proteins, and carbohydrates that provide the energy our bodies require

Meaningful connection: A way of connecting that abandons preconceived notions, agendas, or worries about how one is being seen in order to be fully present in relationship

Medicalization: An overemphasis on medical rather than public health, social, or infrastructure solutions to sources of ill health

mHealth: Term that broadly encompasses medical and public health practices supported by mobile devices, such as mobile phones, patient monitoring devices, personal digital assistants (PDAs), and other wireless devices

Micronutrients: The vitamins and minerals that facilitate the body's metabolic processes

Millennium Development Goals (MDGs): Eight goals, set forth by the United Nations in 2000 and adopted by 189 nations, that responded to the world's main development challenges and were to be achieved by 2015

Mitigation: A strategy that corresponds to primary prevention and aims to stabilize or reduce the production of greenhouse gases

Monitoring and evaluation: A process to help improve performance and achieve results by reviewing and evaluating a program or intervention

Monoculture: The planting of one or few crop types

Morbidity: The incidence or prevalence of disease or disability during a certain period

Mortality rate: The rate at which people die due to a defined cause in a defined population over a defined period of time

National health insurance model: A government-run insurance program that every citizen pays into

Nationally determined contributions (NDCs): The actions countries intend to take to address climate change, both in terms of adaptation and mitigation, which become binding when a country ratifies the Paris Agreement

Non-communicable disease (NCD): A medical condition or disease that is not caused by infectious agents

Ocean acidification: A drop in ocean pH as a result of climate change

One health: The collaborative effort of multiple disciplines working locally, nationally, and globally to obtain optimal health for people, animals, and the environment

Open data: Data that are available for all to access, analyze, and publish without restriction

Oral rehydration solution (ORS): A mixture of salt, sugar, and water widely used to prevent dehydration and death from diarrhea among children; can be prepared by caregivers at home

Organic production: Agricultural activities that integrate cultural, biological, and mechanical practices that foster cycling of resources, promote ecological balance, and conserve biodiversity

Out-of-pocket model: A system in which people pay for health care at cost

Overnutrition: A form of malnutrition that occurs when excess calories create nutritional imbalance and obesity that can lead to poor health outcomes and can increase risk for chronic conditions such as diabetes and heart disease

Paris Agreement: The 2016 Paris climate accord or Paris climate agreement, which is part of the United Nations Framework Convention on Climate Change (UNFCCC), and deals with greenhouse gas emissions mitigation, adaptation, and finance starting in the year 2020, focusing on holding the increase in global average temperature to below 2°C above pre-industrial levels, to increase the ability to adapt to the impacts of climate change, and to direct financial efforts toward low greenhouse gas emissions and climate-resilient development

Passport stamp: A stamp indicating entry or exit from a country

Peer-reviewed journal: A journal that has submitted most of its published articles for review by experts who are not part of the editorial staff

People's Health Assembly: A network of health activists, civil society organizations, and academic institutions from around the world, particularly from low- and middle-income countries, who are committed to comprehensive primary health care and addressing the social, environmental, and economic determinants of health

Performance-based incentive: Paying health care workers, clinics, or hospitals based on utilization rates or health outcomes, providing incentives to increase services rendered and/or quality

Persons with disabilities: Those who have long-term physical, mental, intellectual, or sensory impairments that in interaction with various barriers may hinder these individuals' full and effective participation in society on an equal basis with others

Perspective taking: Taking seriously the perspectives of others, recognizing and acting on the obligation to inform one's own judgment, and engaging diverse and competing perspectives as a resource for learning, citizenship, and work

Place-based knowledge: Knowledge of the context and history that shape the lives of the community

Point-of-use treatment system: Technologies that treat small amounts of water for use in the home

Population health: The health outcomes of a group of individuals, including the distribution of such outcomes within the group

Prevalence: The proportion of disease found to be affecting a particular population

Primary health care: A comprehensive approach based on essential services and broader socio-economic development to address the multiple underlying causes of ill health

Primary source: Original documents (including translations) that were written during an experience or event and that offer a personal testimony or observation, or constitute an official record of the event

Productivity (yield): Amount of food produced per area of land

Psychosis: A symptom of mental illness in which thinking and functioning are so impaired that contact with external reality is lost

Public health: The science and art of preventing disease, prolonging life, and promoting physical health through organized community efforts for the sanitation of the environment, the control of community infections, the education of the individual in principles of personal hygiene, the organization of medical and nursing services for the early diagnosis and preventive treatment of disease, and the development of the social machinery that will ensure for every individual in the community a standard of living adequate for the maintenance of health

Random sample: A sample in which those interviewed are selected at random from a complete set of the population studied, with each member having an equal chance of being selected

Reflection: A mental process through which individuals or groups seek clarity about truth through the integration of experience

Regenerative agriculture: Farming practices informed by knowledge of soil nutrition that intentionally avoids negative environmental impacts and actively seeks to increase soil health and biodiversity in a farm system

Right to health: The right of everyone to the enjoyment of the highest attainable standard of physical and mental health

Right to health impact assessment: An instrument used to analyze the likely effects of policies, programs, and projects across sectors and legal regimes that may significantly affect the right to health, so that these elements can be adjusted to prevent harms and maximize synergies with the right to health

Risk factor: Something that has the potential to cause diseases and injuries, such as poor diet, smoking, or unsafe water

Scaling up: The process of effectively implementing a standardized, low-cost health intervention nationwide to reach the majority of the population

Secondary source: A source that interprets, summarizes, or analyzes a primary source

Selective primary health care: A strategy focused on achievable targets and specific interventions that address treatable diseases

Self-care: Care that is under an individual's control

Service-learning: An educational approach whereby students learn through active participation in thoughtfully organized community service

Shasthya Shebikas: A cadre of community health workers deployed by BRAC

Smallholder: Owner of a small farm

Social determinants of health: The conditions in which people are born, grow, work, live, and age, and the wider set of forces and systems shaping the conditions of daily life

Social-ecological model: A model that accounts for the multiple interrelated factors that facilitate or impede health and well-being; it is based on the fundamental idea that health is not determined solely by biological factors at the individual level, but also produced by interactions at the individual, interpersonal, community, and societal levels

Social injustice: A situation in which the rights of a person or a group of people are ignored

Spontaneous scaling up: A phenomenon that occurs when innovations spread on their own, without any guidance from implementers, due to an organic demand from the population

Stigma: An attribute that is deeply discrediting, often informed by false information, which promotes fear and misunderstanding about the experience of those living with a condition such as mental illness

Subsistence farm: A farm that aims to produce enough food for the same family that works the land

Sustainable Development Goals (SDGs): Created to follow the Millennium Development Goals, which expired in 2015, a universal set of 17 goals along with 169 related targets that UN member states will be expected to use to frame their global development agendas and political policies for the period of 2016 through 2030

Systems thinking: The practice of approaching complex problems with a cross-disciplinary perspective in order to understand linkages and interactions across components of a system or issue

Task-shifting: Policies and practices that enable heath care services to be provided by less specialized health providers, with the aim of maintaining quality and increasing access and/or efficiency of health system performance

Telemedicine: The remote diagnosis and treatment of patients by means of telecommunications technology

Transect walk: See *walk-along*

Transformative engagement and leadership: An approach to activities that identifies a need for a moral or values-based transformation within individuals, communities, and/or societal structures; envisions a path toward said transformation; and engages in relationships and activities in pursuit of such a vision

Triple burden of disease: The disease burden associated with globalization and urbanization

Tropical medicine: A discipline concerned with the diagnosis and treatment of diseases commonly occurring in tropical and subtropical regions, most frequently in the Global South

Undernourishment: The inability to secure enough food to derive sufficient energy from the diet

Undernutrition: A micronutrient deficiency

United Nations Framework Convention on Climate Change: A declaration that sought to stabilize the concentration of greenhouse gases in the atmosphere in order to prevent "dangerous interference" with the earth's climate

U.S.-China Joint Announcement on Climate Change and Clean Energy Cooperation: A 2014 agreement between the United States and China in which the United States would cut emissions to 28% below 2005 levels by 2025, and China pledged to reach a target peak of carbon dioxide by 2030 and increase the share of renewable energy by 20% over the same interval

Value chain: Progressive steps that each add incremental value to a product or process

Values: A set of beliefs, ideals, and morals that an individual or collective considers important, if not essential

Vector-borne diseases: Infectious diseases spread by organisms such as insects or rodents

Vertical scale-up: Term that refers to the building of legal, political, policy, or institutional changes necessary for the large-scale implementation of an intervention

Visa: A document (often adhered to a passport page) that grants permission to enter a country for a designated amount of time

Vision: The belief in or description of a future that an individual or collective would like to see

Voluntourism: A form of tourism in which travelers participate in and often pay to do volunteer work, typically for a charity

Walk-along: A method of inquiry that uses observation, exploration, and accompaniment to enable learning from community members about the natural, built, historical, or cultural environment

Water-based diseases: Infections caused by parasitic pathogens found in aquatic host organisms

Water-borne diseases: Diseases caused by the ingestion of water contaminated by human or animal feces or urine containing pathogens

Water-related insect vector diseases: Diseases caused by insect vectors that either breed in water or bite near water

Water resources: Sources of water that are useful or potentially useful to humans

Water-washed diseases: Diseases caused by inadequate use of water for domestic and personal hygiene

Wellness: The notion of health as a state of complete physical, mental, and social well-being, and not merely the absence of disease or infirmity

Years lived with disability (YLDs): A measure (in years) of the burden of living with a disease or disability

Years of life lost (YLLs): Years lost due to premature mortality, calculated by subtracting the age at death from the life expectancy for a person at that age

Yellow card: Card that provides documentation of a yellow fever vaccine

Yield gap: Disparity between the amount harvested on any given area of land and what could potentially be harvested